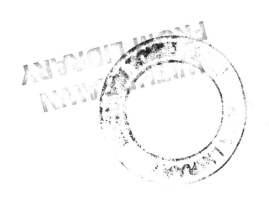

Pediatric and Adolescent Oncofertility

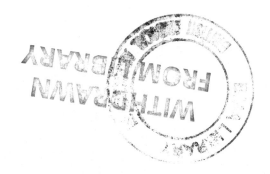

Teresa K. Woodruff • Yasmin C. Gosiengfiao
Editors

Pediatric and Adolescent Oncofertility

Best Practices and Emerging Technologies

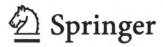 Springer

Editors
Teresa K. Woodruff
Obstetrics and Gynecology
Northwestern University
Chicago, IL, USA

Yasmin C. Gosiengfiao
Northwestern University
Chicago, IL, USA

ISBN 978-3-319-32971-0   ISBN 978-3-319-32973-4   (eBook)
DOI 10.1007/978-3-319-32973-4

Library of Congress Control Number: 2016961253

Printed on acid-free paper

This Springer imprint is published by Springer Nature
The registered company is Springer International Publishing AG Switzerland
The registered company address is Gewerbestrasse 11, 6330 Cham, Switzerland

Preface

We are delighted to publish the fifth book in a series in partnership with Springer about the emerging area of oncofertility now including pediatric and adolescent patients. There has been a remarkable increase in the number of options for adult male and female cancer patients since the publication of our first book *Oncofertility: Fertility Preservation for Cancer Survivors* (ed. Woodruff and Snyder, 2007). The second book *Oncofertility: Ethical, Legal, Social and Medical Perspectives* (eds. Woodruff, Zoloth, Campo-Engelstein, Rodriguez, 2010) addressed complex issues and created a broad dialogue globally around what is possible and needed for cancer patients in a variety of settings. We then turned our attention to a definitive book on medical practice *Oncofertility Medical Practice: Clinical Issues and Implementation* (eds. Gracia and Woodruff, 2012), which provides not only the most up-to-date information on clinical decisioning but also includes the IRB and consent procedures and forms. Since oncofertility is at the intersection of a variety of fields, creating a way to communicate complex ideas across disciplines and patient groups led to a very popular *Oncofertility Communication: Sharing Information and Building Relationships Across Disciplines* (eds. Woodruff, Clayman, and Waimey, 2014). The books have been and are being translated into multiple languages, and, in many ways, I felt we had covered the intellectual terrain for this field. But it became abundantly clear that the emerging issues associated with pediatric and adolescent cancer patients required a fresh look at this topic to inform the field about the concerns, gaps, current solutions, and research that will change the field in the coming years. I'm delighted that Dr. Yasmin Gosiengfiao, M.D., Attending Physician, Division of Hematology, Oncology & Stem Cell Transplantation, Ann & Robert H. Lurie Children's Hospital of Chicago, and Assistant Professor of Pediatrics, Northwestern University Feinberg School of Medicine, joined me in inviting an outstanding group of authors and soliciting diverse subject matter that will ensure that the reader is as up to date as possible.

The chapters in this book start with a "must read" from Drs. Leslie Appiah and Dan Green outlining the "Fertility Risks with Cancer Therapy." If you have time for only one chapter, this is the one to read. We then invited a group of experts in pediatric and adolescent female and male issues ranging from options, sexual function, new research, and testing for gonadal reserve. Even as we think a great deal about oncofertility, this book also covers, for the first time, the emerging area of fertility management for patients with disorders of sex development and sexual minorities and fertility concerns for b-thalassemia patients. Pediatricians, endocrinologists in particular, are seeking information in this area that is contemporary and difficult, thinking about consent, assent, age, ethics, and other core issues.

Finally, we give information on providing fertility preservation consults, the ethics of this field, and insurance and reimbursement issues as well as chapters that address issues that emerge from our Global Oncofertility Network.

We had a great deal of help on this project from Leandra Stevenson, and the editors thank her for ensuring this project could be completed in a timely fashion.

We hope you enjoy *Pediatric and Adolescent Oncofertility - Best Practices and Emerging Technologies* – let us know what you think!

Chicago, IL, USA   Teresa K. Woodruff, PhD
Chicago, IL, USA   Yasmin Gosiengfiao, MD

Contents

Contributors

Teresa Almeida-Santos, MD, Ph.D Faculty of Medicine, University of Coimbra, Coimbra, Portugal

Portuguese Centre for Fertility Preservation, Reproductive Medicine Department, Coimbra Hospital and University Centre, Coimbra, Portugal

Leslie A. Appiah, MD Department of Obstetrics and Gynecology, University of Kentucky College of Medicine, Lexington, KY, USA

Norton Healthcare, Louisville, KY, USA

Mariângela Badalotti, MD, MSc, PhD Fertilitat Centro de Medicina Reprodutiva, Porto Alegre, RS, Brazil

Latin America Oncofertility Netowork – Oncofertility Consortium, Belo Horizonte, MG, Brazil

Linda Ballard, APRN, CPNP Aflac Cancer and Blood Disorders Center, Children's Healthcare of Atlanta, Atlanta, GA, USA

Janie Benoit, MD Pediatric & Adolescent Gynecology, Cincinnati Children's Hospital Medical Center, Cincinnati, OH, USA

Robert E. Brannigan, MD Department of Urology, Northwestern University, Feinberg School of Medicine, Galter Pavilion, Chicago, IL, USA

Lesley Breech, MD Pediatric and Adolescent Gynecology, Cincinnati Children's Hospital Medical Center, Cincinnati, OH, USA

Karen Burns, MD, MS Cancer and Blood Diseases Institute, Cincinnati Children's Hospital Medical Center, Cincinnati, OH, USA

João Pedro Junqueira Caetano, MD, MSc, PhD Pró-Criar Medicina
Reprodutiva, Belo Horizonte, MG, Brazil

Medical Sciences Faculty, Belo Horizonte, MG, Brazil

Latin America Oncofertility Netowork – Oncofertility Consortium,
Belo Horizonte, MG, Brazil

Lisa Campo-Engelstein, PhD Department of Obstetrics & Gynecology,
Alden March Bioethics Institute, Albany Medical College, Albany, NY, USA

Jacira Ribeiro Campos, BSc, MSc, PhD Medical Schooll of Ribeirão Preto,
University of São Paulo, Ribeirao Preto, SP, Brazil

Latin America Oncofertility Netowork – Oncofertility Consortium,
Belo Horizonte, MG, Brazil

Maria Cristina Canavarro, PhD Faculty of Psychology and Educational
Sciences, University of Coimbra, Coimbra, Portugal

Unit of Psychological Intervention, Maternity Dr. Daniel de Matos,
Coimbra Hospital and University Centre, Coimbra, Portugal

Glenn M. Cannon, MD Department of Urology, University of Pittsburgh
School of Medicine, Pittsburgh, PA, USA

Children's Hospital of Pittsburgh, University of Pittsburgh Medical Center,
Pittsburgh, PA, USA

Maurício Barbour Chehin, MD, PhD Huntington Medicina Reprodutiva,
Sao Paulo, SP, Brazil

Latin America Oncofertility Netowork – Oncofertility Consortium,
Belo Horizonte, MG, Brazil

Diane Chen, PhD Division of Adolescent Medicine, Ann & Robert H. Lurie
Children's Hospital of Chicago, Northwestern University Feinberg School of
Medicine, Chicago, IL, USA

Brooke Cherven, MPH, RN, CPON Aflac Cancer and Blood Disorders Center,
Children's Healthcare of Atlanta, Atlanta, GA, USA

Ricardo Marques de Azambuja, BSc, MSc, PhD Fertilitat Centro de Medicina
Reprodutiva, Porto Alegre, RS, Brazil

Latin America Oncofertility Netowork – Oncofertility Consortium,
Belo Horizonte, MG, Brazil

Bruno Ramalho de Carvalho, MD, MSc, PhD Latin America Oncofertility
Netowork – Oncofertility Consortium, Belo Horizonte, MG, Brazil

Ana Carolina Japur de Sá Rosa e Silva, MD, MSc, PhD Medical Schooll of
Ribeirão Preto, University of São Paulo, Ribeirao Preto, SP, Brazil

Latin America Oncofertility Netowork – Oncofertility Consortium,
Belo Horizonte, MG, Brazil

Fernando Marcos dos Reis, MD, MSc, PhD Federal University of Minas Gerais, Belo Horizonte, MG, Brazil

Latin America Oncofertility Netowork – Oncofertility Consortium, Belo Horizonte, MG, Brazil

Courtney A. Finlayson, MD Division of Endocrinology, Department of Pediatrics, Ann and Robert H. Lurie Children's Hospital of Chicago, Chicago, IL, USA

Kathrin Gassei, PhD Department of Obstetrics, Gynecology and Reproductive Sciences, Magee-Womens Research Institute, University of Pittsburgh School of Medicine, Pittsburgh, PA, USA

Veronica Gomez-Lobo, MD Department of Women and Infant Services, Department of Surgery, MedStar Washington Hospital Center, Children's National Medical Center, Washington, DC, USA

Yasmin Gosiengfiao, MD Hematology, Oncology & Stem Cell Transplantation, Ann & Robert H. Lurie Children's Hospital of Chicago, Chicago, IL, USA

Daniel M. Green, MD Department Epidemiology and Cancer Control, Memphis, TN, USA

Division of Cancer Survivorship, Department of Oncology, St. Jude Children's Research Hospital, Memphis, TN, USA

Holly Hoefgen, MD Pediatric & Adolescent Gynecology, Cincinnati Children's Hospital Medical Center, Cincinnati, OH, USA

Jason Jarin, MD Department of Women and Infant Services, Department of Surgery, MedStar Washington Hospital Center, Children's National Medical Center, Washington, DC, USA

Emilie Johnson, MD, MPH Division of Urology Chicago, Department of Urology and Center for Healthcare Studies, Ann & Robert H. Lurie Children's Hospital of Chicago, Northwestern University, Feinberg School of Medicine, Chicago, IL, USA

James A. Kashanian, MD Weill Cornell Medicine – Urology, Weill Cornell Medical Center, New York, NY, USA

Monica M. Laronda, PhD Obstetrics and Gynecology, Northwestern University, Feinberg School of Medicine, Chicago, IL, USA

Jennifer Levine, MD, MSW Obstetrics and Gynecology, Northwestern University, Feinberg School of Medicine, Chicago, IL, USA

Barbara Lockart, DNP, APN/AC-PC, CPON Solid Tumors & Fertility Preservation, Ann & Robert H. Lurie Childrens Hospital of Chicago, Chicago, IL, USA

Joaquim Lopes, MD Cenafert, Salvador, BA, Brazil

Latin America Oncofertility Netowork – Oncofertility Consortium,
Belo Horizonte, MG, Brazil

Ricardo Mello Marinho, MD, MSc, PhD Pró-Criar Medicina Reprodutiva,
Belo Horizonte, MG, Brazil

Medical Sciences Faculty, Belo Horizonte, MG, Brazil

Latin America Oncofertility Netowork – Oncofertility Consortium,
Belo Horizonte, MG, Brazil

Lillian Meacham, MD Aflac Cancer Center/Children's Healthcare
of Atlanta, Pediatrics Emory University, Atlanta, GA, USA

Lillian R. Meacham, MD Department of Pediatrics, Emory University
School of Medicine, Atlanta, GA, USA

Aflac Cancer Center/Children's Healthcare of Atlanta, Atlanta, GA, USA

Cláudia Melo, MSc Faculty of Psychology and Educational Sciences,
University of Coimbra, Coimbra, Portugal

Unit of Psychological Intervention, Maternity Dr. Daniel de Matos,
Coimbra Hospital and University Centre, Coimbra, Portugal

Yoko Miyoshi, MD Department of Pediatrics, Osaka University Graduate
School of Medicine, Osaka, Japan

Steven F. Mullen, PhD Cook Regentec, The Brown School Location,
Bloomington, IN, USA

Simone França Nery, MD, MSc, PhD Federal University of Minas Gerais,
Belo Horizonte, MG, Brazil

Kyle E. Orwig, PhD Department of Obstetrics, Gynecology and Reproductive
Sciences, Magee-Womens Research Institute, University of Pittsburgh
School of Medicine, Pittsburgh, PA, USA

Magee-Womens Research Institute, Pittsburgh, PA, USA

Álvaro Petracco, MD, PhD Fertilitat Centro de Medicina Reprodutiva,
Porto Alegre, RS, Brazil

Latin America Oncofertility Netowork – Oncofertility Consortium,
Belo Horizonte, MG, Brazil

Gwen Quinn, PhD Obstetrics and Gynecology, Northwestern University,
Feinberg School of Medicine, Chicago, IL, USA

H. Lee Moffitt Cancer Center & Research Institute, University of South Florida,
Tampa, FL, USA

Chad Ritenour, MD Division of Men's Health/Infertility and General Urology, Department of Urology Emory University, Atlanta, GA, USA

Jhenifer Kliemchen Rodrigues, BSc, MSc, PhD In Vitro Consultoria, Belo Horizonte, MG, Brazil

Latin America Oncofertility Netowork – Oncofertility Consortium, Belo Horizonte, MG, Brazil

Erin Rowell, MD Obstetrics and Gynecology, Northwestern University, Feinberg School of Medicine, Chicago, IL, USA

Matthew B. Schabath, PhD Obstetrics and Gynecology, Northwestern University, Feinberg School of Medicine, Chicago, IL, USA

H. Lee Moffitt Cancer Center & Research Institute, University of South Florida, Tampa, FL, USA

Peter H. Shaw, MD Department of Pediatrics, University of Pittsburgh School of Medicine, Pittsburgh, PA, USA

Children's Hospital of Pittsburgh, University of Pittsburgh Medical Center, Pittsburgh, PA, USA

Kathleen Shea, MS, CPNP Obstetrics and Gynecology, Northwestern University, Feinberg School of Medicine, Chicago, IL, USA

Sylvia T. Singer, MD UCSF Benioff Children's Hospital Oakland, Oakland, CA, USA

Nao Suzuki, MD, PhD Department of Obstetrics and Gynecology, St. Marianna University School of Medicine, Kawasaki, Japan

Christina Tamargo Obstetrics and Gynecology, Northwestern University, Feinberg School of Medicine, Chicago, IL, USA

H. Lee Moffitt Cancer Center & Research Institute, University of South Florida, Tampa, FL, USA

Alison Y. Ting, PhD Division of Reproductive & Developmental Sciences, Oregon National Primate Research Center, Oregon Health & Science University, Beaverton, OR, USA

Susan T. Vadaparampi, PhD Obstetrics and Gynecology, Northwestern University, Feinberg School of Medicine, Chicago, IL, USA

H. Lee Moffitt Cancer Center & Research Institute, University of South Florida, Tampa, FL, USA

Terri L. Woodard, MD Department of Gynecologic Oncology and Reproductive Medicine, The University of Texas MD Anderson Cancer Center, Houston, TX, USA

Teresa K. Woodruff, PhD Obstetrics and Gynecology, Northwestern University, Feinberg School of Medicine, Chicago, IL, USA

Mary B. Zelinski, PhD Division of Reproductive & Developmental Sciences, Oregon National Primate Research Center, Oregon Health & Science University, Beaverton, OR, USA

Department of Obstetrics & Gynecology, Oregon Health & Science University, Portland, OR, USA

Chapter 1
Fertility Risk with Cancer Therapy

Leslie A. Appiah and Daniel M. Green

Introduction

Advances in cancer treatments have significantly changed the outcome for pediatric cancers with 5-year survival rates approaching 75–80%. With improvements in treatment, 1 in 25 cancer survivors will be of reproductive age [1]. Fertility compromise occurs in 8–12% of female survivors [2] and one-third of adult male survivors of childhood cancer [3]. Manifestations of gonadal injury include disordered puberty from hormonal deficiency, decreased reproductive and sexual function, psychosocial effects, and menopause-related health problems in female survivors such as cardiac, skeletal, and cognitive dysfunction. Standard options for fertility preservation include sperm, oocyte, and embryo banking. Investigational options include testicular, ovarian, and immature oocyte cryopreservation [4, 5]. Most options are invasive and costly, and standard options in females require a minimum of 2 weeks of intervention prior to proceeding with cancer treatment [6]. Estimating risk prior to therapy allows determination and implementation of the appropriate fertility preserving therapies. Identifying agents that protect the ovary prior to and during cancer therapy may mitigate the need for invasive and costly fertility preserving therapies while preserving hormonal function after cancer treatment.

L.A. Appiah, MD (✉)
Department of Obstetrics and Gynecology, University of Kentucky College of Medicine, Lexington, KY, USA

Norton Healthcare, Louisville, KY, USA
e-mail: leslie.appiah@uky.edu

D.M. Green, MD
Department Epidemiology and Cancer Control, Memphis, TN, USA

Division of Cancer Survivorship, Department of Oncology, St. Jude Children's Research Hospital, Memphis, TN, USA

© Springer International Publishing Switzerland 2017
T.K. Woodruff, Y.C. Gosiengfiao (eds.), *Pediatric and Adolescent Oncofertility*,
DOI 10.1007/978-3-319-32973-4_1

Table 1.1 Effects of cancer therapy on male fertility

Treatment		Effect on spermatogenesis and transport	Risk of infertility
Surgery			
	Removal of both testes	Impaired production	100 %
	Removal of one testis		Low
	Damage to hypothalamic/ pituitary gonadotropin producing area		Low – spermatogenesis may be stimulated with exogenous gonadotropin
	Retroperitoneal lymph node dissection	Impaired transport	Variable – retrograde ejaculation; sperm production not impaired
Radiation therapy			
	Irradiation of testes	Impaired production	Fertility very unlikely if testes dose > 7.5 Gy
	Irradiation of hypothalamic/ pituitary gonadotropin producing area		Dose-response relationship unclear; dose < 30 Gy do not appear to produce damage
Chemotherapy	Alkylating agents	Impaired production	Cyclophosphamide equivalent dose (CED): <4 g/m^2 – risk of azoospermia < 15 % >4 g/m^2 – risk of oligo- or azoospermia >50 %

Estimating Risk

Assessment of the risk for impaired fertility after therapy should be undertaken prior to initiation of therapy for optimal fertility preservation outcomes. Surgical procedures, radiation therapy, and chemotherapy can each impair fertility (Table 1.1). Gametogenesis and hormone production are differentially sensitive to treatment exposures in males, whereas these two functions are tightly linked in females. The risk factors for impaired fertility differ for males and females.

Males

Testicular surgery can affect production of sperm and hormones or interfere with transport of sperm [7]. Injury of the gonadotropin-releasing hormone area of the hypothalamus and/or the gonadotropin-producing anterior pituitary can also result in impaired spermatogenesis and sex steroid production [8]. Impaired transport may occur from damage to autonomic nervous system control of urethral sphincters and/or vasodilation secondary to retroperitoneal lymph node dissection or prostatectomy [9].

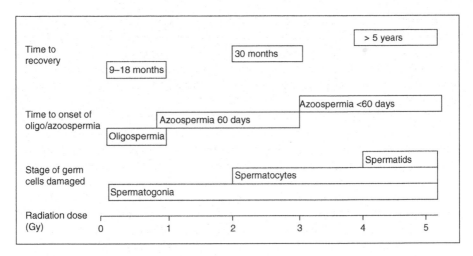

Fig. 1.1 Spermatogenesis following single-dose radiation. Howell. Spermatogenesis after cancer treatment. damage and recovery (*J Natl Cancer Inst Monogr* 2005;34:12–17)

Testicular tissue is extremely radiosensitive with only small amounts of direct radiation required to cause significant impairment in spermatogenesis (Fig. 1.1). The immature stem cells and spermatogonia are most sensitive. Radiation to the testes markedly reduces the number of spermatocytes 2–3 weeks post-therapy with declines in ejaculated sperm counts by approximately 10 weeks. Azoospermia is typically present at 18 weeks post-therapy [10]. Spermatogenesis is significantly impaired at lower direct testicular radiation doses than is hormone production. However, both spermatogenesis and hormone production can be impaired after higher doses of radiation therapy delivered to the hypothalamic/pituitary area.

The effect of chemotherapy on spermatogenesis is dependent on the type of chemotherapeutic agent. Normal sperm count typically recovers by 12 weeks post-therapy in patients treated with non-alkylating agents [11]. However, spermatogenesis is very sensitive to damage by alkylating agents including nitrogen mustard, procarbazine, cyclophosphamide, ifosfamide, chlorambucil, and busulfan, with long-lasting effects on fertility [12]. The risk of azoospermia is approximately 10 % when the cyclophosphamide equivalent dose is less than 4 g/m^2, whereas approximately one-quarter of individuals who receive more than this dose will retain a normal sperm concentration [13].

Females

Surgery for ovarian tumors impairs fertility and hormone production by decreasing the number of follicles present. Fertility-sparing surgery is the standard of care for the management of early-stage, low-grade ovarian tumors in women who have not completed their childbearing. Surgical options include cystectomy for tumors of low malignant potential (borderline tumors) and unilateral oophorectomy for malignancies [14–16]. When cystectomy is performed, the remaining ovary is typically able to compensate if no postoperative chemotherapy or radiation is given. Pelvic surgery for non-gynecologic malignancies can also have a deleterious effect on ovarian function by cytokine production and formation of pelvic adhesions, with subsequent impaired folliculogenesis, ovulation, and tubal transport [17, 18].

All chemotherapeutic agents affect the mature follicle through DNA damage with subsequent apoptosis and temporary amenorrhea [19]. If the primordial follicle pool is unaffected, folliculogenesis will resume after completion of cancer treatment with resumption of menses. Alkylating agents such as cyclophosphamide, busulfan, and nitrogen mustard and heavy metals such as cisplatin have a deleterious effect on the primordial follicles, diminishing the reserve pool [20]. Although patients who receive these therapies may resume menses due to follicular maturation of the remaining follicles, they subsequently experience accelerated folliculogenesis and apoptosis with primary ovarian insufficiency [21].

Radiation injury to the ovaries is dose dependent. Specifically, younger age confers protection from post-therapy infertility because of the larger pool of primordial follicles present at the time of radiation treatment. Radiation doses greater than 2 Gy result in a loss of 50% of ovarian follicles, described as the LD50 [22, 23]. Doses greater than or equal to 15 Gy and 6 Gy in adult and prepubertal patients, respectively, result in infertility. Irreversible damage to the uterus occurs at abdominopelvic doses greater than 30 Gy [24]. Radiation exposure to the hypothalamus and pituitary gland greater than 30 Gy affects production of gonadotropins with decreased folliculogenesis, decreased production of estrogen, and infertility [22].

Risk stratification from chemotherapy is based on the cumulative dose of alkylating agents received due to high risk of gonadotoxicity. The alkylating agent dose (AAD) and the cyclophosphamide equivalent dose (CED) risk-stratification systems allow calculation of risk (Fig. 1.1 and Table 1.2). Using the AAD, a score of 1, 2, or 3 is given for the cumulative dose of each alkylating agent that falls within the first, second, or third cumulative dose tertile, respectively. The scores for individual agents are summed [25]. Patients with a score of 3 or 4 are at increased risk of infertility with a relative risk of pregnancy of 0.72 and 0.65, respectively [26]. The CED is calculated by summing the cyclophosphamide equivalents for cyclophosphamide, ifosfamide, procarbazine, chlorambucil, BCNU, CCNU, melphalan, ThioTEPA, nitrogen mustard, and busulfan [27] (Table 1.2). A CED >7.5g/m^2 is associated with a relative risk of premature menopause of 4.19 (95% is 2.18–8.08).

The AAD is based on drug dose distribution from the specific cohort of patients from which the drug dose distribution was derived, whereas the CED is derived from actual drug doses and therefore has applicability independent of the study population [27]. Risk stratification by alkylating agent should be performed prior to therapy to guide implementation of fertility preservation therapies based on risk. However, treatment regimens may change during the course of therapy, and in such instances, cumulative dose and risk assessment may be recalculated post-therapy.

Table 1.2 Estimating risk: alkylating agent dose (AAD) (Green. *J Clin Oncol.* 27:2677–2685)

Tertile distribution of alkylating agents in cumulative dose

Alkylating agent	Cumulative dose by rertile		
	First	Second	Third
BCNU, mg/m²	1–300	301–529	530–3,370
Busulfan, mg/m²	1–317	318–509	510–6,845
CCNU, mg/m²	1–361	362–610	611–3,139
Chlorambucil, mg/m²	1–165	166–634	635–3,349
Parenteral cyclophosphamide, mg/m²	1–3,704	3,705–9,200	9,201–58,648
Oral cyclophosphamide, mg/m²	1–4,722	4,723–10,636	10,637–143,802
Ifosfamide, mg/m²	1–16,771	16,772–55,758	55,759–192,391
Melphalan, mg/m²	1–39	40–137	138–574
Nitrogen mustard, mg/m²	1–44	45–64	65–336
Procarbazine, mg/m²	1–4,200	4,201–7,000	7,001–58,680
Intrathecal thiotepa, mg	1–80	81–320	321–914
Thiotepa, mg/m²	1–77	78–220	221–3,749

Note: First tertile score is 1; second is 2; and third is 3
Abbreviations: *BCNU* carmustine, *CCNU* lomustine

CED (mg/m²) = 1.0 (cumulative cyclophosphamide dose (mg/m²)) + 0.244 (cumulative ifosfamide dose (mg/m²)) + 0.857 (cumulative procarbazine dose (mg/m²)) + 14.286 (cumulative chlorambucil dose (mg/m²)) + 15.0 (cumulative BCNU dose (mg/m²)) + 16.0 (cumulative CCNU dose (mg/m²)) + 40 (cumulative melphalan dose (mg/m²)) + 50 (cumulative Thio-TEPA dose (mg/m²)) + 100 (cumulative nitrogen mustard dose (mg/m²)) + 8.823 (cumulative busulfan dose (mg/m²)).

Fig. 1.2 Cyclophosphamide equivalent dose calculation

Minimizing Risk

Several agents have been proposed as potentially fertoprotective, or conferring protection against the damaging effects of chemotherapy and radiation (Table 1.3). Gonadotropin-releasing hormone agonists (GnRHa) are the most studied; however, results are conflicting. Several newer agents are currently being evaluated which show some promise. These agents include imatinib, bone marrow-derived mesenchymal stem cells (BMMSC), sphingosine-1-phosphate (S1P), tamoxifen, granulocyte colony-stimulating factor (G-CSF), and AS101. GnRHa, tamoxifen, and G-CSF are the only agents that have been used in humans. Other therapies have shown promise in rodent and primate studies; however, concerns remain about interference with chemotherapeutic efficacy and perpetuation of damaged DNA cell lines with resultant fetal loss and/or malformation. Further studies are required to determine efficacy and safety in humans.

Table 1.3 Potential fertoprotective agents during cancer treatments

Potential fertoprotective agents during cancer treatments Protective agent	Mechanism of action on ovary	Studies demonstrating protective effect	Studies demonstrating no effect	Interactions with cytotoxic treatments
GnRH analog	Direct effect on ovary is unclear; suppresses hypothalamic-pituitary-ovarian axis, possible ovarian quiescence	Rodent: Meirow et al. (2004), Li et al. (2013) Primate: Ataya et al. (1995) Human: Badawy et al. (2009), Severrisdottir et al. (2009), Del Mastro et al. (2011), Demeestere et al. (2013)	Human: Gerber et al. (2011), Munster et al. [28], Elgindy et al. (2013), Demeestere et al. (2013)	No interference with treatment drugs
Imatinib	Inhibit c-Abl kinase apoptosis pathway	Rodent: Gonfolini et al. (2009)	Rodent: Kerr et al. [29]	May interfere with apoptotic action of chemotherapy drugs
Bone marrow mesenchymal stem cells	Tissue differentiation, angiogenesis, anti-apoptosis	Rodent: Kilic et al. (2004), Fu et al. [30], Rabbit: Abd-Allah et al. [31]	NTD	May cause chemotherapy drug resistance with cisplatin
S1P	Inhibit sphingomyelin apoptosis pathway	Rodent: Morita et al. [32], Jurisicova et al. (2009), Hancke et al. [33], Kaya et al. [34] Primate: Zelinski et al. [35] Human xenograft: Zelinski et al. [35]	Rodent: Kaya et al. [34]	May interfere with apoptotic action of chemotherapy drugs

(continued)

Table 1.3 (continued)

Potential fertoprotective agents during cancer treatments Protective agent	Mechanism of action on ovary	Studies demonstrating protective effect	Studies demonstrating no effect	Interactions with cytotoxic treatments
Tamoxifen	Anti-apoptotic activity; antioxidant activity via IGF-1 axis; possible H-P-O axis suppression	Rodent: Ting et al. [36], Mahran et al. [37]	Human: Sverrisdottir et al. [38]	Adjuvant therapy; no interference with treatment drugs
AS101	Inhibits P13K/ PTEN Akt follicle activation pathway; anti-apoptosis	Rodent: Kalich-Philosoph et al. [39]	NTD	No interference w/ treatment drugs May have additive/ synergistic interaction w/treatment drugs
Growth-colony stimulating factor (G-CSF)	Unclear: possibly angiogenesis; anti-apoptosis	Rodent: Skaznik-Wikiel et al. [40]	NTD	No interference with treatment drugs

Gonadotropin-Releasing Hormone Agonist

Gonadotropin-releasing hormone agonist (GnRHa) therapy is the most studied fertoprotective agent, but with conflicting results [41–43]. Reasons include end-points that do not predict long-term ovarian function such as resumption of menstruation, follicle-stimulating hormone (FSH) and estradiol levels, and a lack of data on pregnancy outcomes. Additionally, studies that used different GnRHa therapies had short follow-up periods and few were randomized [28, 44]. A recent prospective study with 257 patients used similar endpoints with inclusion of pregnancy outcome and survival and showed improved pregnancy outcomes with goserelin in hormone receptor negative breast cancer patients receiving adjuvant therapy [45]. Ultimately, meta-analysis of GnRHa therapy has shown ovarian protection in breast cancer patients, but widespread use of GnRHa therapy as an ovarian protective agent in all malignancies cannot be recommended at this time [42]. For this reason, additional agents have been evaluated for efficacy.

Imatinib

Imatinib is a competitive tyrosine kinase inhibitor used for cancer treatment. Chemotherapy induces c-Abl-mediated upregulation of tumor suppressor protein p63 (a homolog of p53) with resultant apoptosis. Rodent studies show that when given prior to cisplatin, imatinib is a potent inhibitor of c-Abl-mediated upregulation and blocks apoptosis of cells. Mice treated with imatinib prior to cisplatin show reduced primordial follicular loss and normal progeny [46, 47]. However, other studies show no protection with imatinib in two independent mice strains [29]. Additionally, the authors show that genetic effects on the oocyte result in early embryonic mortality and marked aneuploidy. There remain concerns regarding whether imatinib- and cisplatin-treated oocytes that do not undergo apoptosis harbor DNA damage that may result in miscarriage or birth defects [48, 49]. The question also remains whether imatinib reduces the efficacy of cisplatin on the primary tumor target while upregulating the effects of cisplatin in other cell types [50].

Bone Marrow-Derived Mesenchymal Stem Cells

Bone marrow-derived mesenchymal stem cells (MSC) have been used to treat various diseases because of their self-renewal capacity and multi-potency [51, 52]. For example, stem cells have been successfully employed for tissue repair after spinal, renal, and myocardial injury [53, 54]. The potential benefit of stem cell therapy after acute tissue damage appears to be related to tissue integration and differentiation to replace damaged cells, angiogenesis, and anti-apoptosis. Adult MSC have not been unequivocally proven to differentiate into follicles; however, several rodent studies have been conducted to assess the role of MSC as an ovarian protective agent from chemotherapy. Kilic et al. showed preservation of primordial and primary follicles in in vivo rat MSC studies, suggesting that MSC may preferentially migrate to the injured follicular cells and repair the ovarian tissue by decreased programmed cell death [55]. Similarly, Fu et al. demonstrated an increase in follicle number as well as a normalization of FSH and estradiol levels after several weeks in rodents treated with MSC after cyclophosphamide therapy [30]. They also illustrated in vitro production of angiogenic and anti-apoptotic cytokines, including vascular endothelial growth factor (VEGF), insulin-like growth factor (IGF-1), and hepatocyte growth factor (HGF) from MSC. Effects of therapy on progeny were not assessed in either study. Abd-Allah et al. further demonstrated MSC protection of ovarian follicles in rabbit studies and were able to show in vivo cytokine production [31]. Despite the potential promise of MSC as an ovarian protection agent, studies of MSC injected intravenously in rodent models have shown that MSC may mediate tumor resistance to cisplatin [56]. Therefore, route, dose, and efficacy of MSC as an ovarian protective agent in primates and humans are warranted.

Sphingosine-1-phosphate (S1P)

There are several apoptotic pathways, including the pathway which triggers apoptosis of ovarian follicles. In the pathway, sphingomyelin is degraded to ceramide which has pro-apoptotic effects. Ceramide is subsequently degraded to sphingosine and then sphingosine-1-phosphate (S1P) through hydrolysis. Sphingosine-1-phosphate regulates proliferative cellular processes, including cell growth and cell differentiation, and inhibits apoptosis [33]. In vivo mice studies of ovarian tissue xenografts treated with S1P show increased vascular density and angiogenesis with reduced follicular apoptosis. However, in mice treated with S1P pre-chemotherapy, the evidence is inconclusive, with some studies showing a protective effect in the presence of dacarbazine [33] and others showing no effect in the presence of cyclophosphamide [34]. Conversely, S1P treatment prior to radiation therapy has been shown to be effective in a dose-dependent manner with preservation of both primordial and primary follicles in rats, primates, and xenografted ovarian tissue [32, 34, 35]. Male mice who received local treatment with S1P prior to radiation were also shown to have protection of early stages of spermatogenesis [57]. Limitations of S1P are that it must be injected into tissue rather than administered systemically, thus limiting its clinical usefulness. A benefit of this targeted treatment is that it may minimize interference with cancer therapy efficacy in other tissues. This has not been adequately studied, however. Lastly, consistent with concerns with other fertoprotective agents, inhibition of follicular apoptosis with S1P may result in transmission of genetically damaged DNA. Studies of offspring in mice and primates treated with S1P prior to radiation showed no propagation of DNA damage and no abnormalities in the offspring [58].

Tamoxifen

Tamoxifen is a selective estrogen receptor modulator (SERM) with agonist-antagonist properties used as adjuvant treatment of hormone sensitive breast cancer. Rodent studies have shown ovarian protection with tamoxifen administered prior to cyclophosphamide [36]. Tamoxifen has also been shown to be protective when given prior to radiation treatment in rats with a reduction in loss of primordial follicles and increase in AMH [37]. Human studies with tamoxifen given post-chemotherapy have shown no protection [38]. Human studies evaluating the effects of tamoxifen as an ovarian protective agent have been conflicting due to study design and use of different endpoints [59]. Furthermore, the postulated mechanism of action remains unclear. Studies suggest that the protective effects of tamoxifen may be due to the anti-apoptotic and antioxidant effects of its estrogen-agonist properties [60, 61]. Protection may also result from increased transcription and translation of IGF-1 which has been shown to augment granulosa cell FSH receptor expression in the ovary and potentiate FSH action. Lastly, antagonist effects of tamoxifen are similar to GnRHa with downregulation of the H-P-O axis and ovarian quiescence which may also have a protective role. Well-designed human studies are warranted to assess the protective effect of tamoxifen on ovarian function during chemotherapy and radiation.

AS101

AS101 is a tellurium-based immunomodulator that inhibits the P13K/PTEN/Akt pathway and has anti-apoptotic and anti-inflammatory properties [62, 63]. AS101 has been shown to be protective against hematopoietic damage in mice treated with cyclophosphamide without adversely affecting treatment outcome [64–67]. It has also been shown to have antitumor effects in mice and human studies and synergistic effects with cyclophosphamide [64, 67–69]. Studies of gonadal protection in mice have similarly shown AS101 to protect against chemotherapy-induced follicular damage and reduce sperm DNA damage without interfering with cancer treatments [39, 70]. The proposed mechanism of action is inhibition of activation and loss of dormant primordial follicles during chemotherapy as well as reduced apoptosis in the granulosa cells of growing follicles of particular benefit, AS101 can be administered systemically. Human studies further evaluating the effect on gonadal protection are warranted.

Granulocyte Colony-Stimulating Factor (G-CSF)

Granulocyte colony-stimulating factor (G-CSF) is a polypeptide with growth factor and cytokine properties that stimulates granulocyte and stem cell production from the bone marrow and promotes neovascularization following ischemia [71, 72]. In mice studies, G-CSF has been shown to prevent damage to microvessels and significantly reduce destruction of primordial follicles caused by the alkylators cyclophosphamide and busulfan [40]. Additionally, next-generation breeding showed no adverse effects in the offspring. G-CSF has also been shown to be protective against the effects of cisplatin in mice models with improvement in follicular number and AMH levels [73]. It is postulated that with neovascularization, G-CSF decreases chemotherapy-related blood vessel loss and the associated focal ischemia seen in chemotherapy-related follicle loss [20]. Potential direct effects on the follicle remain unclear; however, anti-apoptotic mechanistic action of G-CSF has been proposed [74, 75]. The advantage of G-CSF over other agents is that it is currently used in breast cancer patients and patients undergoing autologous bone marrow transplantation for prevention of chemotherapy-induced neutropenia and has been shown not to reduce the efficacy of chemotherapeutic agents [76]. Further studies are warranted to establish the specific mechanism of action and optimal timing and dosage of G-CSF during chemotherapy in humans.

In the future, different fertoprotective agents may be tailored to cancer treatment regimens. To achieve this goal, rodent and primate studies that demonstrate safety and efficacy need to be translated into human studies. Agents currently used in humans for other indications need to be evaluated in prospective studies to better assess efficacy as a fertoprotective agent. To adequately study these treatments, lessons from GnRHa studies are helpful: endpoints must be accurately defined and reproductive and survival outcome measured. Accurate endpoints may include posttreatment follicular number and reliable and reproducible markers of ovarian reserve. Lastly and most importantly, therapies must show that administration during cancer treatment does not affect treatment outcome or result in propagation of DNA damage leading to fetal loss and/or malformation. Identification of successful fertoprotective agents will enhance therapeutic options to preserve fertility and restore hormonal function after cancer treatment.

Conclusion

Improved quality of life in survivorship must now be our collective goal as oncofertility specialists. As we protect the vital cardiac, pulmonary, renal, and cognitive functions of our patients, so also must we protect reproductive and sexual function. Without this protection, we leave a very significant proportion of society without the ability to fulfill a very basic and fundamental human need. Estimating risk prior to cancer treatment allows identification of harm with stratification of those most at risk. Minimizing risk through the development of fertoprotective agents decreases the need for invasive, costly, and time-consuming fertility preservation therapies. Standardizing care to incorporate both risk-reducing strategies provides the best care for our patients and will allow us to achieve our gold standard of comprehensive and timely care.

References

1. American Cancer Society. Cancer treatment and survivorship facts & figures. Atlanta, Georgia; 2014.
2. Geenen MM, Cardous-Ubbink MC, Kremer LCM, van den Bos C, van der Pal HJH, Heinen RC, et al. Medical assessment of adverse health outcomes in long-term survivors of childhood cancer. J Am Med Assoc. 2007;297(24):2705–15.
3. Rendtorff R, Hohmann C, Reinmuth S, Muller A, Dittrich R, Beyer M, et al. Hormone and sperm analyses after chemo- and radiotherapy in childhood and adolescence. Klin Padiatr. 2010;222(3):145–9.

4. Ayensu-Coker L, Bauman D, Lindheim SR, Breech L. Fertility preservation in pediatric, adolescent and young adult female cancer patients. Pediatr Endocrinol Rev. 2012;10(1):174–87.
5. Osterberg EC, Ramasamy R, Masson P, Brannigan RE. Current practices in fertility preservation in male cancer patients. Urol Ann. 2014;6(1):13–7.
6. Coyne K, Purdy M, O'Leary K, Yaklic JL, Lindheim SR, Appiah LA. Challenges and considerations in optimizing ovarian stimulation protocols in oncofertility patients. Front Public Health. 2014;2:246.
7. Djaladat H. Organ-sparing surgery for testicular tumours. Curr Opin Urol. 2015;25(2):116–20.
8. Ntali G, Karavitaki N. Efficacy and complications of pituitary irradiation. Endocrinol Metab Clin N Am. 2015;44(1):117–26.
9. Pettus JA, Carver BS, Masterson T, Stasi J, Sheinfeld J. Preservation of ejaculation in patients undergoing nerve-sparing postchemotherapy retroperitoneal lymph node dissection for metastatic testicular cancer. Urology. 2009;73(2):328–31.
10. Meistrich ML. Effects of chemotherapy and radiotherapy on spermatogenesis in humans. Fertil Steril. 2013;100(5):1180–6.
11. Meistrich ML, Wilson G, Mathur K, Fuller LM, Rodriguez MA, McLaughlin P, et al. Rapid recovery of spermatogenesis after mitoxantrone, vincristine, vinblastine, and prednisone chemotherapy for hodgkin's disease. J Clin Oncol. 1997;15(12):3488–95.
12. Howell SJ, Shalet SM. Spermatogenesis after cancer treatment: damage and recovery. J Natl Cancer Inst Monogr. 2005;34:12–7.
13. Green DM, Liu W, Kutteh WH, Ke RW, Shelton KC, Sklar CA, et al. Cumulative alkylating agent exposure and semen parameters in adult survivors of childhood cancer: a report from the St Jude Lifetime Cohort Study. Lancet Oncol. 2014;15(11):1215–23.
14. Zhang M, Jiang W, Li G, Xu C. Ovarian masses in children and adolescents – an analysis of 521 clinical cases. J Pediatr Adolesc Gynecol. 2014;27(3):e73–7.
15. Cass DL, Hawkins E, Brandt ML, Chintagumpala M, Bloss RS, Milewicz AL, et al. Surgery for ovarian masses in infants, children, and adolescents: 102 consecutive patients treated in a 15-year period. J Pediatr Surg. 2001;36(5):693–9.
16. Grigsby TJ, Kent EE, Montoya MJ, Sender LS, Morris RA, Ziogas A, et al. Attitudes toward cancer clinical trial participation in young adults with a history of cancer and a healthy college student sample: a preliminary investigation. J Adolesc Young Adult Oncol. 2014;3(1):20–7.
17. diZerega GS. The peritoneum and its response to surgical injury. Prog Clin Biol Res. 1990;358:1–11.
18. Practice Committee of the American Society for Reproductive Medicine, Society of Reproductive Surgeons. Pathogenesis, consequences, and control of peritoneal adhesions in gynecologic surgery. Fertil Steril. 2007;88(1):21–6.
19. Meirow D, Nugent D. The effects of radiotherapy and chemotherapy on female reproduction. Hum Reprod Update. 2001;7(6):535–43.
20. Meirow D, Dor J, Kaufman B, Shrim A, Rabinovici J, Schiff E, et al. Cortical fibrosis and blood-vessels damage in human ovaries exposed to chemotherapy. Potential mechanisms of ovarian injury. Hum Reprod. 2007;22(6):1626–33.
21. Larsen EC, Muller J, Rechnitzer C, Schmiegelow K, Andersen AN. Diminished ovarian reserve in female childhood cancer survivors with regular menstrual cycles and basal fsh < 10 iu/i. Hum Reprod. 2003;18(2):417–22.
22. Green DM, Kawashima T, Stovall M, Leisenring W, Sklar CA, Mertens AC, et al. Fertility of female survivors of childhood cancer: a report from the childhood cancer survivor study. J Clin Oncol. 2009;27(16):2677–85.
23. Wallace WHB, Thomson AB, Saran F, Kelsey TW. Predicting age of ovarian failure after radiation to a field that includes the ovaries. Int J Radiat Oncol Biol Phys. 2005;62(3):738–44.
24. Larsen EC, Schmiegelow K, Rechnitzer C, Loft A, Muller J, Andersen AN. Radiotherapy at a young age reduces uterine volume of childhood cancer survivors. Acta Obstet Gynecol Scand. 2004;83(1):96–102.

25. Tucker MA, Dangio GJ, Boice JD, Strong LC, Li FP, Stovall M, et al. Bone sarcomas linked to radiotherapy and chemotherapy in children. N Engl J Med. 1987;317(10):588–93.
26. Green DM, Nolan VG, Srivastava DK, Leisenring W, Neglia JP, Sklar CA, et al. Quantifying alkylating agent exposure: evaluation of the cyclophosphamide equivalent dose-a report from the childhood cancer survivor study. J Clin Oncol. 2011;29(15):9547.
27. Green DM, Nolan VG, Goodman PJ, Whitton JA, Srivastava D, Leisenring WM, et al. The cyclophosphamide equivalent dose as an approach for quantifying alkylating agent exposure: a report from the childhood cancer survivor study. Pediatr Blood Cancer. 2014;61(1):53–67.
28. Munster PN, Moore AP, Ismail-Khan R, Cox CE, Lacevic M, Gross-King M, et al. Randomized trial using gonadotropin-releasing hormone agonist triptorelin for the preservation of ovarian function during (neo)adjuvant chemotherapy for breast cancer. J Clin Oncol. 2012;30(5):533–8.
29. Kerr JB, Hutt KJ, Cook M, Speed TP, Strasser A, Findlay JK, et al. Cisplatin-induced primordial follicle oocyte killing and loss of fertility are not prevented by imatinib. Nat Med. 2012;18(8):1170–2. author reply 2–4.
30. Fu X, He Y, Xie C, Liu W. Bone marrow mesenchymal stem cell transplantation improves ovarian function and structure in rats with chemotherapy-induced ovarian damage. Cytotherapy. 2008;10(4):353–63.
31. Abd-Allah SH, Shalaby SM, Pasha HF, El-Shal AS, Raafat N, Shabrawy SM, et al. Mechanistic action of mesenchymal stem cell injection in the treatment of chemically induced ovarian failure in rabbits. Cytotherapy. 2013;15(1):64–75.
32. Morita Y, Perez GI, Paris F, Miranda SR, Ehleiter D, Haimovitz-Friedman A, et al. Oocyte apoptosis is suppressed by disruption of the acid sphingomyelinase gene or by sphingosine-1-phosphate therapy. Nat Med. 2000;6(10):1109–14.
33. Hancke K, Strauch O, Kissel C, Gobel H, Schafer W, Denschlag D. Sphingosine 1-phosphate protects ovaries from chemotherapy-induced damage in vivo. Fertil Steril. 2007;87(1):172–7.
34. Kaya H, Desdicioglu R, Sczik M, Ulukaya E, Ozkaya O, Yimaztepe A, et al. Does sphingosine 1-phosphate have a protective effect on cyclophosphamide- and irradiation-induced ovarian damage in the rat model? Fertil Steril. 2008;89(3):732–5.
35. Zelinski MB, Murphy MK, Lawson MS, Jurisicova A, Pau KYF, Toscano NP, et al. In vivo delivery of fty720 prevents radiation-induced ovarian failure and infertility in adult female nonhuman primates. Fertil Steril. 2011;95(4):1440–U289.
36. Ting AY, Petroff BK. Tamoxifen decreases ovarian follicular loss from experimental toxicant dmba and chemotherapy agents cyclophosphamide and doxorubicin in the rat. J Assist Reprod Genet. 2010;27(11):591–7.
37. Mahran YF, El-Demerdash E, Nada AS, Ali AA, Abdel-Naim AB. Insights into the protective mechanisms of tamoxifen in radiotherapy-induced ovarian follicular loss: impact on insulin-like growth factor 1. Endocrinology. 2013;154(10):3888–99.
38. Sverrisdottir A, Nystedt M, Johansson H, Fornander T. Adjuvant goserelin and ovarian preservation in chemotherapy treated patients with early breast cancer: results from a randomized trial. Breast Cancer Res Treat. 2009;117(3):561–7.
39. Kalich-Philosoph L, Roness H, Carmely A, Fishel-Bartal M, Ligumsky H, Paglin S, et al. Cyclophosphamide triggers follicle activation and "burnout"; as101 prevents follicle loss and preserves fertility. Sci Transl Med. 2013;5(185):185ra62.
40. Skaznik-Wikiel ME, McGuire MM, Sukhwani M, Donohue J, Chu TJ, Krivak TC, et al. Granulocyte colony-stimulating factor with or without stem cell factor extends time to premature ovarian insufficiency in female mice treated with alkylating chemotherapy. Fertil Steril. 2013;99(7):2045–54.
41. Turner NH, Partridge A, Sanna G, Di Leo A, Biganzoli L. Utility of gonadotropin-releasing hormone agonists for fertility preservation in young breast cancer patients: the benefit remains uncertain. Ann Oncol. 2013;24(9):2224–35.
42. Del Mastro L, Ceppi M, Poggio F, Bighin C, Peccatori F, Demeestere I, et al. Gonadotropin-releasing hormone analogues for the prevention of chemotherapy-induced premature ovarian

failure in cancer women: systematic review and meta-analysis of randomized trials. Cancer Treat Rev. 2014;40(5):675–83.

43. Oktay K, Sonmezer M, Oktem O, Fox K, Emons G, Bang H. Absence of conclusive evidence for the safety and efficacy of gonadotropin-releasing hormone analogue treatment in protecting against chemotherapy-induced gonadal injury. Oncologist. 2007;12(9):1055–66.

44. Loibl S, Gerber B. Gonadotropin-releasing hormone analogue for premenopausal women with breast cancer. JAMA. 2011;306(16):1760. author reply -1.

45. Moore HC, Unger JM, Phillips KA, Boyle F, Hitre E, Porter D, et al. Goserelin for ovarian protection during breast-cancer adjuvant chemotherapy. N Engl J Med. 2015;372(10):923–32.

46. Gonfloni S, Di Tella L, Caldarola S, Cannata SM, Klinger FG, Di Bartolomeo C, et al. Inhibition of the c-abl-tap63 pathway protects mouse oocytes from chemotherapy-induced death. Nat Med. 2009;15(10):1179–85.

47. Morgan S, Lopes F, Gourley C, Anderson RA, Spears N. Cisplatin and doxorubicin induce distinct mechanisms of ovarian follicle loss; imatinib provides selective protection only against cisplatin. PLoS One. 2013;8(7):e70117.

48. Cherry SM, Hunt PA, Hassold TJ. Cisplatin disrupts mammalian spermatogenesis, but does not affect recombination or chromosome segregation. Mutat Res Genet Toxicol Environ Mutagen. 2004;564(2):115–28.

49. Woodruff TK. Preserving fertility during cancer treatment. Nat Med. 2009;15(10):1124–5.

50. Wang-Rodriguez J, Lopez JP, Altuna X, Chu TS, Weisman RA, Ongkeko WM. Sti-571 (gleevec) potentiates the effect of cisplatin in inhibiting the proliferation of head and neck squamous cell carcinoma in vitro. Laryngoscope. 2006;116(8):1409–16.

51. Prockop DJ. Marrow stromal cells as stem cells for nonhematopoietic tissues. Science. 1997;276(5309):71–4.

52. Dawn B, Stein AB, Urbanek K, Rota M, Whang B, Rastaldo R, et al. Cardiac stem cells delivered intravascularly traverse the vessel barrier, regenerate infarcted myocardium, and improve cardiac function. Proc Natl Acad Sci U S A. 2005;102(10):3766–71.

53. Eliopoulos N, Zhao J, Forner K, Birman E, Young YK, Bouchentouf M. Erythropoietin gene-enhanced marrow mesenchymal stromal cells decrease cisplatin-induced kidney injury and improve survival of allogeneic mice. Mol Ther. 2011;19(11):2072–83.

54. Villanueva PD, Sanz-Ruiz R, Garcia AN, Santos MEF, Sanchez PL, Fernandez-Aviles F. Functional multipotency of stem cells: what do we need from them in the heart? Stem Cells Int. 2012;2012:817364.

55. Kilic S, Pinarli F, Ozogul C, Tasdemir N, Naz Sarac G, Delibasi T. Protection from cyclophosphamide-induced ovarian damage with bone marrow-derived mesenchymal stem cells during puberty. Gynecol Endocrinol. 2014;30(2):135–40.

56. Roodhart JML, Daenen LGM, Stigter ECA, Prins HJ, Gerrits J, Houthuijzen JM, et al. Mesenchymal stem cells induce resistance to chemotherapy through the release of platinum-induced fatty acids. Cancer Cell. 2011;20(3):370–83.

57. Otala M, Suomalainen L, Pentikainen MO, Kovanen P, Tenhunen M, Erkkila K, et al. Protection from radiation-induced male germ cell loss by sphingosine-1-phosphate. Biol Reprod. 2004;70(3):759–67.

58. Paris F, Perez GI, Fuks Z, Haimovitz-Friedman A, Nguyen H, Bose M, et al. Sphingosine 1-phosphate preserves fertility in irradiated female mice without propagating genomic damage in offspring. Nat Med. 2002;8(9):901–2.

59. Rose DP, Davis TE. Effects of adjuvant chemohormonal therapy on the ovarian and adrenal-function of breast-cancer patients. Cancer Res. 1980;40(11):4043–7.

60. Dubey RK, Tyurina YY, Tyurin VA, Gillespie DG, Branch RA, Jackson EK, et al. Estrogen and tamoxifen metabolites protect smooth muscle cell membrane phospholipids against peroxidation and inhibit cell growth. Circ Res. 1999;84(2):229–39.

61. Nathan L, Chaudhuri G. Antioxidant and prooxidant actions of estrogens: potential physiological and clinical implications. Semin Reprod Endocrinol. 1998;16(4):309–14.

62. Hayun M, Naor Y, Weil M, Albeck M, Peled A, Don J, et al. The immunomodulator as101 induces growth arrest and apoptosis in multiple myeloma: association with the akt/survivin pathway. Biochem Pharmacol. 2006;72(11):1423–31.
63. Indenbaum V, Bin H, Makarovsky D, Weil M, Shulman LM, Albeck M, et al. In vitro and in vivo activity of as101 against west nile virus (wnv). Virus Res. 2012;166(1–2):68–76.
64. Kalechman Y, Albeck M, Oron M, Sobelman D, Gurwith M, Horwith G, et al. Protective and restorative role of as101 in combination with chemotherapy. Cancer Res. 1991;51(5):1499–503.
65. Kalechman Y, Albeck M, Sotnikbarkai I, Sredni B. As101 protection of bone-marrow stromal cells function from adverse-effects of cyclophosphamide treatment in vivo or asta-z in vitro. Exp Hematol. 1992;20(6):728.
66. Kalechman Y, Sotnikbarkai I, Albeck M, Sredni B. The protective role of as101 in combination with cytotoxic drugs acting by various mechanisms of action. J Immunol. 1993;150(8):A131.
67. Sredni B, Weil M, Khomenok G, Lebenthal I, Teitz S, Mardor Y, et al. Ammonium trichloro(dioxoethylene-o, o')tellurate (as101) sensitizes tumors to chemotherapy by inhibiting the tumor interleukin 10 autocrine loop. Cancer Res. 2004;64(5):1843–52.
68. Kalechman Y, Rushkin G, Nerubay J, Albeck M, Sredni B. Effect of the immunomodulator as101 on chemotherapy-induced multilineage myelosuppression, thrombocytopenia, and anemia in mice. Exp Hematol. 1995;23(13):1358–66.
69. Sredni B, Tichler T, Shani A, Catane R, Kaufman B, Strassmann G, et al. Predominance of th1 response in tumor bearing mice and cancer patients treated with as101. J Natl Cancer Inst. 1996;88(18):1276–84.
70. Carmely A, Meirow D, Peretz A, Albeck M, Bartoov B, Sredni B. Protective effect of the immunomodulator as101 against cyclophosphamide-induced testicular damage in mice. Hum Reprod. 2009;24(6):1322–9.
71. Demetri GD, Griffin JD. Granulocyte colony-stimulating factor and its receptor. Blood. 1991;78(11):2791–808.
72. Bussolino F, Wang JM, Defilippi P, Turrini F, Sanavio F, Edgell CJS, et al. Granulocyte-colony and granulocyte-macrophage-colony stimulating factors induce human-endothelial cells to migrate and proliferate. Nature. 1989;337(6206):471–3.
73. Akdemir A, Zeybek B, Akman L, Ergenoglu AM, Yeniel AO, Erbas O, et al. Granulocyte-colony stimulating factor decreases the extent of ovarian damage caused by cisplatin in an experimental rat model. J Gynecol Oncol. 2014;25(4):328–33.
74. Solaroglu I, Tsubokawa T, Cahill J, Zhang JH. Anti-apoptotic effect of granulocyte-colony stimulating factor after focal cerebral ischemia in the rat. Neuroscience. 2006;143(4):965–74.
75. Harada M, Qin YJ, Takano H, Minamino T, Zou YZ, Toko H, et al. G-csf prevents cardiac remodeling after myocardial infarction by activating the jak-stat pathway in cardiomyocytes. Nat Med. 2005;11(3):305–11.
76. Smith TJ, Khatcheressian J, Lyman GH, Ozer H, Armitage JO, Balducci L, et al. 2006 update of recommendations for the use of white blood cell growth factors: an evidence-based clinical practice guideline. J Clin Oncol. 2006;24(19):3187–205.

Chapter 2
Fertility Preservation Options for Female Pediatric and Adolescent Oncology Patients

Kathleen Shea and Jennifer Levine

Introduction

Maintaining the ability to have biologic children has been identified as an important component to post cancer quality of life in survivors [1, 2]. Achieving this in younger cancer patients has become more feasible secondary to improvements in reproductive technology [3]. Healthcare providers are now increasingly called upon to be familiar with the indications and options for fertility preservation in female pediatric and adolescent cancer patients [4]. Type of cancer, age, pubertal development, severity of illness at time of diagnosis, and type of treatment all impact decision making related to fertility preservation [5]. Patients at high risk include those receiving high-dose alkylating agents and pelvic radiation which lead to depletion of ovarian reserve and radiation to the brain that may interfere with the hypothalamic-pituitary-gonadal axis and those requiring surgical resection of reproductive structures. Patients receiving alkylating agents combined with pelvic radiation or total body irradiation and those that are older age at time of treatment are also at high risk for infertility [6]. This chapter will give an overview of current options for fertility preservation for female pediatric and adolescent cancer patients.

K. Shea, MS, CPNP • J. Levine, MD, MSW (✉)
Pediatric Hematology/Oncology/Stem Cell Transplantation, Columbia University Medical Center, 161 Fort Washington Ave IP7, New York, NY, USA
e-mail: Kas10@cumc.columbia.edu; jl175@cumc.columbia.edu

© Springer International Publishing Switzerland 2017
T.K. Woodruff, Y.C. Gosiengfiao (eds.), *Pediatric and Adolescent Oncofertility*,
DOI 10.1007/978-3-319-32973-4_2

Protection of Ovarian Function

Ovarian Transposition

Ovarian transposition, also known as oophoropexy, involves surgically relocating the ovaries out of the field of radiation. By decreasing exposure to radiation, transposition can reduce the incidence of premature ovarian failure [7]. Rhabdomyosarcoma of the bladder, vagina, or uterus or soft tissue or pelvic bone sarcomas, such as Ewing's sarcoma, are the main diagnostic indications for ovarian transposition in children. The procedure can be done laparoscopically or with concomitant laparotomy. The optimal timing is just prior to radiation therapy, as the ovaries can migrate back to the pelvis. If placed correctly, radiation exposure can be reduced by 90–95 %. However, patients need to be made aware that due to radiation scatter, ovaries are not always protected, and this technique is not always successful. Results are dependent on other variables such as age of patient, dose of radiation, degree of scatter, whether ovaries were shielded, and if gonadotoxic chemotherapy was also used [8].

An additional procedure to reverse the transposition may be necessary to facilitate either spontaneous pregnancy or assisted reproduction if the ovary is not in close proximity to the fallopian tube [9]. Alternatively, transabdominal monitoring and harvesting of oocytes during assisted reproduction may be utilized. Transabdominal harvesting may result in fewer oocytes obtained compared to use of transvaginal ultrasound, but equal efficacy in terms of fertilization rates, embryo number and quality, and pregnancy rates [10]. Although ovarian transposition is generally well tolerated, potential side effects include pelvic pain, necrosis, and ovarian torsion [11]. While few long-term results in adults are available, transposition has been reported to be effective at maintaining endocrine function, although it has had less success as a fertility preservation procedure [8]. The American Society of Clinical Oncology (ASCO) 2013 Guidelines for adults recommend discussing the option of ovarian transposition when pelvic radiation therapy is performed as cancer treatment [12]. For children, ASCO recommends providing information on methods that are investigational, and some would recommend ovarian transposition be discussed at a multidisciplinary meeting at the time of cancer diagnosis [8].

Ovarian Suppression

Strategies to protect the ovaries during chemotherapy include the use of gonadotropin-releasing hormone (GnRH) analogues. Though widely studied, efficacy of this approach has been conflicting; ASCO currently advises that there is insufficient evidence to support GNRH analogues as a means to preserve fertility [12]. Following the publication of the ASCO guidelines, the use of goserelin for ovarian suppression during chemotherapy for breast cancer appeared to protect against ovarian failure, reduce the risk of early menopause, and improve prospects for fertility [13]. Well-designed studies in the pediatric population across a variety of diagnoses and ages remain necessary to ascertain the effectiveness of this strategy in this population.

Assisted Reproductive Endocrinology

Embryo and Oocyte Cryopreservation

Embryo and oocyte cryopreservation are considered standard of care fertility preservation options in postpubertal patients at risk of ovarian failure [12]. Oocyte cryopreservation was designated nonexperimental by the American Society for Reproductive Medicine (ASRM) in 2012 [14]. Embryo cryopreservation is an established fertility preservation method with live birth rates of 30–40 % per embryo transferred in the general US population, with only slightly lower rates of live births from cryopreserved oocytes [15]. Furthermore, there is good evidence that fertilization and pregnancy rates are similar to in vitro fertilization/intracytoplasmic sperm injection (IVF/ICSI) with fresh oocytes when vitrified/warmed oocytes are used as part of IVF/ICSI for young women [14]. Although data are limited, no increase in chromosomal abnormalities, birth defects, and developmental deficits has been reported in the offspring born from cryopreserved oocytes when compared to pregnancies from conventional IVF/ICSI and the general population [14].

Both embryo and oocyte cryopreservation require controlled ovarian stimulation (COS) with daily injectable gonadotropins, traditionally beginning on the third day of the menstrual cycle and continuing daily for 10–12 days on average. The potential risks of COS include mild to severe ovarian hyperstimulation syndrome or intraabdominal bleeding. It is estimated that severe hyperstimulation syndrome will occur in 0.4–2.0 % of women during ovarian stimulation [16]. Ovulation is triggered by a single dose of human chorionic gonadotropin, and transvaginal oocyte retrieval is performed 34–36 h later under sedation. Newer, more flexible protocols have been developed where ovarian stimulation is not dependent on the timing of the menstrual cycle, resulting in fewer delays and shorter time to treatment initiation [17–20]. The number of total and mature oocytes retrieved, oocyte maturity rate, mature oocyte yield, and fertilization rates has been reported to be similar in random- ($n = 35$) and conventional-start ($n = 93$) COS cycles [19]. However, even if the process may be completed in 2–3 weeks, this may still be too long of a delay for patients that urgently require the start of treatment.

In those who can delay the start of treatment, oocyte cryopreservation may be preferred by younger pubertal patients, patients without partners, those who do not wish to use donor sperm, and/or those who have religious or ethical objections to embryo freezing [21, 22]. For those individuals who do wish to preserve embryos, harvested oocytes are fertilized in vitro either with partner or donor sperm and then cryopreserved. Intracytoplasmic sperm injection (ICSI) may be recommended to offset the risk of fertilization failure. Newer cryopreservation techniques such as vitrification have been shown to result in higher survival, fertilization, implantation, and pregnancy rates than slow-freezing techniques [23–26].

Despite the technical availability of these procedures, barriers continue to exist in their practical clinical application. Far more medical practitioners believe that pubertal female patients should be referred to a fertility specialist at diagnosis than those that actually make such a referral [27]. As noted above, the time to complete an embryo or oocyte cryopreservation cycle often exceeds the timeframe that patients and medical practitioners are willing to delay the start of therapy [28]. For many patients, the cost of oocyte or embryo cryopreservation and future IVF cycle may be prohibitive with fees in the USA between approximately $7,000 and $15,000 for a cycle [29]. Many insurance companies will not cover the cost of fertility preservation procedures as cancer patients do not meet the criteria of infertility, i.e., they have not been trying to achieve pregnancy for more than 1 year [30].

Ovarian Tissue Cryopreservation and Transplantation

An experimental option that is increasingly being performed, ovarian tissue cryopreservation, involves surgically removing all or part of the cortex of the ovary. The tissue, which contains thousands of primordial follicles, is cut into strips and cryopreserved. As the process does not require hormonal stimulation, it is the only fertility preservation technique involving gonadal tissue that is available to prepubertal girls or pubertal girls in whom initiation of treatment cannot be delayed [31, 32]. Following completion of treatment, when fertility is desired, the ovarian tissue can be thawed and transplanted orthotopically, i.e., at the site of the ovaries, or heterotopically, i.e., at another location. Once transplanted, the follicles within the ovary have the potential to mature when appropriately stimulated. Approximately 40 live births have been reported utilizing orthotopic re-transplantation in individuals who were postpubertal at the time of retrieval [5, 33]. No live births have been reported in individuals who were prepubescent at the time of tissue cryopreservation. However, a live birth has been reported after autograft of ovarian tissue in a patient who had initiated puberty but was premenarchal at the time of the cryopreservation. The patient, who had sickle cell disease, had developed primary ovarian failure after a myeloablative conditioning regimen as part of a hematopoietic stem cell transplantation [33].

Because of its investigational nature, ovarian tissue cryopreservation should be performed in centers with clinical expertise under IRB-approved protocols that include follow-up for recurrent cancer [12]. Obtaining tissue requires a surgical procedure with anesthesia, although ideally this could be coordinated with other procedures required for evaluation or treatment [34]. Maturation of immature follicles retrieved from ovarian tissue remains an area of critical research. The capacity for in vitro maturation would negate the need to autotransplant the ovarian tissue in vivo [35] and would prevent the risk of reintroducing cancerous cells that may be present in transplanted ovarian tissue [36].

Assessment of Ovarian Reserve

Discussions about reproduction should continue posttreatment and during survivorship for all patients. Patients who have developed acute ovarian failure (AOF) following the completion of cancer-directed therapy can be identified by lack of entry into puberty or sustained amenorrhea and sustained elevations of FSH in the menopausal range in pubertal patients. These patients should be referred to an endocrinologist for consideration of hormone replacement. Determining which patients have experienced a decrease in their ovarian reserve insufficient to result in AOF, referred to as premature menopause (PM), has remained a much more elusive goal. The Children's Oncology Group (COG) currently recommends screening patients exposed to gonadotoxic therapy for Tanner stage and pubertal, menstrual, and pregnancy history. Current guidelines recommend screening follicle-stimulating hormone (FSH), luteinizing hormone (LH), and estradiol levels beginning at age 13 [37]; however, these measures are very inexact and are likely to become abnormal only once ovarian reserve is significantly compromised. Early follicular phase FSH, anti-Mullerian hormone (AMH) (a product of antral follicles), and ultrasound assessments of antral follicle count are utilized in the reproductive endocrinology community to evaluate fertility and potential response to fertility interventions [38] and show promise as better surrogate measures of remaining ovarian reserve. Refining this estimate is crucial to allowing more accurate counseling of pediatric and adolescent cancer survivors about their reproductive options post therapy.

Reproductive Options Post Therapy

Donor Oocytes and Embryos

Patients who are in AOF may consider options such as utilization of donor oocytes or embryos if their uterus has not been impaired by cancer-directed therapy such as radiation. Oocytes from another woman (either a non-anonymous or anonymous donor) may be fertilized with the recipient's partner's sperm or with donor sperm and placed in the recipient's uterus. The oocyte donor receives the same ovarian stimulation regimen used during an IVF cycle. The recipient receives hormonal medication to modify her cycle in preparation for the embryo transfer. If pregnancy is achieved, hormonal treatment continues through at least the twelfth week of pregnancy. Woman without ovaries may achieve pregnancy with the use of exogenous hormones [39]. The use of donated embryos may also be considered in couples with infertility affecting both partners, infertility in a single woman, or couples with genetic disorders. IVF cycles may result in unused embryos that may be destroyed, donated to research, or donated to another woman to achieve pregnancy. Recipients need to be counseled and informed of the complexities involved in potential relationships between donors and recipients and individual state laws regarding parentage during pregnancy and after birth. Rates of success are dependent on the age of the donor woman, quality of embryos at the time of freezing, and number of embryos transferred [39].

Fertility Preservation Post Therapy

Many patients who are treated with gonadotoxic agents as children and adolescents will retain reproductive potential post treatment but will be at risk of premature menopause [40]. For these patients, it is important to conduct conversations regarding their plan for starting a family. While it remains virtually impossible to determine the remaining reproductive window for a given individual, cryopreserving oocytes or embryos post completion of therapy may be of interest to individuals who are not certain when they might want to start a family. Recent evidence also suggests that even individuals with evidence of premature menopause can achieve pregnancies with the use of assisted reproduction such as IVF/ICSI [41].

Gestational Carrier

A gestational carrier or gestational surrogate is an arrangement between a woman who carries and delivers a baby for another person that is the intended parent. This option may be considered by a woman who does not have a uterus, has uterine damage or scarring, or has a condition that prevents her from carrying a pregnancy to term. This option involves an IVF cycle with embryos made from donors or the intended parent and not the gestational carrier. Medical and psychological screening is required for gestational carriers. Intended parents have genetic, medical, and psychological evaluations. Intended parents need to obtain legal counsel regarding state laws and gestational carrier contracts [42].

Adoption

Patients not able to have biologic children may consider adoption as a means of family building. Cancer survivors may face more challenges such as additional medical documentation of their health status and a required 5-year off treatment waiting period [43]. Individuals and couples would need to explore the various scenarios surrounding adoption such as domestic or international origins, open or closed adoption, and comfort level accepting an infant or older child, siblings, or medically fragile children. Many agencies and individual countries have age, income, and marital status requirements. Birth mothers choosing adoptive parents may have ethnic and/or religious preferences. Adoption agencies and lawyers guide candidates through the adoption process. Adoption is costly with fees ranging from $29,000 to $49,000 for domestic adoption and $17,000 to $28,000 for international adoptions. The Internal Revenue Service offers a federal tax credit (maximum $13,400) for adoptive families. Some states may have programs for adoption of children from foster care systems that may be less costly.

Access to Fertility Preservation

First and foremost in ensuring access to fertility preservation procedures for pediatric and adolescent cancer patients and their families is establishing notification of risks to fertility and possible fertility preservation options as standard of care. Multiple publications have demonstrated that this is not currently the case [44–46] . Despite ASCO guidelines advising oncologists to discuss fertility risks and preservation strategies and make referrals to reproductive endocrinologists, over half are not doing so. Often cited barriers are lack of proper training and knowledge about referrals and perception that patients could not delay treatment to pursue options and patients were not interested in discussing fertility because it was not mentioned [47]. Female oncologists and those with favorable attitudes toward fertility preservation and those with patients that ask about fertility preservation are more likely to refer to reproductive specialists [48]. In 2013, ASCO updated its guidelines to include other physicians as well as nurses, psychologists, and other nonphysician providers as candidates for disseminating information to patients regarding fertility preservation [12].

Institutions are increasingly developing fertility programs that provide guidance about the elements necessary to effectively inform patients about their risks and options and create workflows and infrastructure to provide timely referrals to reproductive endocrinology. The key elements include developing institutional policies that demonstrate a commitment to fertility preservation, creating a team of individuals who "champion" the provision of these services, developing educational resources for patients and families as well as clinical staff, and developing established relationships with reproductive endocrinologists [49–51]. Programs such as LIVESTRONG provide assistance to financially eligible patients with the cost of medication and contract with agencies across the USA to provide services as reduced cost for cancer patients (http://www.livestrong.org/we-can-help/fertility-services).

Ethical Considerations

As outlined above, there are numerous concerns that appropriate access to fertility preservation options exists. Despite significant study in the area of gonadotoxicity, it remains extremely difficult to assess the risk for AOF or PM in a given individual prior to the start of cancer-directed therapy. Because there is also limited data related to the overall efficacy of the various fertility cryopreservation techniques specifically in the pediatric oncology population clinicians, patients and parents must often make decisions about expensive, invasive procedures with limited information during an already emotional time [52]. Given that there is no standardization of coverage of these procedures by insurance companies, there is also the concern that socioeconomic disparities may exist based upon who is able to pay and therefore access interventions [22].

In the pediatric population, minors will be asked to provide their assent for procedures that are related to issues, i.e., family planning, that they may be ill-saited to consider. Disposition of stored ovarian tissue, oocytes, or embryos in the setting of a patient's death remains an issue of concern, particularly in the pediatric setting where a patient is under the age of 18 and is not legally able to determine disposition of stored tissue. While there are mechanisms by which stored tissue would not be able to be utilized unless the patient has reached maturity and consented to the use of the tissue, controversies remain [52]. In the setting of embryos, the situation is further complicated by the wishes and desires of the individual who provided the sperm. Disposition of unused tissue, oocytes, or embryos can also present moral and religious conflicts if the patient is able to become pregnant via intercourse or assisted reproduction and does not require use of the stored tissue.

Future Directions

Generation of Gametes from Somatic Cells

Ovarian tissue cryopreservation followed by orthotopic or heterotopic transplantation is currently the only method of fertility preservation for prepubertal girls and the only method available to pubertal girls and adolescents that cannot delay therapy to do oocyte cryopreservation. Research studying the development of ovarian follicles in vitro is underway. This presents significant challenges given the complex systems involved in oocyte development and maturation. Researchers are exploring ways to apply current culture systems to the growth and development of cryopreserved-thawed follicles for clinical use in patients who have banked ovarian tissue. This would eliminate the need for additional reimplantation surgery, eliminate the risk of reintroduction of potentially diseased ovarian tissue into a healthy recipient, and present an option when treatment cannot be delayed [53–55].

Coverage of Fertility Preservation by Insurance

As noted above, fertility preservation costs are generally not covered by most insurance companies as most cancer patients do not fit the insurance companies' definition of infertility that is being unable to achieve pregnancy after 1 year of trying. Arguments have been made that given the iatrogenic nature of infertility among patients with cancer, different eligibility criteria should be applied to these patients when considering fertility preservation interventions [56].

Conclusion

Increased knowledge about the importance of fertility preservation for pediatric and adolescent patients with cancer and improvements in assisted reproduction techniques has increased the likelihood that meeting the family planning goals for survivors of cancer has and will continue to improve over time. Fully meeting this goal means refining risk, developing the institutional infrastructure to identify patients at risk in a timely fashion, streamlining referrals to the appropriate subspecialists, advocating for insurance coverage for fertility preservation procedures, and continuing to move the research agenda forward to advance the efficacy of available options.

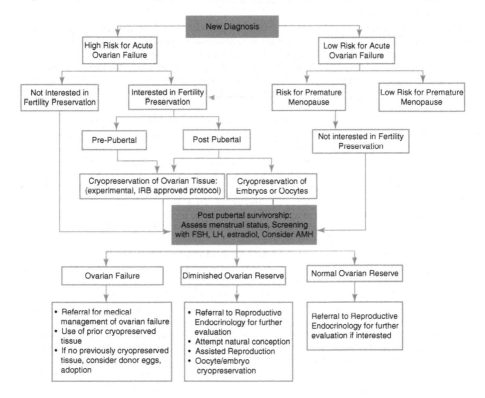

References

1. Jeruss JS, Woodruff TK. Preservation of fertility in patients with cancer. N Engl J Med. 2009;360(9):902–11. doi:10.1056/NEJMra0801454. PubMed PMID: 19246362; PMCID: 2927217.
2. Schover LR. Psychosocial aspects of infertility and decisions about reproduction in young cancer survivors: a review. Med Pediatr Oncol. 1999;33(1):53–9.
3. Ginsberg JP. New advances in fertility preservation for pediatric cancer patients. Curr Opin Pediatr. 2011;23(1):9–13. doi:10.1097/MOP.0b013e3283420fb6. PubMed PMID: 21157350; PMCID: 3095100.
4. Caserta D, Ralli E, Matteucci E, Marci R, Moscarini M. Fertility preservation in female cancer patients: an emerging challenge for physicians. Panminerva Med. 2014;56(1):85–95.

5. Anderson RA, Mitchell RT, Kelsey TW, Spears N, Telfer EE, Wallace WH. Cancer treatment and gonadal function: experimental and established strategies for fertility preservation in children and young adults. Lancet Diabetes Endocrinol. 2015;3(7):556–67. doi:10.1016/S2213-8587(15)00039-X.

6. Levine JM, Kelvin JF, Quinn GP, Gracia CR. Infertility in reproductive-age female cancer survivors. Cancer. 2015;121(10):1532–9. doi:10.1002/cncr.29181.

7. Terenziani M, Piva L, Meazza C, Gandola L, Cefalo G, Merola M. Oophoropexy: a relevant role in preservation of ovarian function after pelvic irradiation. Fertil Steril. 2009;91(3):935 e15–6. doi:10.1016/j.fertnstert.2008.09.029.

8. Irtan S, Orbach D, Helfre S, Sarnacki S. Ovarian transposition in prepubescent and adolescent girls with cancer. Lancet Oncol. 2013;14(13):e601–8. doi:10.1016/S1470-2045(13)70288-2.

9. Noyes N, Knopman JM, Long K, Coletta JM, Abu-Rustum NR. Fertility considerations in the management of gynecologic malignancies. Gynecol Oncol. 2011;120(3):326–33. doi:10.1016/j.ygyno.2010.09.012.

10. Barton SE, Politch JA, Benson CB, Ginsburg ES, Gargiulo AR. Transabdominal follicular aspiration for oocyte retrieval in patients with ovaries inaccessible by transvaginal ultrasound. Fertil Steril. 2011;95(5):1773–6. doi:10.1016/j.fertnstert.2011.01.006.

11. Gomez-Hidalgo NR, Darin MC, Dalton H, Jhingran A, Fleming N, Brown J, Ramirez PT. Ovarian torsion after laparoscopic ovarian transposition in patients with gynecologic cancer: a report of two cases. J Minim Invasive Gynecol. 2015;22(4):687–90. doi:10.1016/j.jmig.2015.02.009.

12. Loren AW, Mangu PB, Beck LN, Brennan L, Magdalinski AJ, Partridge AH, Quinn G, Wallace WH, Oktay K, American Society of Clinical Oncology. Fertility preservation for patients with cancer: American Society of Clinical Oncology clinical practice guideline update. J Clin Oncol Off J Am Soc Clin Oncol. 2013;31(19):2500–10. doi:10.1200/JCO.2013.49.2678.

13. Moore HC, Unger JM, Phillips KA, Boyle F, Hitre E, Porter D, Francis PA, Goldstein LJ, Gomez HL, Vallejos CS, Partridge AH, Dakhil SR, Garcia AA, Gralow J, Lombard JM, Forbes JF, Martino S, Barlow WE, Fabian CJ, Minasian L, Meyskens Jr FL, Gelber RD, Hortobagyi GN, Albain KS, Investigators PS. Goserelin for ovarian protection during breast-cancer adjuvant chemotherapy. N Engl J Med. 2015;372(10):923–32. doi:10.1056/NEJMoa1413204. PubMed PMID: 25738668; PMCID: 4405231.

14. Practice Committees of American Society for Reproductive Medicine, Society for Assisted Reproductive Technology. Mature oocyte cryopreservation: a guideline. Fertil Steril. 2013;99(1):37–43. doi:10.1016/j.fertnstert.2012.09.028.

15. Practice Committee of American Society for Reproductive Medicine. Fertility preservation in patients undergoing gonadotoxic therapy or gonadectomy: a committee opinion. Fertil Steril. 2013;100(5):1214–23. doi:10.1016/j.fertnstert.2013.08.012.

16. Practice Committee of American Society for Reproductive Medicine. Ovarian hyperstimulation syndrome. Fertil Steril. 2008;90(5 Suppl):S188–93. doi:10.1016/j.fertnstert.2008.08.034.

17. Sonmezer M, Turkcuoglu I, Coskun U, Oktay K. Random-start controlled ovarian hyperstimulation for emergency fertility preservation in letrozole cycles. Fertil Steril. 2011;95(6):2125. e9–11. doi:10.1016/j.fertnstert.2011.01.030.

18. Keskin U, Ercan CM, Yilmaz A, Babacan A, Korkmaz C, Duru NK, Ergun A. Random-start controlled ovarian hyperstimulation with letrozole for fertility preservation in cancer patients: case series and review of literature. JPMA J Pak Med Assoc. 2014;64(7):830–2.

19. Cakmak H, Katz A, Cedars MI, Rosen MP. Effective method for emergency fertility preservation: random-start controlled ovarian stimulation. Fertil Steril. 2013;100(6):1673–80. doi:10.1016/j.fertnstert.2013.07.1992.

20. Kim JH, Kim SK, Lee HJ, Lee JR, Jee BC, Suh CS, Kim SH. Efficacy of random-start controlled ovarian stimulation in cancer patients. J Korean Med Sci. 2015;30(3):290–5. doi:10.3346/jkms.2015.30.3.290. PubMed PMID: 25729252; PMCID: 4330484.

21. Noyes N, Knopman JM, Melzer K, Fino ME, Friedman B, Westphal LM. Oocyte cryopreservation as a fertility preservation measure for cancer patients. Reprod Biomed Online. 2011;23(3):323–33. doi:10.1016/j.rbmo.2010.11.011.

22. Ayensu-Coker L, Essig E, Breech LL, Lindheim S. Ethical quandaries in gamete-embryo cryo-preservation related to oncofertility. J Law Med Ethics J Am Soc Law Med Ethics. 2013;41(3):711–9. doi:10.1111/jlme.12081.
23. Martinez-Burgos M, Herrero L, Megias D, Salvanes R, Montoya MC, Cobo AC, Garcia-Velasco JA. Vitrification versus slow freezing of oocytes: effects on morphologic appearance, meiotic spindle configuration, and DNA damage. Fertil Steril. 2011;95(1):374–7. doi:10.1016/j.fertnstert.2010.07.1089.
24. Cao YX, Xing Q, Li L, Cong L, Zhang ZG, Wei ZL, Zhou P. Comparison of survival and embryonic development in human oocytes cryopreserved by slow-freezing and vitrification. Fertil Steril. 2009;92(4):1306–11. doi:10.1016/j.fertnstert.2008.08.069.
25. Smith GD, Serafini PC, Fioravanti J, Yadid I, Coslovsky M, Hassun P, Alegretti JR, Motta EL. Prospective randomized comparison of human oocyte cryopreservation with slow-rate freezing or vitrification. Fertil Steril. 2010;94(6):2088–95. doi:10.1016/j.fertnstert.2009.12.065.
26. Fadini R, Brambillasca F, Renzini MM, Merola M, Comi R, De Ponti E, Dal Canto MB. Human oocyte cryopreservation: comparison between slow and ultrarapid methods. Reprod Biomed Online. 2009;19(2):171–80.
27. Kohler TS, Kondapalli LA, Shah A, Chan S, Woodruff TK, Brannigan RE. Results from the survey for preservation of adolescent reproduction (SPARE) study: gender disparity in delivery of fertility preservation message to adolescents with cancer. J Assist Reprod Genet. 2011;28(3):269–77. doi:10.1007/s10815-010-9504-6. PubMed PMID: 21110080; PMCID: 3082660.
28. Burns KC, Boudreau C, Panepinto JA. Attitudes regarding fertility preservation in female adolescent cancer patients. J Pediatr Hematol Oncol. 2006;28(6):350–4.
29. Hirshfeld-Cytron J, Grobman WA, Milad MP. Fertility preservation for social indications: a cost-based decision analysis. Fertil Steril. 2012;97(3):665–70. doi:10.1016/j.fertnstert.2011.12.029.
30. Basco D, Campo Engelstein L, Rodriguez S. Insuring against infertility: expanding state infertility mandates to include fertility preservation technology for cancer patients. J Law Med Ethics J Am Soc Law Med Ethics. 2010;38(4):832–9. doi:10.1111/j.1748-720X.2010.00536.x. PubMed PMID: 21105946; PMCID: 3097090.
31. Gracia CR, Chang J, Kondapalli L, Prewitt M, Carlson CA, Mattei P, Jeffers S, Ginsberg JP. Ovarian tissue cryopreservation for fertility preservation in cancer patients: successful establishment and feasibility of a multidisciplinary collaboration. J Assist Reprod Genet. 2012;29(6):495–502. doi:10.1007/s10815-012-9753-7. PubMed PMID: 22466745; PMCID: 3370042.
32. Kim SS. Fertility preservation in female cancer patients: current developments and future directions. Fertil Steril. 2006;85(1):1–11. doi:10.1016/j.fertnstert.2005.04.071.
33. Demeestere I, Simon P, Dedeken L, Moffa F, Tsepelidis S, Brachet C, Delbaere A, Devreker F, Ferster A. Live birth after autograft of ovarian tissue cryopreserved during childhood. Hum Reprod. 2015. doi:10.1093/humrep/dev128.
34. Babayev SN, Arslan E, Kogan S, Moy F, Oktay K. Evaluation of ovarian and testicular tissue cryopreservation in children undergoing gonadotoxic therapies. J Assist Reprod Genet. 2013;30(1):3–9. doi:10.1007/s10815-012-9909-5. PubMed PMID: 23242649; PMCID: 3553347.
35. Smitz J, Dolmans MM, Donnez J, Fortune JE, Hovatta O, Jewgenow K, Picton HM, Plancha C, Shea LD, Stouffer RL, Telfer EE, Woodruff TK, Zelinski MB. Current achievements and future research directions in ovarian tissue culture, in vitro follicle development and transplantation: implications for fertility preservation. Hum Reprod Update. 2010;16(4):395–414. doi:10.1093/humupd/dmp056. PubMed PMID: 20124287; PMCID: 2880913.
36. Dolmans MM, Marinescu C, Saussoy P, Van Langendonckt A, Amorim C, Donnez J. Reimplantation of cryopreserved ovarian tissue from patients with acute lymphoblastic leukemia is potentially unsafe. Blood. 2010;116(16):2908–14. doi:10.1182/blood-2010-01-265751.
37. Metzger ML, Meacham LR, Patterson B, Casillas JS, Constine LS, Hijiya N, Kenney LB, Leonard M, Lockart BA, Likes W, Green DM. Female reproductive health after childhood, adolescent, and young adult cancers: guidelines for the assessment and management of female

reproductive complications. J Clin Oncol Off J Am Soc Clin Oncol. 2013;31(9):1239–47. doi:10.1200/JCO.2012.43.5511.

38. Practice Committee of the American Society for Reproductive Medicine. Testing and interpreting measures of ovarian reserve: a committee opinion. Fertil Steril. 2012;98(6):1407–15. doi:10.1016/j.fertnstert.2012.09.036.

39. American Society for Reproductive Medicine. [Cited 2015 August 7th]. Available from: https://www.asrm.org/BOOKLET_Third-party_Reproduction/.

40. Sklar CA, Mertens AC, Mitby P, Whitton J, Stovall M, Kasper C, Mulder J, Green D, Nicholson HS, Yasui Y, Robison LL. Premature menopause in survivors of childhood cancer: a report from the childhood cancer survivor study. J Natl Cancer Inst. 2006;98(13):890–6. doi:10.1093/jnci/djj243.

41. Barton SE, Najita JS, Ginsburg ES, Leisenring WM, Stovall M, Weathers RE, Sklar CA, Robison LL, Diller L. Infertility, infertility treatment, and achievement of pregnancy in female survivors of childhood cancer: a report from the Childhood Cancer Survivor Study cohort. Lancet Oncol. 2013;14(9):873–81. doi:10.1016/S1470-2045(13)70251-1. PubMed PMID: 23856401; PMCID: 3845882.

42. Armour KL. An overview of surrogacy around the world: trends, questions and ethical issues. Nurs Women Health. 2012;16(3):231–6. doi:10.1111/j.1751-486X.2012.01734.x.

43. Quinn GP, Zebrack BJ, Sehovic I, Bowman ML, Vadaparampil ST. Adoption and cancer survivors: findings from a learning activity for oncology nurses. Cancer. 2015. doi:10.1002/cncr.29322.

44. Shnorhavorian M, Harlan LC, Smith AW, Keegan TH, Lynch CF, Prasad PK, Cress RD, Wu XC, Hamilton AS, Parsons HM, Keel G, Charlesworth SE, Schwartz SM, AHSC Group. Fertility preservation knowledge, counseling, and actions among adolescent and young adult patients with cancer: a population-based study. Cancer. 2015. doi:10.1002/cncr.29328.

45. Quinn GP, Block RG, Clayman ML, Kelvin J, Arvey SR, Lee JH, Reinecke J, Sehovic I, Jacobsen PB, Reed D, Gonzalez L, Vadaparampil ST, Laronga C, Lee MC, Pow-Sang J, Eggly S, Franklin A, Shah B, Fulp WJ, Hayes-Lattin B. If you did not document it, it did not happen: rates of documentation of discussion of infertility risk in adolescent and young adult oncology patients' medical records. J Oncol Pract Am Soc Clin Oncol. 2015;11(2):137–44. doi:10.1200/JOP.2014.000786.

46. Bastings L, Baysal O, Beerendonk CC, Braat DD, Nelen WL. Referral for fertility preservation counselling in female cancer patients. Hum Reprod. 2014;29(10):2228–37. doi:10.1093/humrep/deu186.

47. Quinn GP, Vadaparampil ST, King L, Miree CA, Wilson C, Raj O, Watson J, Lopez A, Albrecht TL. Impact of physicians' personal discomfort and patient prognosis on discussion of fertility preservation with young cancer patients. Patient Educ Couns. 2009;77(3):338–43. doi:10.1016/j.pec.2009.09.007.

48. Quinn GP, Vadaparampil ST, Lee JH, Jacobsen PB, Bepler G, Lancaster J, Keefe DL, Albrecht TL. Physician referral for fertility preservation in oncology patients: a national study of practice behaviors. J Clin Oncol Off J Am Soc Clin Oncol. 2009;27(35):5952–7. doi:10.1200/JCO.2009.23.0250.

49. Kim J, Kim KH, Mersereau JE. Building a successful fertility preservation program at a major cancer center. J Gynecol Oncol. 2014;25(2):148–54. doi:10.3802/jgo.2014.25.2.148. PubMed PMID: 24761219; PMCID: 3996265.

50. Reinecke JD, Kelvin JF, Arvey SR, Quinn GP, Levine J, Beck LN, Miller A. Implementing a systematic approach to meeting patients' cancer and fertility needs: a review of the Fertile Hope Centers of Excellence program. J Oncol Pract Am Soc Clin Oncol. 2012;8(5):303–8. doi:10.1200/JOP.2011.000452. PubMed PMID: 23277768; PMCID: 3439231.

51. Oncorfertility Consortium. Implementation of a fertility preservation program [cited 2015 August 8th]. Available from: http://oncofertility.northwestern.edu/implementation-fertility-preservation-program.

52. Stegmann BJ. Unique ethical and legal implications of fertility preservation research in the pediatric population. Fertil Steril. 2010;93(4):1037–9. doi:10.1016/j.fertnstert.2009.11.047.
53. Telfer EE, Zelinski MB. Ovarian follicle culture: advances and challenges for human and nonhuman primates. Fertil Steril. 2013;99(6):1523–33. doi:10.1016/j.fertnstert.2013.03.043. PubMed PMID: 23635350; PMCID: 3929501.
54. Shea LD, Woodruff TK, Shikanov A. Bioengineering the ovarian follicle microenvironment. Annu Rev Biomed Eng. 2014;16:29–52. doi:10.1146/annurev-bioeng-071813-105131. PubMed PMID: 24849592; PMCID: 4231138.
55. De Vos M, Smitz J, Woodruff TK. Fertility preservation in women with cancer. Lancet. 2014;384(9950):1302–10. doi:10.1016/S0140-6736(14)60834-5. PubMed PMID: 25283571; PMCID: 4270060.
56. Campo-Engelstein L. Consistency in insurance coverage for iatrogenic conditions resulting from cancer treatment including fertility preservation. J Clin Oncol Off J Am Soc Clin Oncol. 2010;28(8):1284–6. doi:10.1200/JCO.2009.25.6883. PubMed PMID: 20142588; PMCID: 2834493.

Chapter 3
Assessing Ovarian Reserve

Yasmin Gosiengfiao and Veronica Gomez-Lobo

Background

Female cancer survivors are known to be at risk for decreased fertility and early menopause. Fertility is defined as the ability to produce young [1–3]. Conversely, infertility is defined by the failure to achieve a clinical pregnancy after 12 months or more of regular unprotected sexual intercourse [4]. Having pregnancies thus would be the best measure of fertility. Using pregnancies as a measure of fertility, however, limits one to waiting until a childhood cancer survivor has grown into an adult and has attempted to get pregnant. Even among adults, not all adult women attempt to get pregnant. Thus, surrogate measures of fertility are necessary to assess the effect of chemotherapy/radiation/surgery on fertility.

Most cancer survivors experience infertility due to direct effects of treatment on the ovary or testes. The initial number of follicles in humans is established in utero at 5 months gestation with approximately ten million primordial follicles. This number of follicles (or ovarian reserve) diminishes in utero and after birth to nearly 500,000 at menarche and continues to decline thereafter until these fall below a certain threshold and menopause appears [5]. Ovarian reserve is the concept that views reproductive potential as a function of the number and quality of oocytes. Radiation and other gonadotoxic agents are thought to affect the number of follicles by possibly accelerating this process of attrition [2, 6–8]. The effect of treatment on an individual patient's ovarian reserve depends on many factors including: the age at the time of gonadotoxic treatment, the type and dose

Y. Gosiengfiao, MD (✉)
Hematology, Oncology & Stem Cell Transplantation, Ann & Robert H. Lurie Children's Hospital of Chicago, 225 E. Chicago Ave Box 30, Chicago, IL, USA
e-mail: ygosiengfiao@luriechildrens.org

V. Gomez-Lobo, MD
Women and Infant Services (MWHC)/Surgery (CNMC), MedStar Washington Hospital Center/Children's National Medical Center, 110 Irving St NW, Washington, DC 20010, USA

© Springer International Publishing Switzerland 2017
T.K. Woodruff, Y.C. Gosiengfiao (eds.), *Pediatric and Adolescent Oncofertility*,
DOI 10.1007/978-3-319-32973-4_3

of therapy, genetic factors, previous illnesses, and prior infertility. It is important to note that even before menopause (or the cessation of menses) is noted, the number and/or quality of the follicles may preclude pregnancy [9]. Infertility may be caused by decreased ovarian reserve or sperm production, but other causes such as tubal, uterine, and cervical factors may influence fertility. Thus, surrogate measures of ovarian or testicular reserve do not fully measure fertility potential.

Assessing Ovarian Reserve

There are several markers that have been used to assess ovarian reserve (OR). It should be noted, however, that most of the research regarding these markers has been performed in healthy ovarian aging and women seeking treatment for infertility and debate still remains regarding the ability of these markers to predict oocyte quality, quantity, and fecundity in healthy women. Furthermore, it is important to note that these tests are "screening" tests that would be helpful only if they predict ovarian reserve prior to menopause or ovarian insufficiency [6]. Thus, these markers may not be good measures of fertility for young women treated with gonadotoxic agents [10].

Menstrual Cycles

In 2006 the American College of Obstetrics and Gynecology (ACOG) and the American Academy of Pediatrics (AAP) issued a Committee Opinion stating that the menstrual cycle is a vital sign, thus stressing the importance of menses [11]. The average age of menarche in the western world declined rapidly in the last two centuries but has been stable since the 1950s in the developed world. Normal menstrual cycles in young females include a median age of menarche of 12 years, mean cycle interval of 32 days with a range of 21–45 days, and flow length of 7 days. Primary amenorrhea is defined as the absence of menses by age 15, and secondary amenorrhea has been defined as the absence of cycles for more than 6 months [11]. Early menopause has been defined as cessation of menses prior to age 40, and the average age of menopause in the United States is 51. Adult female survivors of childhood cancers have been noted to have earlier age of menopause and a higher rate or premature menopause than the general population [3].

The presence or absence of menses has traditionally been used as the primary measure of fertility and ovarian function in cancer survivors, but it should be noted that there are many common causes of amenorrhea including pregnancy, polycystic ovary syndrome, structural issues (scarring of the uterus), and disturbances of the central gonadotropin-releasing hormone pulse generator. These disturbances are often referred to as hypogonadotropic hypogonadism and may be caused by significant weight loss, strenuous exercise, substantial changes in sleeping or eating habits, as well as severe stressors [11]. For example, a young cancer survivor may have absence of menses due to hypothalamic disturbances caused by the stress of treatment or ovarian insufficiency due to gonadotoxic agents. In addition, women may continue to have regular menses even in the presence of diminished ovarian reserve (such as occurs in the perimenopause). Thus, the presence of menses is a poor predictor of ovarian reserve and other markers should be used to assess OR.

Antral Follicle Counts and Ovarian Volume

Antral follicle counts and ovarian volume have traditionally been measured using transvaginal ultrasound in adult women. Both of these undergo an age-related decline and are good predictors of the number of eggs that can be retrieved with ovarian stimulation in women undergoing in vitro fertilization. Antral follicle count (AFC) is the number of small follicles (2–9 mm) that are observed in both ovaries during the early follicular phase of the cycle [6]. AFC is noted to have good inter-cycle and interobserver reliability and thus is considered promising as a screening test for ovarian reserve. Again tests revealing low AFC (three to six total antral follicles) correlate with poor response to ovarian stimulation but does not reliably predict failure to conceive [6]. Ovarian volume in general correlates with a number of follicles but has been noted in some studies to have poor inter-cycle reliability [6]. Though interobserver variability can be minimized with the use of three-dimensional sonography, this test is poor at predicting diminished ovarian reserve [6]. In children, AFC and ovarian volume can be performed transabdominally but requires a radiologist skilled in this technique and has not been well studied in this age group. Thus, antral follicle counts may help in predicting decreased ovarian reserve but deserves further study in cancer populations and children.

Endocrine Hormones

Biochemical tests for ovarian reserve in adult women include basal measurements such as follicle-stimulating hormone (FSH), estradiol, inhibin B, and anti-Mullerian hormone as well as stimulated tests such as the clomiphene citrate challenge test [6]. The latter cannot be performed in children but the former should be further studied.

Follicle-Stimulating Hormone (FSH), Inhibin B, and Estradiol

FSH is secreted by the pituitary in order to stimulate follicular growth and varies throughout the menstrual cycle. When ovarian reserve is decreased, FSH begins to rise earlier in the cycle and lead to earlier follicular growth and increase in estradiol concentrations. As follicles further decrease in number, the FSH continues to rise and estradiol levels fall. Inhibin B is secreted by preantral follicles, and as follicles decrease so does inhibin B which in turn lowers central nervous system feedback and thus further increases FSH [12–14].

Serum FSH assays have significant inter- and intra-cycle variability, the absolute values differ depending on which one is used, and the sensitivity in identifying poor responders to ovarian stimulation in women varies widely [6]. In addition, children have low FSH due to hypothalamic suppression. It should be noted that in spite of these limitations, consistently high levels of FSH are predictive of diminished ovarian reserve, and levels above 40 IU/L are diagnostic for premature ovarian insufficiency or menopause [6]. Estradiol assays also have poor intra- and inter-cycle variability, and basal levels do not differ between women with and without diminished ovarian reserve [6]. Furthermore, in prepubertal children, estradiol levels are also low due to hypothalamic suppression. Inhibin B has also been noted to not be a reliable measure of ovarian reserve. Thus, the use of FSH, inhibin B, and estradiol levels in assessing fertility potential of cancer patients is limited by variation with the menstrual cycles, poor sensitivity, and the low to undetectable levels in prepubertal children. Furthermore, combined ovarian reserve test models have not been shown to be superior to single tests in predicting ovarian reserve [6].

Anti-Mullerian Hormone (AMH)

AMH is a hormone produced by the granulosa cells, which acts as a follicular gatekeeper and is independent of FSH or gonadotropin. This marker is an indirect marker of antral follicle counts and thus ovarian reserve [15]. In childhood and adolescence, there is a complex rise in AMH level, which likely reflects the different stages of follicle development. It then peaks in a woman's early 20s before declining to menopause, correlating positively with nongrowing follicle recruitment [20].

Interest in the use of AMH as a measure of ovarian reserve to measure the gonadotoxic effect of chemotherapy/radiotherapy is growing, especially for children in whom FSH and inhibin B are not useful. When compared with other ovarian reserve markers, AMH levels reflect changes in ovarian function earlier, and there is no significant fluctuation of AMH during the menstrual cycle, and it is highly predictive for timing of menopause [16–18], suggesting that it may be the most useful marker for monitoring the decline of reproductive capacity. Moreover, serum AMH levels are detectable in healthy females from birth to menopause [19, 20], making it suitable as a marker even in prepubertal girls. Studies of AMH screening have noted an association with poor results with in vitro fertilization (IVF), but levels are not necessarily predictive [6]. Low AMH cut points are associated with sensitivities in general IVF populations of 40–97 % with specificities of 78–92 %, and low levels of AMH are specific for poor ovarian response but not pregnancy [6]. Furthermore, it should be noted that there are limited data correlating AMH and natural fertility at different stages of reproductive life and especially in children and adolescents. In addition, AMH assays continue to evolve and there are no international standards [6]. Therefore, more long-term data is needed to ascertain the use of AMH to evaluate fertility preservation strategies as well as predict long-term ovarian function after cancer therapy (Fig. 3.1).

Current Data on AMH in Children Receiving Cancer Therapy

In women treated with mechlorethamine, vincristine, procarbazine, and prednisone (MOPP) chemotherapy for Hodgkin lymphoma during childhood, AMH was noted to be lower compared with healthy women and women treated without MOPP [21]. In a larger series of 185 childhood cancer survivors, although the cohort's median

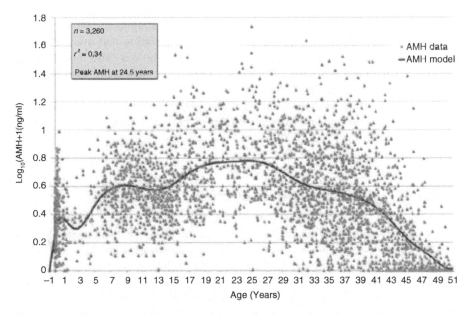

Fig. 3.1 A validated model of serum AMH from conception to menopause [20]

AMH concentration was no different from controls, the AMH levels were lower than the 10th percentile of normal values in 27 % of the survivors. Survivors treated with three or more procarbazine containing chemotherapy cycles and those treated with abdominal or total body irradiation had significantly lower AMH levels than controls [22]. In adult women with cancer, AMH declines during treatment followed by recovery in some patients, with the rate of recovery determined by the pretreatment AMH level [23].

Ovarian Reserve Testing as a Predictor of Menstrual Pattern and Fertility

Ovarian reserve testing to predict the risk of acute ovarian failure and early menopause and future fertility in females prior to cancer therapy would allow us to better target patients for ovarian preservation procedures [24]. In adults, one small series in breast cancer survivors demonstrated that inhibin B and AMH prior to therapy were significantly lower in the women who went on to develop amenorrhea after treatment [25]. Similarly, in 46 adolescent and young adult women with a new cancer diagnosis requiring chemotherapy, pretreatment AMH levels were associated with the rate of recovery of AMH after treatment. Participants with a pretreatment AMH level >2 ng/mL had a faster rate of recovery of AMH after chemotherapy compared to participants with pretreatment AMH levels </= 2 ng/mL [23].

In addition, the ability of ovarian reserve testing to predict time to menopause and ovarian insufficiency on survivors who are menstruating would be very useful in order for them to plan posttreatment fertility preservation and other therapies [24]. In a prospective study of breast cancer survivors who were still menstruating, the patients who had cessation of menses 2 years later were more likely to have lower AMH and higher FSH at study entry [24].

To date there is no data regarding the ability of ovarian reserve testing to predict risk of premature menopause in prepubertal girls before therapy or in survivors of childhood cancer.

Effect of Female Hormones on Ovarian Reserve Testing

Many young women who receive cancer therapy are placed on birth control pills to regulate menses or estrogen replacement therapy when ovarian insufficiency is suspected. It is important to understand the effect of this treatment on ovarian reserve testing. A study evaluating ovarian reserve testing in 887 healthy women, 18–46 years old, found that AMH, antral follicle counts, and ovarian volume were all significantly decreased in oral contraception users when compared to nonusers [26]. In a small study comparing young cancer survivors on birth control pills with control women on the pills during the third week of pills (while taking active pills), there were no differences noted in FSH, inhibin B, estradiol, or AMH, but the AFC was lower in the cancer survivors [27].

Several studies have evaluated ovarian reserve testing during the placebo or pill-free week comparing survivors with spontaneous menses and those on birth control pills. Results from these studies are contradictory, use small samples, and compare populations exposed to cancer therapy to each other and not healthy age-matched controls [21, 28]. In addition, there are no studies which evaluate whether ovarian reserve testing in women on female hormones is predictive of menstrual function or fertility.

Conclusions

Ovarian reserve testing has been extensively studied in healthy women who seek infertility treatment but not in young girls receiving cancer therapy. This population would benefit significantly from rigorous data regarding ovarian reserve testing which may predict their risk of early menopause and assess the risk and benefits of fertility preservation options. Research in this population is limited by the fact that the numbers of girls at individual institutions are low as well as the fact that the outcome of interest (the ability to achieve successful pregnancy) may be far in the future [27]. Future multicenter studies with collaborative efforts of reproductive specialists, oncologists, and patient advocates will need to be performed.

References

1. Byrne J, et al. Early menopause in long-term survivors of cancer during adolescence. Am J Obstet Gynecol. 1992;166(3):788–93.
2. Green DM, et al. Ovarian failure and reproductive outcomes after childhood cancer treatment: results from the Childhood Cancer Survivor Study. J Clin Oncol. 2009;27(14):2374–81.
3. Thomas-Teinturier C, et al. Age at menopause and its influencing factors in a cohort of survivors of childhood cancer: earlier but rarely premature. Hum Reprod. 2013;28(2):488–95.
4. Zegers-Hochschild F, et al. International Committee for Monitoring Assisted Reproductive Technology (ICMART) and the World Health Organization (WHO) revised glossary of ART terminology, 2009. Fertil Steril. 2009;92(5):1520–4.
5. Faddy MJ, Gosden RG. A model conforming the decline in follicle numbers to the age of menopause in women. Hum Reprod. 1996;11(7):1484–6.
6. Practice committee of the american society for reproductive medicine. Testing and interpreting measures of ovarian reserve: a committee opinion. Fertil Steril. 2015;103(3):e9–17.
7. Goodwin PJ, et al. Risk of menopause during the first year after breast cancer diagnosis. J Clin Oncol. 1999;17(8):2365–70.
8. Bines J, Oleske DM, Cobleigh MA. Ovarian function in premenopausal women treated with adjuvant chemotherapy for breast cancer. J Clin Oncol. 1996;14(5):1718–29.
9. Koyama H, et al. Cyclophosphamide-induced ovarian failure and its therapeutic significance in patients with breast cancer. Cancer. 1977;39(4):1403–9.

10. Domingues TS, Rocha AM, Serafini PC. Tests for ovarian reserve: reliability and utility. Curr Opin Obstet Gynecol. 2010;22(4):271–6.
11. ACOG Committee Opinion No. 349, November 2006: menstruation in girls and adolescents: using the menstrual cycle as a vital sign. Obstet Gynecol. 2006;108(5):1323–8.
12. Burger HG. The endocrinology of the menopause. Maturitas. 1996;23(2):129–36.
13. Richardson SJ, Senikas V, Nelson JF. Follicular depletion during the menopausal transition: evidence for accelerated loss and ultimate exhaustion. J Clin Endocrinol Metab. 1987;65(6):1231–7.
14. Burger HG, et al. The endocrinology of the menopausal transition: a cross-sectional study of a population-based sample. J Clin Endocrinol Metab. 1995;80(12):3537–45.
15. La Marca A, et al. Anti-Mullerian hormone (AMH) as a predictive marker in assisted reproductive technology (ART). Hum Reprod Update. 2010;16(2):113–30.
16. Tsepelidis S, et al. Stable serum levels of anti-Mullerian hormone during the menstrual cycle: a prospective study in normo-ovulatory women. Hum Reprod. 2007;22(7):1837–40.
17. van Rooij IA, et al. Serum antimullerian hormone levels best reflect the reproductive decline with age in normal women with proven fertility: a longitudinal study. Fertil Steril. 2005;83(4):979–87.
18. Broer SL, et al. Anti-mullerian hormone predicts menopause: a long-term follow-up study in normoovulatory women. J Clin Endocrinol Metab. 2011;96(8):2532–9.
19. Hagen CP, et al. Serum levels of anti-Mullerian hormone as a marker of ovarian function in 926 healthy females from birth to adulthood and in 172 Turner syndrome patients. J Clin Endocrinol Metab. 2010;95(11):5003–10.
20. Kelsey TW, et al. A validated model of serum anti-Mullerian hormone from conception to menopause. PLoS One. 2011;6(7):e22024.
21. van Beek RD, et al. Anti-Mullerian hormone is a sensitive serum marker for gonadal function in women treated for Hodgkin's lymphoma during childhood. J Clin Endocrinol Metab. 2007;92(10):3869–74.
22. Lie Fong S, et al. Assessment of ovarian reserve in adult childhood cancer survivors using anti-Mullerian hormone. Hum Reprod. 2009;24(4):982–90.
23. Dillon KE, et al. Pretreatment antimullerian hormone levels determine rate of posttherapy ovarian reserve recovery: acute changes in ovarian reserve during and after chemotherapy. Fertil Steril. 2013;99(2):477–83.
24. Su HI. Measuring ovarian function in young cancer survivors. Minerva Endocrinol. 2010;35(4):259–70.
25. Anders C, et al. A pilot study of predictive markers of chemotherapy-related amenorrhea among premenopausal women with early stage breast cancer. Cancer Invest. 2008;26(3):286–95.
26. Birch Petersen K, et al. Ovarian reserve assessment in users of oral contraception seeking fertility advice on their reproductive lifespan. Hum Reprod. 2015;30(10):2364–75.
27. Bath LE, et al. Depletion of ovarian reserve in young women after treatment for cancer in childhood: detection by anti-Mullerian hormone, inhibin B and ovarian ultrasound. Hum Reprod. 2003;18(11):2368–74.
28. Larsen EC, et al. Reduced ovarian function in long-term survivors of radiation- and chemotherapy-treated childhood cancer. J Clin Endocrinol Metab. 2003;88(11):5307–14.

Chapter 4
Contraception and Menstrual Suppression for Adolescent and Young Adult Oncology Patients

Janie Benoit and Holly Hoefgen

According to the 2013 National Youth Risk Behavior Survey [1], 47% of high school students in the United States (USA) admitted to previous sexual intercourse, and of those, 14% did not use any method of pregnancy prevention [1]. An unintended pregnancy during cancer treatments may result in delay in therapy, teratogenic exposure, and/or pregnancy termination [2]. For many of these patients, unintended pregnancy is associated with an unacceptable health risk. Therefore, an open and early discussion about contraceptive needs and options is essential to the overall care of the adolescent and young adult oncology patient. Choosing a contraceptive method is an important decision with many involved factors for both patients and physicians. We must consider the efficacy and safety profile of each method, as well as how the method fits into each patient's lifestyle, including technical, social, and religious factors, among others. In the adolescent oncology patient, these issues can compound quickly. Medically, these patients' present increased challenges due to their underlying diagnoses and the increased risk of thrombotic disease associated with all malignancy. A thorough discussion of indicated contraceptive methods should be undertaken with each patient, with focus placed on efficacy and safety. An added benefit (or alternative use) of contraceptive medications during cancer treatment has been to elicit menstrual lightening and suppression, especially in patients with low blood count, menorrhagia, and/or risk of bone marrow suppression. Additionally, every social situation is unique and we must remember to ensure confidentiality in our adolescent patients seeking sexual health counseling and contraception.

The Centers for Disease Control and Prevention adapted the World Health Organization (WHO) guidance to create the US Medical Eligibility Criteria (MEC)

J. Benoit, MD • H. Hoefgen, MD (✉)
Pediatric & Adolescent Gynecology, Cincinnati Children's Hospital Medical Center,
Cincinnati, OH, USA
e-mail: Janie.benoit@cincinnatichildrens.org; Holly.Hoefgen@cchmc.org

© Springer International Publishing Switzerland 2017
T.K. Woodruff, Y.C. Gosiengfiao (eds.), *Pediatric and Adolescent Oncofertility*,
DOI 10.1007/978-3-319-32973-4_4

for Contraceptive Use, 2010 [3] (with updates occurring in 2011 and 2012), for use by healthcare providers. It can be found in its complete form on the CDC website in the reproductive health section (see Appendix) (www.cdc.gov/reproductivehealth/ UnintendedPregnancy/USMEC.htm). The US MEC ranks contraceptive methods based on a four-point scale for a large number of medical conditions [3].

Categories of medical eligibility criteria for contraceptive use
1. A condition for which there is no restriction for the use of the contraceptive method
2. A condition for which the advantages of using the method generally outweigh the theoretical or proven risks
3. A condition for which the theoretical or proven risks usually outweigh the advantages of using the method
4. A condition that represents an unacceptable health risk if the contraceptive method is used

The only cancers outlined specifically are ovarian, cervical, breast, gestational trophoblastic neoplasia, and malignant hepatoma. However, there is a special designation under high risk of DVT/PE for active cancer (metastatic, on therapy, or within 6 months of clinical remission, excluding non-melanoma skin cancer) that is also of great importance in the oncology patient population.

The WHO also classifies contraception based on efficacy into four tiers [4]:

- Tier 1 (most effective): Sterilization, implants, intrauterine devices (IUD)
- Tier 2: Depot medroxyprogesterone acetate (DMPA), combined hormonal methods
- Tier 3: Barrier methods
- Tier 4: Behavioral methods

Below we will outline all available methods of contraception and discuss their efficacy, safety profiles, ease of use, and common side effects. We will also note any particular concerns in the oncology population (see also Table 4.1).

Contraception

1. Behavioral methods

    (a) Abstinence

        (i) Abstinence is a wise and safe choice at any life stage, particularly for young patients who do not feel ready for a sexual relationship. However, abstinence-only programs are ineffective in delaying sexual debut or in reducing sexual risk behaviors among teens that are already sexually active [5]. Comprehensive sexual education has been shown to significantly decrease teen pregnancy rates, increase age at first intercourse, and significantly increase the likelihood of contraception use at first intercourse [5–7]. Furthermore, female participants in comprehensive

Table 4.1 Contraception options

Category	Contraception	Medication names	Failure rate[a] (%)		Continued use at 1 year (%)	ADRs	Cancer-specific issues/contraindications
			Best use	Common use			
Behavioral methods	Abstinence/no method		0	0–85			These methods are especially ineffective for patients undergoing cancer treatments. Discussions should focus on counseling more effective methods
	Timing		3–5	24	47		
	Withdraw		4	22	46		
Barrier methods	Male condom		2	18	43	Latex or spermicide sensitivities can be seen	Condoms should be advised in ALL sexually active AYA patients to decrease the risk of STI transmission
	Female condom		5	21	41		Diaphragm may be a viable option in hormone-sensitive cancer patients who cannot have copper IUD
	Diaphragm		6	12	57		

(continued)

Table 4.1 (continued)

| Category | Contraception | Medication names | Failure rate[a] (%) | | Continued use at 1 year (%) | ADRs | Cancer-specific issues/ contraindications |
			Best use	Common use			
Estrogen progesterone methods	Pills	Lutera, Levora, Yaz, Sprintec, Ortho-Cyclen …	0.3	9	67	Increased risk of VTE	Should be avoided in cancer pts if possible due to increased risk of VTE
						Nausea/vomiting	Advantageous for bone health
	Transdermal patch	Xulane Ortho Evra	0.3	9	67	Serum EE levels higher than 35 EE COC	Advantageous for bone health
						VTE risk similar to 35 EE COC	Not recommended for patients >90 kg
						Transient skin reactions	
						More initial BTB than COCs	
	Transvaginal ring	Nuva ring	0.3	9	67	Serum EE levels lower than most COCs	May not have positive effect on bone health
						Headache	
						Vaginal wetness	

Short- or intermediate-acting progesterone methods	Progesterone-only pills	Norethindrone (Ortho Micronor)	0.3	9	67	Breakthrough bleeding	
						Headache	
						Nausea	
						Breast tenderness	
						Acne	
	Injectable progesterone	DMPA (Depo-Provera)	0.2	6	56	Irregular vaginal bleeding	Not recommended in treatments resulting in osteopenia/osteoporosis
						Amenorrhea	
						Weight gain	
						Transient decrease in bone mineral density	
LARC – progesterone based	Progesterone implant	Implanon Nexplanon	0.05	0.05	84	May cause unpredictable vaginal bleeding	Irregular bleeding pattern may not be the best choice in patients with concerns for anemia
	LNG IUD	Mirena Skyla	0.2	0.2	80	Chance for amenorrhea	Used for treatment of endometrial hyperplasia and low-grade cancer
							May be considered for select breast cancer patients on tamoxifen

(continued)

Table 4.1 (continued)

Category	Contraception	Medication names	Failure rate[a] (%)		Continued use at 1 year (%)	ADRs	Cancer-specific issues/ contraindications
			Best use	Common use			
LARC – nonhormonal	Copper IUD	ParaGard	0.8	0.6	78	May increase menstrual blood flow	First line for breast cancer patients Not recommended if Concern for anemia
Emergency contraception	Combined OCPs LNG methods ulipristal copper IUD	Yuzpe method Plan B/Next Choice Ella ParaGard			NA	N/V, Irregular vaginal bleeding. Some breast tenderness, abdominal pain, dizziness, HA, fatigue	There are absolutely no situations in which risks outweigh the benefits of EC

[a]Percentage of women experiencing unintended pregnancy within the first year

sexual education programs were more likely to choose age-appropriate sexual partners, less likely to note first intercourse as an unwanted event, and more likely to express overall healthier partnerships associated with their first sexual encounter. Sexual education has not been shown to be associated with an earlier onset of sexual debut [5]. Therefore, although a patient who notes abstinence as their form of contraception should be encouraged to continue, sexual health should always be part of the discussion.

(b) Noncoital sexual behaviors

    (i) Noncoital sexual behavior includes mutual masturbation, oral sex, and anal sex and is a common expression of sexuality. The National Survey of Family Growth found that 45 % of females aged 15–19 years have had oral sex with an opposite-sex partner, but these numbers have remained stable over the past two decades. Compared with oral or vaginal sex, which are common in more than 90 % of males and females by age 25 years, anal sex is less common (10 % of female adolescents aged 15–19 years) and often is initiated later. Noncoital sexual behavior commonly coexists with coital behavior. The prevalence of oral sex among adolescents jumps dramatically in the first 6 months after initiation of vaginal intercourse, suggesting that both are often initiated around the same time and with the same partner. Although there is little risk of pregnancy with strictly noncoital activities, given this association, contraceptive discussion is warranted. Sexually transmitted infections, including HIV, HSV, HPV, hepatitis virus, syphilis, gonorrhea, and chlamydia, can be transmitted through noncoital sexual activity, and patients should be strongly counseled regarding safe sexual practices [8].

(c) Coitus interruptus/withdrawal method

    (i) This method involves the withdrawing of the penis from the vagina and away from the external genitalia prior to ejaculation. It is mentioned here as a point of discussion, as it is practiced widely, with 55 % of adolescent women aged 15–19 years reporting having used the method before [9]. The failure rate of such technique is high (22 % with typical use) and it does not provide protection against sexually transmitted infections [9].

2. Barrier methods

  (a) Male condoms

    (i) The male condom acts as a physical barrier, covering the penis and blocking the passage of sperm into the vagina. According to the 2013 YRBS, 41 % of US high school students did not use a condom during the last sexual intercourse [1]. All sexually active adolescents should be encouraged on regular condom use for the prevention of sexually transmitted infections including HIV, as well as increased contraceptive efficacy. In the general population, condom use has an overall reassuring failure rate of 2 %. However, in typical use, the male condom alone has a failure rate of 18 % [9]. For this reason, a more reliable form of contraception should be counseled as first line.

(b) Vaginal barriers/spermicides

   (i) Female condom

      1. The female condom is a soft, loose polyurethane sheath with two rings, one on either end. One ring is placed in the vagina; the other is placed outside the introitus. These devices are available over the counter. Efficacy is poor, with a typical use failure rate in the general population of 21 % [9].

   (ii) Diaphragm

      1. The diaphragm is a dome-shaped flexible rubber cup. Spermicide is applied to the dome, and the device is inserted into the vagina prior to intercourse so that the posterior rim rests in the posterior fornix and the anterior rim fits behind the pubic bone with the dome of the device covering the cervix. The diaphragm must be sized and prescribed by a physician. Once in position, it can provide contraceptive protection for up to 6 h before additional spermicide is required. After intercourse, it should be left in place for at least 6 h but should not be left in place for a combined duration of longer than 24 h due to a rare risk of toxic shock syndrome. The diaphragm also has a lower efficacy rating with typical use failure rates of 12 %. However, this may be a good option in a very select subset of patients with hormone-sensitive cancers and an aversion or contraindication to the copper intrauterine device (IUD) [9].

   (iii) Spermicides

      1. Spermicidal gels, creams, and foams are available for use with the diaphragm but can also be used individually for contraception. Spermicidal suppositories can be used alone or with condoms. However, efficacy is low with a typical use failure rate of 28 % in the general population, when used alone for contraception [9]. Given the difficulty of correct usage and high failure rate, we would not commonly recommend this method for use in the adolescent population. However, it may be useful in the subset of patient for whom the diaphragm would be indicated.

3. Estrogen-containing contraceptives

   The current options for combined estrogen and progesterone contraceptive methods are the oral *p*ill, the transdermal *p*atch, and the vaginal *r*ing (PPR). There are many non-contraceptive benefits of using a combined regimen, including but not limited to regulation of menstrual cycles, treatment of menorrhagia/

dysmenorrhea, and treatment of acne and pelvic pain [10]. Studies are variable on the possible improvement of bone mineral density in premenopausal women. These regimens have also been shown to decrease the risk of endometrial, ovarian, and colorectal cancers, and modern formulations have no increase in breast cancer risk [11]. As a class, all estrogen-based contraceptives are tier 2 efficacy, with a typical use first-year failure rate of 9%. The continuation rates of these methods at 1 year are also the same, at 67% [9].

As a class, there is an increased risk of venous thromboembolism (VTE) that is dependent on the estrogen dose and duration. Although the relative risk of VTE is increased, the absolute risk for each individual user is low, as thrombosis is a rare event in the healthy young female population that commonly uses this contraceptive method. However, these combined regimens may pose a high risk of VTE if patients are not carefully selected [9].

For the malignant diagnoses specifically listed in the MEC, PPR are noted as a category 4 (unacceptable risk) for relationship to elevated DVT/VTE risk (active cancer, or within 6 months after clinical remission, excluding non-melanoma skin cancers), current breast cancer, and malignant liver tumors. They are classified as a category 1 for gestational trophoblastic disease and a category 2 for cervical cancer awaiting treatment. It is important to take the overall medical condition into consideration, as other conditions such as obesity, hyperlipidemia, diabetes, and liver and renal failure may be part of the medical history in chronically ill children. Similarly, it is important to note that any patient with a complicated solid organ transplant is not a candidate for estrogens (category 4), but for an uncomplicated transplant patient, estrogen-containing contraceptives are considered a category 2.

(a) Pills

  (i) Combined oral contraceptive pills (COCs) are available in a wide variety of formulations. The choice of pill should be determined by the patient and physician based on clinical picture, medical history, and patient preference. The basic mechanisms of action are the same for all formulations and include both inhibition of ovulation and folliculogenesis and thickening of cervical mucus. COCs are taken daily and depending on the cycling pattern chosen can be given between 21 and 90 days with a 4–7-day pill-free interval for withdrawal bleeding. Use among adolescents is popular, with 19% of sexually active US high school students endorsing use of COCs to prevent pregnancy prior to their last act of sexual intercourse [1]. However, compliance and continuation may prove challenging in this age group.

(b) Patch

  (i) The contraceptive transdermal patch is a thin, flexible patch that contains 6 mg of norelgestromin (active metabolite of norgestimate) and 0.75 mg of ethinyl estradiol (EE). The patch releases 150 mcg of norelgestromin and 20 mcg of EE daily. The patch provides serum levels of EE that are higher than the common 35 mcg EE COC formulations; however, the VTE risk of the patch is equivalent to a 35EE/norgestimate oral contraceptive pill. The patch is applied to the buttocks, upper arm, lower abdomen, or upper torso and changed once weekly for 3 weeks. The fourth week is a hormone-free interval to allow for cycling. Its mechanism of action is the same as that of oral contraceptive pills. In some studies, the patch appears to enhance consistent and correct use as compared to COCs; however, their overall continuation rates and failure rates are the same. Patch users may note a transient skin reaction and more initial breakthrough bleeding than COCs users; the latter effect improves with use. Patients greater than 90 kg may have a higher risk of pregnancy when using the patch [9].

(c) Ring

   (i) A soft, transparent flexible ring that releases 120 mcg of etonogestrel (major metabolite of desogestrel) and 15 mcg of EE daily. Although several cases of VTE have been reported in vaginal ring users, the serum EE levels are two and threefold lower than that found in 35EE COCs and the birth control patch. However, there have been studies linking the progesterone component of the ring to an increased risk of VTE. Possibly due to the lower estrogen output, studies have not shown improvement in bone mineral density using the ring, even after 24 months of use [9].

   The ring is placed vaginally once every 28 days, with the last 7 days being a ring-free time frame to allow for withdrawal bleeding. The mechanism of action is mostly ovulation suppression, similar to oral contraceptive pills. In theory, the ease of once-monthly use should improve patient compliance and improve method success rates. However, in randomized comparative trials, the ring and COCs showed similar compliance and continuation rates. The vaginal ring has excellent cycle control, even in the first few cycles. It can be removed for up to 3 h without compromising effectiveness and is safe to use with tampons or during intercourse. The most commonly reported side effects are headache and vaginal wetness [9].

4. Progesterone-only contraceptives

   All of the progesterone-only contraceptives are approved for patients at higher risk of deep venous thrombosis and pulmonary embolism (DVT/PE), such as patients with active or of history of malignancies (MEC category 2). They are not associated with an increased risk of high blood pressure or cardiovascular disease. An added benefit is menstrual lightening or suppression, to different degrees depending on the formulation used. The only absolute contraindications to progesterone-based medications are pregnancy and a personal history of hormone-dependent breast cancer. Progesterone-only contraception may be provided as an oral medication, injectable form, or an implant. Their mechanisms of action for contraception are through increased viscosity of cervical mucus, ovulatory suppression, and endometrial thinning.

(a) Progesterone-only pills (norethindrone 35 mcg)

   (i) Progesterone-only pills must be taken at the same time every day. This regimen's efficacy depends on compliance with a typical use failure rate in the general population of 9 % [12]. Efficacy strongly depends on strict compliance, taking the medication at the same time or within 3 h after that time every day, making it less than ideal for adolescents. Up to 10 % of users will develop amenorrhea after 1 year of use [13]. Side effects are uncommon but may include breakthrough bleeding, headaches, nausea, acne, and breast tenderness. The risks are minimal [9].

(b) Injectable contraceptive (depot medroxyprogesterone acetate)

   (i) (DMPA is most commonly given as a 150 mg intramuscular injection, administered every 12 weeks. It is also available in a 104 mg subcutaneous injection with identical dosing intervals [9]. Its efficacy relies on compliance with a typical use failure rate in the general population of 3–6 % [8, 12]. Up to 50 % of users will develop amenorrhea after 1 year of use. Side effects include initial breakthrough bleeding, weight gain, headaches, nausea, breast tenderness, acne, and mood disorder [9, 14].

   In 2004, the FDA issued a black box warning stating that prolonged use of DMPA may result in significant loss of bone mineral density (BMD). Following this event, the WHO collected expert reviews concluding that DMPA is associated with a risk of reversible BMD reduction during treatment, which has not been proven to increase fracture risk [15]. The American College of Obstetricians and Gynecologists released a Committee Opinion stating that healthcare providers should inform women and adolescents considering initiating DMPA or continuing to use the method about the benefits and the risks of DMPA and should discuss the FDA "black box" warning. However, the effect of DMPA on BMD should not prevent practitioners from prescribing DMPA or continuing use beyond 2 years. The use of routine DXA scans or supplemental estrogen was not recommended in adolescent and young adult populations taking DMPA. However, discussing and recommending long-acting reversible contraception (LARC) methods that are both more efficacious and have no effect on BMD were suggested [12].

   On average, patients on DMPA have a weight gain of less than 2 kg per year [16]. However, it has also been shown that certain populations, such as those that are obese or more sedentary, are more at risk for weight gain with DMPA [17, 18].

(c) Long-acting reversible contraception (LARC)

   LARC methods are the most effective birth control methods with a failure rate of <1 %. In September 2014, the AAP (American Academy of Pediatrics) published a new recommendation stating that the first-line contraceptive choice for adolescents who choose not to be abstinent should be a LARC method. Their safety and efficacy in adolescents has been well demonstrated and these methods are recommended for teenagers [19].

LARCs include the intrauterine device (IUD) and the contraceptive implant. In the Contraceptive CHOICE project, all contraceptive options were counseled and provided to participants at no cost for the duration of the 2–3 year project. Seventy-five percent of participants in the CHOICE project chose LARC methods; this is astounding compared to the national average of 8.5 % at the time [20]. Adolescents chose LARC at similar rates to their adult counterparts (69–71 %); however, the younger adolescent population appeared to favor the etonogestrel implant system [21]. A recent analysis of the CHOICE project evaluated contraception continuation in teenagers and young women and demonstrated high rates of continuation and satisfaction with LARC, similar to that in the older adult population [22, 23]. It has also been shown that adolescents are more likely to continue LARC than non-LARC contraceptive methods [24]. The continuation rate of LARC methods in teenagers and young women has been shown to be 81 % [23]. However, the use of these devices continues to be low with only 1.6 % of sexually active high school students reporting the use of LARC methods in themselves or their partner [1].

(i) Contraceptive implants

The subdermal rod, marketed currently as Nexplanon, measures 4 cm by 2 mm and has a constant release of etonogestrel. It is currently approved for contraception at 3-year duration. The device is inserted superficially in the upper arm during a simple office procedure by a trained physician or licensed provider requiring only local anesthesia [25]. The risks of the procedure are rare but include bleeding, hematoma formation, and infection. The main side effects are irregular, unpredictable vaginal bleeding (50 %), acne (12 %), headaches (16 %), weight gain (12 %), and mood disturbance (6 %). About 11 % of patients become amenorrheic after 1 year of use [26]. Removal requires a second small office procedure with local anesthetic and a small incision with similar risks. Removal can be challenging due to an inability to palpate the rod, breakage of the implant, or encapsulation of the device in subcutaneous tissue.

Continuation rates have been shown to be higher than 80 % after 1 year of use in one study [23]. Other studies have found higher discontinuation rates averaging 35 %, with persistent bleeding irregularities cited as the most frequent reason for discontinuation [26].

(ii) *Levonorgestrel IUDs*

This device, the most common of which is marketed as the Mirena, is T shaped and contains a barrel with 52 mg of levonorgestrel. It is inserted into the uterine cavity through the cervix using a speculum and indicated instruments. This is a simple office procedure in most instances.

Levonorgestrel (LNG) is released at an initial rate of 20 mcg/day that decreases to 10–14 mcg per day over the course of its currently approved 5-year duration of use [9]. The main risks are IUD expulsion (6%) [23], a slight increase risk of pelvic inflammatory disease (PID) in the 20 days following insertion (1%), and uterine perforation (1/1000) [27] [28]. It is important to clarify that overall, IUD use in teenagers is encouraged and that it does not increase risk of PID, sexually transmitted infections (STI), or infertility. Cervical screening for chlamydia and gonorrhea should be performed on all women at high risk for STIs, including all adolescents. Side effects of the LNG IUD are minimal but include limited irregular vaginal bleeding, acne, headaches, and mood disturbance. Other benefits include menstrual lightening (up to 90% of flow) or suppression (in 50% of patients at 24 months of use), alleviation of dysmenorrhea and pelvic pain, and reduction of risk of endometrial cancer. There is limited evidence for or against IUD use in cancer-related immunocompromised patients; however, the CDC and WHO both support its use and are reassuring about its safety based on other types of immunocompromised patient data [12].

A lower-dose levonorgestrel IUD became available in the United States in 2013, marketed as Skyla. This IUD contains 13.5 mg of levonorgestrel, which is initially released at a rate of 14 mcg/day that decreases to 5 mcg/day over its approved 3-year duration of use. It has a slightly smaller size and diameter, which theoretically may make it more suitable for placement in certain populations with a small uterine cavity or cervical stenosis. The low-dose levonorgestrel IUD is not currently approved for the treatment of menorrhagia and has a lower likelihood of amenorrhea (13% vs 24%) compared with the higher-dose IUD [29].

Overall, the levonorgestrel IUDs have been proven to be a highly effective birth control method that is both beneficial and safe. Nonsexually active teenagers and young adults usually tolerate insertion in the office well. In patients who are unable to tolerate in-office placement, such as those with special needs, the IUD can be placed under general anesthesia. In our practice, we attempt to bundle this procedure with an otherwise required anesthesia whenever possible, such as may be needed for central line placement or biopsy. However, IUD insertion under anesthesia can be scheduled independently.

5. Nonhormonal LARC

(a) Copper IUD

The copper IUD, marketed in the United States as Copper T 380A (ParaGard), is approved for a duration of 10 years. It is the only highly effective nonhormonal contraceptive method, with a perfect and typical use failure rate of less 1% [9]. A variety of different copper IUD types are available in other countries; in Canada, for example, the Mona Lisa N, Mona Lisa 5, and Mona Lisa 10 are each approved for 3, 5, or 10 years, respectively.

Table 4.2 Emergency contraception treatment regimens

Method	Dosing	Efficacy
Estrogen plus progesterone (Yuzpe regimen)	100–120 mcg ethinyl estradiol plus 500–600 mcg levonorgestrel in each dose, given twice, 12 h apart	47–89 % pregnancy prevention
Levonorgestrel	0.75 mg given twice, 12 h apart, *or* 1.5 mg given as a single dose	59–94 % pregnancy prevention
Ulipristal	30 mg dose orally ×1	98–99 %
Copper intrauterine device	Inserted within 120 h after intercourse	At least 99 %

The Copper T 380A is a T-shaped device, with thin copper wire wound around the stem and each arm. It is inserted into the uterine cavity through the cervix using a speculum and indicated instruments. This is a simple office procedure in most instances. Cervical screening for chlamydia and gonorrhea should be performed on all women at high risk for STIs, including all adolescents. The copper IUD's mechanisms of action include local intrauterine inflammatory reaction, which creates an environment toxic to sperm and ova, causing decreased sperm motility and viability and preventing fertilization and implantation of the embryo [9]. Common side effects are irregular breakthrough bleeding, heavier menstrual cycles (up to 50 %), and dysmenorrhea, all of which should improve with time. The primary benefit is providing a reliable but rapidly reversible birth control method. The main risks are uterine perforation (1/1,000) [27], expulsion (5 %), and increased risk of pelvic infection limited to the first 20 days after placement of IUD. Copper IUD is approved for and shown to be safe in adolescents. It may have additive benefit in the oncology population, as a safe and reliable form of contraception in patients with hormone-dependent malignancies.

6. Emergency contraception

There is no single mechanism of action of emergency contraception (EC) [30] as it depends on the time in the menstrual cycle the medication is taken and what method is chosen. Options for emergency contraception range from high-dose combined oral contraceptive pills (the Yuzpe method), single- or multidose progesterone methods (levonorgestrel or ulipristal), or placement of a copper IUD. Specific regimens can be found in Table 4.2 [31] and are most effective 0–72 h after intercourse with moderate efficacy up to 5 days [30]. According to the US MEC, given the associated complications and comorbidities of pregnancy and the short-term use of EC methods, there are absolutely no instances in which the risks outweigh the benefits of use. Therefore, this option should always be considered and discussed in adolescent oncology patients. Given the urgency of timing for effective treatment following unprotected intercourse, it is imperative to begin this conversation before the need arises, such as during a general sexual health discussion. Several barriers to the use of EC have been noted in adolescents including knowledge of the option of EC in general, understanding of the use and safety of the medications, and cost barriers. Further barriers relate to difficulty of accessing medications from providers and pharmacies, where staff may not approve of or understand the laws regarding EC use in younger patients [32]. It is important to understand the exact prescribing laws for EC and adolescents as they apply in your particular state (http://www.guttmacher.org/statecenter/spibs/spib_EC.pdf).

Survivors

It has been shown that, in general, centers caring for adolescent and young adult (AYA) oncology patients do not routinely discuss sexual health with their patients; therefore, survivors have limited awareness of the contraceptive options available to them. Even though specific data is not available for unintended pregnancy among cancer survivors, we do know that survivors in the 15–30-year-old range are more likely than their peers to terminate a pregnancy. For patients who have been cancer-free for at least 6 months and are without a history of chest wall radiation, hormonally mediated cancers, anemia, osteoporosis, or VTE, the use of all of the above-noted contraception options is available. Patients with a history of chest wall radiation are at an increased risk of breast cancer and may not be candidates for exogenous hormones; therefore, the copper IUD would be first line in these patients. However, some physicians will allow modern hormone formulations, as they no longer show an increased risk of breast cancer in the general population. In general, the important point to note is that AYA individuals with cancer need to be aware of their sexual health options during all stages of their diagnosis and treatment, and all healthcare providers should become comfortable with, at a minimum, asking the relevant questions [4].

Menstrual Regulation and Suppression

In oncology patients, suppression of menses is mainly used to prevent anemia and thrombocytopenia but can also be used to provide relief of menstrual-related symptoms. Patients with thrombocytopenia are at increased risk for hemorrhage; therefore, cessation of menses is crucial. However, depending on the platelet levels, intramuscular injections may be contraindicated due to an elevated risk of hematoma formation. The overall aim of treatment is for high efficacy without causing any harm. Common regimens are discussed below and summarized in Table 4.3.

Per WHO definitions, amenorrhea is defined as absence of bleeding or spotting within a 90-day time interval.

Table 4.3 Menstrual suppression regimens

Medications	% of amenorrhea	Dosing and frequency	Side effect profile	Other benefits	Contraceptive failure rates	Risks	Contraindications
GnRh agonists (leuprolide-acetate)	73–96 % w rapid onset	11.25 mg IM typically q 8–12 weeks / Also option of SC or IV daily	Menopause-like sx (ex. hot flashes)	Possible protection of ovarian fct	Not approved for BC	Hematoma, ↓ BMD	Severe thrombocytopenia for IM
Oral progestins	76 % w high dose	Norethindrone acetate 5 mg daily to 10 mg twice a day	Irregular BTB	↓ dysmenorrhea	(Only Micronor approved for BC)		Pregnancy
High-dose (norethindrone acetate, medroxyprogesterone)	10 % w low dose	Medroxyprogesterone acetate 10 mg daily to twice a day	Weight gain, acne, headache, depression	↓ endometrial cancer risk	8 % typical use		Breast cancer
Low-dose (norethindrone)		Norethindrone 0.35 mg one daily			<1 % perfect use		
Depot medroxyprogesterone acetate	50–60 % at 1 year	150 mg IM every 12 weeks 104 mg SQ every 12 weeks	Initial irregular BTB	↓ dysmenorrhea	3–6 % typical use	Reversible ↓ BMD	Pregnancy
	70 % at 2 years		Weight gain, headache, depression	↓ endometrial cancer risk	<1 % perfect use		Breast cancer
IUD-containing levonorgestrel	50 % at 6–12 months	52 mg levonorgestrel IUD insertion every 5 years	Initial irregular BTB	↓ dysmenorrhea	<1 %	Uterine perforation	Pregnancy
	60 % at 5 years		Rare: acne, headache	↓ endometrial cancer risk		↑PID for 20 days after insertion / IUD expulsion	Breast cancer

Medications	% of amenorrhea	Dosing and frequency	Side effect profile	Other benefits	Contraceptive failure rates	Risks	Contraindications
Danazol	High (?)	200 mg PO daily to twice a day	Hirsutism, weight gain, acne, menopausal-like sx	↓ dysmenorrhea	Not approved for BC	Nonreversible androgenic changes	Pregnancy
Continuous combined hormonal treatment	Great variation		Initial BTB	↓acne, ↓ dysmenorrhea	8–9 % typical use	DVT, pulmonary embolism	Pregnancy
Pill	88 % at 12 months	Daily oral intake	Nausea, breast tenderness,	↓ ovarian cancer risk	<1 % Perfect use		Thrombophilia, Hx DVT/EP/stroke
Patch		Weekly patch change		↓ erdometrial cancer risk			Breast cancer, migraines w aura, severe HTN
Vaginal ring		Monthly ring change		↓ovarian cyst			

GnRH Agonist

GnRH agonists for the purpose of menstrual suppression are given as an injectable medication, which offer a high amenorrhea rate (73–97 %) [33]. These medications have been proven to be superior to DMPA in preventing moderate to severe bleeding in young women undergoing myelosuppressive chemotherapy with subsequent severe thrombocytopenia [34]. They can be given intravenous (IV), subcutaneous (SC), or intramuscular (IM) with a frequency ranging from daily to every 8–12 weeks according to the route of administration. In our practice, 11.25 mg leuprolide depot is typically chosen and given every 8–12 weeks IM. Alternatively if the patient is thrombocytopenic, leuprolide IV can be given daily until platelet counts are safe for an IM injection to be given.

Breakthrough bleeding for the first 2–3 weeks after initial injection is common as a result of the initial increase in FSH and LH secretion. At roughly 2 weeks, a hypogonadal effect is achieved through receptor downregulation. This "flare effect" should be expected and planned for within the course of disease or therapy. Possible side effects of treatment are hot flushes, insomnia, joint pain, weight gain, and mood disturbance. The main risks of GnRH agonists are a decrease in bone mineral density (BMD) and local contusion or hematoma at the injection site. Patients should be offered immediate add-back therapy to prevent vasomotor symptoms and negative impact on BMD. Options of add-back therapies include norethindrone acetate 5–10 mg daily or very low-dose estradiol with progestin. Norethindrone acetate is a progestin with estrogenic action, which has been shown to be as effective as low-dose estradiol in prevention of BMD decreases and vasomotor symptoms, without an increased thromboembolic risk [35, 36].

Due to its side effect profile, it is recommended that menstrual suppression using GnRH agonists should only be given for a limited time during chemotherapy treatment and/or during the time frame that the patient is at elevated risk for decreasing blood count secondary to treatment or malignancy.

Progestin-Only Pills

High-dose progestin-only pills (POP) can be given for menstrual lightening or suppression. Typically, amenorrhea can be achieved in a short period of time (1–3 days), and this method is very safe and effective. Possible side effects are acne, weight gain, headache, lipid profile changes, and mood disturbance. Due to the need for daily oral medication, the success of this treatment relies on compliance. There are a few options for treatment regimens with high-dose progestin pills, including norethindrone acetate, medroxyprogesterone acetate, megestrol, and danazol. Medication side effect profiles should be discussed with patients.

Dosages:

- Norethindrone acetate 5 mg daily to 10 mg twice a day
- Medroxyprogesterone acetate 10 mg daily to twice a day
- Megestrol 80 mg daily
- Danazol 200 mg daily to twice a day

Low-dose POP (norethindrone 0.35 mg) given continuously is also an option for menstrual suppression. The rate of amenorrhea with low-dose POP is 10 % [13], which is lower than with high-dose POP, but side effects are decreased.

Depot Medroxyprogesterone Acetate

This injectable hormonal contraceptive is a popular birth control method, which can also be used for menstrual lightening and amenorrhea. Rates of amenorrhea are about 50 % after 1 year of use, though initial irregular vaginal bleeding is common [37, 38]. About 12 % of DMPA users report being amenorrheic 3 months after their initial injection [37]. In one study involving teenagers, nearly two thirds of DMPA users endorsed amenorrhea with DMPA use [14]. Similar rates of amenorrhea have been noted with DMPA-SC as with DMPA-IM [14].

DMPA has some theoretical association with a possible increased risk of deep venous thrombosis and pulmonary embolism, although benefits usually outweigh this risk in women with active cancer [10]. Patients who have a high risk of low blood count, including anemia and thrombocytopenia, due to their malignancy or chemotherapy regimen may not tolerate initial irregular bleeding.

Combined Hormonal Contraception (Pill, Patch, Ring)

Combined hormonal contraceptives can be taken in extended regimens without taking the hormone-free intervals. There is an increased risk of breakthrough bleeding with these protocols. It is suggested to stop hormonal pills for roughly 5 days when breakthrough bleeding occurs to allow for withdraw bleed. About 70 % of women become amenorrheic after 1 year of use [39].

In patients with malignancy, the estrogen contained in combined hormonal contraceptives increases the risk of deep venous thrombosis and pulmonary embolism. In addition, it is important to consider that some patients might experience nausea and emesis during the course of their malignancy and treatment, and combined hormonal contraceptives may exacerbate these symptoms leading to a need for discontinuation. In addition, there are a number of drugs or medications that may interact with combined hormonal contraceptives, either altering serum levels of the given medication or COC.

Levonorgestrel IUD for Menstrual Suppression

The 52 mg levonorgestrel IUD can be used for menstrual lightening and suppression; however, these desired side effects develop over time in a subset of users. Menstrual lightening (up to 90 % of flow) is identified in a majority of patients with suppression noted in 50 % of patients at 24 months of use [37]. There is an initial risk of light irregular menstrual bleeding for the first 3–6 months after insertion. If a patient has established menstrual lightening or suppression with a levonorgestrel IUD in place at the time of her diagnosis of malignancy, it is recommended to leave the device in place [38].

Appendix: Medical Eligibility Criteria for Contraceptive Use

PDF file saved as MEC Appendix A

Summary Chart of U.S. Medical Eligibility Criteria for Contraceptive Use

Summary Chart of U.S. Medical Eligibility Criteria for Contraceptive Use

References

1. Brener ND, Kann L, Shanklin S, et al. Methodology of the youth risk behavior surveillance system – 2013. MMWR Recomm Rep (Morbidity and Mortality Weekly Report Recommendations and Reports/Centers for Disease Control). 2013;62(RR-1):1–20.
2. Committee Opinion No. 607: Gynecologic concerns in children and adolescents with cancer. Obstet Gynecol. 2014;124(2 Pt 1):403–8.
3. WHO. Medical eligibility criteria for contraceptive use. 5th ed. Geneva: WHO; 2015. Available at http://apps.who.int/iris/bitstream/10665/172915/1/WHO_RHR_15.07_eng.pdf.
4. Patel A, Schwarz EB. Cancer and contraception. Release date May 2012. SFP Guideline #20121. Contraception. 2012;86(3):191–8.
5. Lindberg LD, Maddow-Zimet I. Consequences of sex education on teen and young adult sexual behaviors and outcomes. J Adolesc Health Off Publ Soc Adolesc Med. 2012;51(4):332–8.
6. Kohler PK, Manhart LE, Lafferty WE. Abstinence-only and comprehensive sex education and the initiation of sexual activity and teen pregnancy. J Adolesc Health Off Publ Soc Adolesc Med. 2008;42(4):344–51.
7. Mueller TE, Gavin LE, Kulkarni A. The association between sex education and youth's engagement in sexual intercourse, age at first intercourse, and birth control use at first sex. J Adolesc Health Off Publ Soc Adolesc Med. 2008;42(1):89–96.
8. Committee Opinion No. 582: addressing health risks of noncoital sexual activity. Obstet Gynecol. 2013;122(6):1378–82.
9. Hatcher RA, Trussell J, Nelson AL, Cates W, Kowal D, Policar MS. Contraceptive technology. 20th ed. Ardent Media Inc., New York, NY 2011.
10. ACOG Practice Bulletin No. 110: noncontraceptive uses of hormonal contraceptives. Obstet Gynecol. 2010;115(1):206–18.
11. Sorensen K, Aksglaede L, Petersen JH, Juul A. Recent changes in pubertal timing in healthy Danish boys: associations with body mass index. J Clin Endocrinol Metab. 2010;95(1): 263–70.

12. U.S. Medical Eligibility Criteria for Contraceptive Use, 2010. MMWR Recomm Rep (Morbidity and Mortality Weekly Report Recommendations and Reports/Centers for Disease Control). 2010;59(RR-4):1–86.
13. Black A, Francoeur D, Rowe T, et al. Canadian contraception consensus. J Obstet Gynaecol Can JOGC J Obstet Gynecol Can JOGC. 2004;26(4):347–87. 89–436.
14. Cromer BA, Smith RD, Blair JM, Dwyer J, Brown RT. A prospective study of adolescents who choose among levonorgestrel implant (Norplant), medroxyprogesterone acetate (Depo-Provera), or the combined oral contraceptive pill as contraception. Pediatrics. 1994;94(5):687–94.
15. Committee Opinion No. 602: depot medroxyprogesterone acetate and bone effects. Obstet Gynecol. 2014;123(6):1398–402.
16. Lopez LM, Edelman A, Chen M, Otterness C, Trussell J, Helmerhorst FM. Progestin-only contraceptives: effects on weight. Cochrane Database Syst Rev. 2013;7:CD008815.
17. Bonny AE, Ziegler J, Harvey R, Debanne SM, Secic M, Cromer BA. Weight gain in obese and nonobese adolescent girls initiating depot medroxyprogesterone, oral contraceptive pills, or no hormonal contraceptive method. Arch Pediatr Adolesc Med. 2006;160(1):40–5.
18. Bonny AE, Lange HL, Rogers LK, Gothard DM, Reed MD. A pilot study of depot medroxyprogesterone acetate pharmacokinetics and weight gain in adolescent females. Contraception. 2014;89(5):357–60.
19. Committee Opinion No. 539: adolescents and long-acting reversible contraception: implants and intrauterine devices. Obstet Gynecol. 2012;120(4):983–8.
20. Secura GM, Madden T, McNicholas C, et al. Provision of no-cost, long-acting contraception and teenage pregnancy. N Engl J Med. 2014;371(14):1316–23.
21. Mestad R, Secura G, Allsworth JE, Madden T, Zhao Q, Peipert JF. Acceptance of long-acting reversible contraceptive methods by adolescent participants in the Contraceptive CHOICE Project. Contraception. 2011;84(5):493–8.
22. Eisenberg D, McNicholas C, Peipert JF. Cost as a barrier to long-acting reversible contraceptive (LARC) use in adolescents. J Adolesc Health Off Publ Soc Adolesc Med. 2013; 52(4 Suppl):S59–63.
23. Rosenstock JR, Peipert JF, Madden T, Zhao Q, Secura GM. Continuation of reversible contraception in teenagers and young women. Obstet Gynecol. 2012;120(6):1298–305.
24. Deans EI, Grimes DA. Intrauterine devices for adolescents: a systematic review. Contraception. 2009;79(6):418–23.
25. McNicholas C, Peipert JF. Long-acting reversible contraception for adolescents. Curr Opin Obstet Gynecol. 2012;24(5):293–8.
26. Darney P, Patel A, Rosen K, Shapiro LS, Kaunitz AM. Safety and efficacy of a single-rod etonogestrel implant (Implanon): results from 11 international clinical trials. Fertil Steril. 2009;91(5):1646–53.
27. Heinemann K, Reed S, Moehner S, Do Minh T. Risk of uterine perforation with levonorgestrel-releasing and copper intrauterine devices in the European Active Surveillance Study on Intrauterine Devices. Contraception. 2015;91(4):274–9.
28. Farley TM, Rosenberg MJ, Rowe PJ, Chen JH, Meirik O. Intrauterine devices and pelvic inflammatory disease: an international perspective. Lancet. 1992;339(8796):785–8.
29. Dean G, Goldberg AB. Intrauterine contraception (IUD): overview. 2014. http://www.uptodate.com/contents/intrauterine-contraception-iud-overview?source=search_result&search=Intrauterine+contraception+%28IUD%29%3A+Overview&selectedTitle=1%7E150.
30. ACOG Practice Bulletin No. 112: emergency contraception. Obstet Gynecol. 2010;115(5):1100–9.
31. Zieman M. Emergency contraception. 2014. http://www.uptodate.com/contents/emergency-contraception?source=search_result&search=Emergency+contraception&selectedTitle=1%7E137.
32. ACOG Committee Opinion Number 542: Access to emergency contraception. Obstet Gynecol. 2012;120(5):1250–3.
33. Quaas AM, Ginsburg ES. Prevention and treatment of uterine bleeding in hematologic malignancy. Eur J Obstet Gynecol Reprod Biol. 2007;134(1):3–8.

34. Meirow D, Rabinovici J, Katz D, Or R, Shufaro Y, Ben-Yehuda D. Prevention of severe menorrhagia in oncology patients with treatment-induced thrombocytopenia by luteinizing hormone-releasing hormone agonist and depo-medroxyprogesterone acetate. Cancer. 2006;107(7):1634–41.
35. Friedman AJ, Daly M, Juneau-Norcross M, Gleason R, Rein MS, LeBoff M. Long-term medical therapy for leiomyomata uteri: a prospective, randomized study of leuprolide acetate depot plus either oestrogen-progestin or progestin 'add-back' for 2 years. Hum Reprod. 1994; 9(9):1618–25.
36. Divasta AD, Laufer MR, Gordon CM. Bone density in adolescents treated with a GnRH agonist and add-back therapy for endometriosis. J Pediatr Adolesc Gynecol. 2007;20(5):293–7.
37. Hubacher D, Lopez L, Steiner MJ, Dorflinger L. Menstrual pattern changes from levonorgestrel subdermal implants and DMPA: systematic review and evidence-based comparisons. Contraception. 2009;80(2):113–8.
38. Committee Opinion No. 606: options for prevention and management of heavy menstrual bleeding in adolescent patients undergoing cancer treatment. Obstet Gynecol. 2014;124(2 Pt 1): 397–402.
39. Miller L, Hughes JP. Continuous combination oral contraceptive pills to eliminate withdrawal bleeding: a randomized trial. Obstet Gynecol. 2003;101(4):653–61.

Chapter 5
Female Sexual Function in Childhood, Adolescent, and Young Adult Cancer Survivors

Terri L. Woodard

Scope of the Problem

For most individuals, healthy sexual functioning represents an important component of overall health and quality of life. Previous studies have demonstrated a positive association between sexual function and overall health status [1, 2].

Cancer and its treatment affect multiple facets of life, including sexual well-being. Sexual functioning may be impacted through physiologic and/or psychosocial mechanisms. Unfortunately, it appears that survivors of cancer are at risk for persistent or worsening sexual problems [3]. As the number of survivors increases, the recognition of sexual well-being as an important quality-of-life issue continues to become more pressing [4, 5].

While there is growing literature on sexual function in adults diagnosed with cancer, research that addresses the sexual concerns of young adult and childhood cancer survivors is severely lacking [6], even though it is a priority concern in this population. In 2010, LIVE**STRONG** conducted a survey of more than 3000 cancer survivors, of which over 30% of respondents were adolescent and young adult (AYA) cancer survivors. Sexual functioning and satisfaction was one of the three top physical concerns reported, with 46% of people experiencing problems in this area. Unfortunately, the majority of these survivors (71%) reported that they did not receive care for sexual problems [7].

While many survivors of childhood cancer do not report problems with sexual functioning, there is evidence that there is a higher risk of impairment in this population. A survey of 599 young men and women aged 18–39 who were diagnosed with cancer at age 21 or younger revealed that 42.7% reported at least one

T.L. Woodard, MD
Department of Gynecologic Oncology and Reproductive Medicine, The University of Texas MD Anderson Cancer Center, 1155 Pressler Street, Unit 1362,
Houston, TX 77030-3721, USA
e-mail: tlwoodard@mdanderson.org

© Springer International Publishing Switzerland 2017
T.K. Woodruff, Y.C. Gosiengfiao (eds.), *Pediatric and Adolescent Oncofertility*,
DOI 10.1007/978-3-319-32973-4_5

problematic sexual symptom, with women having significantly higher symptom scores (21.6) than men (10.6) [8]. In a separate cohort study of adult female survivors of childhood cancer, women with a history of childhood cancer had poorer overall sexual functioning and significantly lower levels of sexual interest, desire, arousal, and satisfaction compared with their healthy siblings. Survivors with ovarian failure reported lower sexual functioning scores compared with those who had normal menses, though interestingly, sexual functioning scores did not improve with the addition of hormonal therapy (such as oral contraceptives or traditional hormone replacement therapy) [9].

As healthcare providers who strive to optimize the survivorship experience of patients, it is important to acknowledge how sexual functioning interfaces with other quality-of-life measures. Young adult survivors of childhood cancer with sexual dysfunction report decreased physical functioning, poorer general health, greater fatigue, and poorer mental health [10]. Sexual dysfunction is also correlated with lower life satisfaction and more distress [8].

Barriers to Care

There are a number of barriers that make addressing sexual concerns in this patient population challenging. Sex and sexuality are sensitive topics that are difficult for many people to discuss; they may be especially difficult for younger people who may feel embarrassed and/or lack the knowledge and vocabulary to speak freely about sexual problems. In addition, some providers experience discomfort talking with younger patients about sexual issues because they are not certain of what is "age appropriate" or, in the case of minors, they fear offending parents by bringing up the discussion [11]. Additionally, time constraints and a lack of knowledge of providers also influence whether providers address sexual concerns in their patients [12].

Many young people desire information about sexual health and sexual concerns, but most are not getting the counseling and care that they need, even though they represent an especially vulnerable group that may be more at risk for sexual problems. Patients who were diagnosed and treated at a very young age may have never grasped a complete understanding of how their treatment has impacted their reproductive health. Thus, it is important that providers are equipped with the confidence and skills that enable them to discuss sexual issues with patients in an age-appropriate manner [13].

Sexual Development

When considering sexual function and well-being in the adolescent and young adult population, it is important to do so in a developmental context. Normal sexual development is variable between individuals, and it is influenced not only by age but by culture and personal experiences. Sexual development begins at birth. It includes the physical changes that occur with growing older as well as the beliefs and behaviors that people exhibit about sex.

Infancy and Childhood

In infancy, children are curious about their genitals and may touch them in private and/or public. They are completely uninhibited. During early childhood, children remain openly curious about their own bodies and start to develop a curiosity about other's bodies. As they become a little older and have more interaction with peers, they begin to develop an awareness of the "differences" between boys and girls. It is generally at this time that they become aware of the concept of "gender" and adopt a stable sense of gender identity. They also begin to ask questions about sex.

Upon reaching school age, children begin to grasp a better understanding of societal norms with regard to sex and sexuality. They tend to become more modest and may desire more privacy, such as when changing their clothing. They remain curious about sex, but are often more reluctant to talk about it with adults. It is not uncommon for them to develop a sexual attraction and interest in other people during this stage.

Preadolescence

Puberty begins during preadolescence. Preadolescents may become even more self-conscious as they experience physical changes in their bodies. Masturbation becomes more common. Although they generally do not have a lot of sexual experience, they are aware of different types of sexual activity as well as differences in sexual preferences and orientation. It is during this period when "group dating" often begins; some may even start to partner off as "boyfriend and girlfriend." Sexual exploration and experience varies, but often involves "making out."

Adolescence

Adolescence is a complex time when the individual transitions from a child to an adult. Important developmental milestones include establishing autonomy, solidifying identity, and sexual emergence. While there is a wide range of diversity in development and life experiences during this developmental period, it is generally characterized by an increased interest in romantic and sexual relationships.

Adolescents can and do form emotional attachments to romantic partners. There is also an increase in genital sex behaviors, such as sexual intercourse.

Sexual Development in Survivors of Childhood Cancer

Young adult survivors of childhood cancer may not reach sexual development milestones at the same rate as their peers as a result of medical and psychosocial challenges that are the result of their cancer experience. For example, cancer treatment can cause failed puberty, which is characterized by delayed or absent physical maturation. When a patient's disease isolates and alienates her from peers and the "normal" developmental experience, her psychosexual identity may not be well established and romantic relationships may not have the opportunity to form. As a result, the individual may not have ample opportunity to learn and adopt normal healthy sexual behaviors.

Childhood cancer survivors experience a delay in dating and initiation of social contacts compared with their peers [14]. Not only are they more likely to marry later [15–17], they are also significantly more likely to be unmarried than their siblings [9]. They exhibit a later time of first sexual intercourse [14, 18, 19] and are less likely to be sexually active in general. They also report lower satisfaction with sexual experiences [14].

Risk Factors for Sexual Dysfunction

Since altered sexual development may influence sexual function in survivors of childhood cancer, multiple studies have attempted to identify specific risk factors for sexual dysfunction. Older age, being female, and having health problems are factors that have been associated with sexual dysfunction in this population [8]. In a separate study, older age at the time of sexual function assessment, having ovarian failure at a younger age, a history of treatment with cranial radiation, and having a cancer diagnosis during adolescence were identified as risk factors for poorer sexual functioning [9].

Long-Term and Late Effects of Cancer Treatment on Sexual Functioning

Cancer and its treatment can have profound effects on long-term sexual functioning. These effects can be the result of physiologic factors, psychosocial factors, or, most frequently, a combination of both [20].

Physiologic Effects

Cancer treatment modalities such as surgery, chemotherapy, irradiation, and hormonal therapy can cause hormonal, vascular, and/or neurologic changes that affect sexual function [20]. Primary hypogonadism (ovarian failure) can result from treatment with chemotherapy (particularly alkylating agents), surgery (bilateral oophorectomy), and abdominal/pelvic irradiation. Ovarian failure results in hypoestrogenemia; if survivors were prepubertal at the time of failure, puberty will not occur. In such instances, hormone replacement therapy must be given to promote normal development of adult height and secondary sexual characteristics. If failure occurs postpuberty, hypoestrogenism can result in menopausal symptoms such as hot flashes and vaginal dryness.

Central hypogonadism can occur when patients receive cranial radiation that affects the hypothalamic-pituitary axis. As a result, the pituitary does not release the gonadotropins (FSH and LH) that direct ovarian function. In these cases, patients also may experience pubertal failure that can be treated with gonadotropin and/or hormone replacement. Conversely, cranial irradiation that includes the hypothalamus may lead to premature activation of the hypothalamic-pituitary-gonadal axis, resulting in precocious puberty.

Surgery that affects the vulva and vagina can cause dryness, sensory changes, and pain. Pelvic irradiation often leads to decreased blood flow that may lead to complications such as vaginal strictures and fistulas [21]. Survivors that receive these therapies may experience diminished sensation, pain, postcoital bleeding, and difficulties with vaginal penetration. Both pelvic surgery and radiation can cause nerve damage, resulting in weakening of the pelvic musculature that leads to discomfort during intercourse as well as urine and/or fecal incontinence. Patients who receive hematopoietic stem cell transplants are at risk for graft versus host disease of the vagina, which is associated with vaginal dryness, shortening, and pain [22].

Psychosocial Effects

Sexual functioning is also influenced by psychological and social factors. A diagnosis of cancer is life changing and often introduces challenges in peoples' lives beyond the obvious medical consequences. Distress, depression, or anxiety related to a cancer diagnosis will negatively affect a woman's sexual functioning. Treatment-related bodily disfigurement (as a result of a mastectomy [23], presence of a stoma, [24]) and hair loss [25] have been shown to be associated with emotional distress and poorer quality of life in cancer survivors in general, but may be less of a problem in childhood cancer survivors [26]. However, these physical changes can negatively influence body image and self-esteem, decreasing one's confidence in engaging in sexual activity and/or sexual relationships.

Cancer-related infertility is also intertwined with sexual health; a woman might be reluctant to pursue and/or maintain romantic relationships because she believes that a potential partner might reject her because of her inability to have a biological child.

Social Effects

Personal relationships are also affected by cancer and cancer therapy. For young people, feelings of alienation and isolation are common. They may avoid dating and going out. Friendships may wane if the patient is unable to "keep up" with the developmental and social milestones of her peers. Often, there are changes in existing romantic relationships, as the partner's role expands to being a caregiver. Both the patient and her partner may no longer fully see her as a sexual being. Finally, the financial impact of cancer and cancer therapy can be an additional stressor that influences sexual functioning.

Female Sexual Dysfunction

Since women who are survivors of childhood and adolescent cancer are at risk for sexual problems, it is important that they are screened for female sexual dysfunction (FSD). Accurate diagnosis is vital so that proper care can be given.

A sexual complaint is diagnosed as a dysfunction when the criteria from the American Psychiatric Association's Diagnostic and Statistical Manual (DSM) [27] for sexual dysfunctions are met and the complaint results in significant distress. The newly published *Diagnostic and Statistical Manual of Mental Disorders*, 5th edition (DSM-5), created new diagnostic classifications including female sexual interest/arousal disorder (FSIAD), female orgasmic disorder, and genito-pelvic pain/penetration disorder (GPPPD) (see Table 5.1). Along with information obtained from a thorough clinical interview, physical examination, and indicated laboratory testing, DSM-5 criteria should be used to establish the diagnosis and etiology of sexual dysfunction in women.

Female Sexual Interest/Arousal Disorder (FSIAD)

The diagnosis of female sexual interest/arousal disorder is characterized by a lack of or significantly reduced sexual interest/arousal. It must be manifested by at least three of the following (in any combination): (1) absent/reduced interest in sexual

Table 5.1 DSM-5 classification of female sexual dysfunction

Disorder	Diagnostic criteria
Female orgasmic disorder (FOD)	(1) A marked delay in, marked infrequency of, or absence of orgasm and/or (2) a markedly reduced intensity of orgasmic sensations
Female sexual interest/arousal disorder (FSIAD)	Requires at least three of the following (in any combination): (1) absent/reduced interest in sexual activity, (2) absent/reduced sexual/erotic thoughts or fantasies, (3) no or reduced initiation of sexual activity and being unreceptive to a partner's attempts to initiate sex, (4) absent or reduced sexual excitement/pleasure during sex in all or almost all (approximately 75–100%) of sexual encounters, (5) absent or reduced sexual interest/arousal in response to any internal or external sexual/erotic cues (e.g., verbal, visual), and (6) absent or reduced genital or nongenital sensations during sexual activity during sex in almost all or all (approximately 75–100%) of sexual encounters
Genito-pelvic pain/penetration disorder (GPPPD)	Persistent or recurrent difficulties with one or more of (1) vaginal penetration during intercourse; (2) marked vulvovaginal or pelvic pain during intercourse or penetration attempts; (3) marked fear of anxiety about vulvovaginal or pelvic pain in anticipation of, during, or as a result of vaginal penetration; and (4) marked tensing or tightening of the pelvic floor muscles during attempted vaginal penetration

activity, (2) absent/reduced sexual/erotic thoughts or fantasies, (3) no or reduced initiation of sexual activity and being unreceptive to a partner's attempts to initiate sex, (4) absent or reduced sexual excitement/pleasure during sex in all or almost all (approximately 75–100%) of sexual encounters, (5) absent or reduced sexual interest/arousal in response to any internal or external sexual/erotic cues (e.g., verbal, visual), and (6) absent or reduced genital or nongenital sensations during sexual activity during sex in almost all or all (approximately 75–100%) of sexual encounters.

Female Orgasmic Disorder

The diagnosis of female orgasmic disorder (FOD) requires the presence of (1) a marked delay in, marked infrequency of, or absence of orgasm and/or (2) a markedly reduced intensity of orgasmic sensations.

Genito-pelvic Pain/Penetration Disorder (GPPPD)

The diagnosis of genito-pelvic pain/penetration disorder (GPPPD) requires persistent or recurrent difficulties with one or more of (1) vaginal penetration during intercourse; (2) marked vulvovaginal or pelvic pain during intercourse or penetration attempts; (3) marked fear of anxiety about vulvovaginal or pelvic pain in anticipation of, during, or as a result of vaginal penetration; and (4) marked tensing or tightening of the pelvic floor muscles during attempted vaginal penetration.

> The DSM-5 requires that a woman must have symptoms 75–100 % of the time to make a diagnosis of sexual disorder, except when there is a substance or medication-induced disorder. The symptoms have to be present for at least 6 months and should not be better explained by a nonsexual mental disorder, a consequence of severe relationship distress (e.g., partner violence) or other significant stressors.

> Each of the sexual dysfunction categories can be further described by using specifiers such as "lifelong versus acquired "and "generalized versus situational." The severity of the problem should also be documented—specifically, whether it is mild, moderate, or severe. Finally, associated features should be noted, including the presence of (1) partner factors (partner sexual problem and/or health status); (2) relationship factors (difficult communication, differences in desire for sexual activity); (3) individual vulnerability factors (poor body image, history of sexual or emotional abuse), psychiatric comorbidity (depression and/or anxiety), or stressors (job loss, bereavement); (4) cultural or religious factors (attitudes about sexuality); and (5) medical factors relevant to prognosis, course, or treatment.

Screening and Assessment

The Children's Oncology Group Long-Term Follow-Up Guidelines for Survivors of Childhood, Adolescent, and Young Adult Cancer (COG-LTFU Guidelines) provide evidence-based recommendations for screening and management of late effects of cancer treatment, including psychosexual dysfunction [28].

It has been recommended that sexual health status in women cancer survivors should be assessed at regular intervals and at least annually [29, 30] as well as anytime a woman voices a sexual concern. To facilitate screening and assessment, office intake forms can include screening questions that prompt patients to provide information about sexual functioning. There are a number of screening instruments that can be used in an office setting that will allow quick identification, some of which have been developed and/or validated for use in cancer survivors [31–33]. Simply asking the patient about her sexual function and activity validates that it is an important part of overall health.

When introducing the topic of sexual functioning, it is important to communicate with the patient in a comfortable, nonjudgmental manner. Some providers find it is helpful to "normalize" the presence of sexual concerns, which lets the patient know that she is not the only person experiencing her problem. Questions should start as open ended and become more directed. No assumptions should be made about her sexuality or sexual behaviors (i.e., assuming sexual orientation or practice of monogamy).

A complete history should be elicited with special emphasis on the gynecologic and sexual history. Medication should be thoroughly reviewed, as many can have negative effects on sexual function [34]. The physical examination should include a thorough pelvic examination [35]. Both external and internal genitalia should be evaluated for abnormalities, such as atrophy, scarring, and strictures. Laboratory evaluation (such as sex hormones and thyroid function tests) can be added as indicated.

Although the focus of this article is on sexual functioning of adolescent and young adult female cancer survivors, it is imperative that other aspects of sexual health are discussed. Discussions about pregnancy and STI prevention are particularly important in this population, as they are vulnerable to reproductive health complications as it relates to immune compromise, incompatibility between desired contraception methods and treatment, and pregnancy complications [11].

Treatment

Some specialty cancer centers have recognized that women with a history of cancer have unique needs with regard to sexual functioning and have developed supportive services that can help patients anticipate and manage sexual issues before, during, and after cancer treatment. Often, these expert teams are multidisciplinary and may include gynecologists, reproductive psychologists, sex therapists, and pelvic floor physical therapists who can assess patients and provide a comprehensive treatment plan to optimize sexual functioning.

Treatment plans should be tailored to the individual patient and focus on the physical, psychological, and social factors that contribute to her sexual problem [29]. While there are few FDA-approved treatments for sexual dysfunction in women, there are still a considerable number of treatments that can be utilized to improve women's sexual satisfaction and well-being.

Education and Setting of Expectations

Healthcare providers can play a major role in helping women with sexual concerns or sexual dysfunction by providing accurate, unbiased sexual health education. Women who were diagnosed at a very young age might have some educational deficits in this area. It is not uncommon for some to have erroneous knowledge and beliefs about sex, including basic anatomy and physiology. Furthermore, societal influences of what "normal" sex and sexuality are can promote unrealistic expectations about how an individual woman's sex life should be. It is imperative to educate women that "normal" sexual functioning is variable between women and even throughout an individual woman's life. It should also be emphasized that the overall goal of healthy sexual functioning should be the achievement of sexual satisfaction and that she should be encouraged to define what that means for her as an individual and as part of a couple.

Lifestyle modification should be encouraged, as overall well-being influences sexual functioning. Women should be counseled to adopt healthy lifestyle behaviors, such as smoking cessation, limiting alcohol consumption, exercising most days of the week, getting adequate sleep, eating a healthy diet, and reducing stress as much as possible. The conditions surrounding sexual experiences should be optimized as well. Women should be informed of the importance of adequate sexual stimulation and arousal, which can be achieved with prolonged foreplay and the use of sexual aids. If patients experience difficulty with sexual intercourse, they should be encouraged to explore alternative means of expressing sexual intimacy and incorporate sexual activities that don't require intercourse. If intercourse is desired, the use of vaginal lubricants and moisturizers can make sexual activity easier and more comfortable.

Non-pharmacologic Therapies

Significant improvements in sexual function after intervention with traditional sex therapy and/or cognitive-behavioral therapy have been observed [36]. Traditional sex therapy is a behavioral treatment that aims to improve an individual/couple's erotic experiences while reducing anxiety and self-consciousness about sexual activity [37]. Cognitive-behavioral sex therapy includes traditional behavioral sex therapy components but places a greater emphasis on modifying thought patterns or beliefs that interfere with intimacy and sexual pleasure [37]. Directed masturbation has been demonstrated to be efficacious in the treatment of orgasmic disorders [38–40]. Mindfulness-based cognitive-behavioral treatments have also shown excellent promise for sexual desire problems [41]. Brotto et al. demonstrated that a brief mindfulness-based cognitive-behavioral intervention was successful in improving sexual desire and arousal problems in gynecologic cancer survivors [41]. Finally, a two-session counseling intervention that included education and support regarding cancer and reproductive issues was found to lessen anxiety about sexual and romantic relationships in adolescents and young adults with cancer [41].

Pelvic floor therapy is a type of physical therapy that can help strengthen the muscles of the pelvic floor and increase blood supply and innervation to the pelvic floor muscles. A pelvic floor exercise program has been shown to improve pelvic floor strength and sexual functioning in survivors of gynecologic cancers [42]. Dilator therapy is often recommended to selected patients for the prevention of vaginal stenosis in patients who received pelvic radiotherapy [43]; however, evidence that it prevents vaginal stenosis or improves quality of life is mixed [44]. Adherence to long-term use is often poor [45]. Data on the use of dilators for the treatment of sexual dysfunction in the adolescent population and younger is nonexistent.

Pharmacologic Therapies

For women who are prematurely postmenopausal as a result of their cancer treatment, hormonal replacement therapy can restore the normal hormonal milieu. However, only conjugated equine estrogen and ospemifene are FDA approved for the specific treatment of female sexual dysfunction. Vaginal estrogen can be prescribed in a variety of forms and is effective in the treatment of vulvovaginal atrophy (VVA), a common cause of painful intercourse. However, the use of estrogen in any form in patients with a history of hormone-sensitive cancer is controversial. Ospemifene is a selective estrogen receptor modulator that acts directly on the vulvovaginal tissues to reverse atrophy without exerting estrogenic effects on the uterus and breast; however, it has not been specifically studied in cancer survivors [46]. Finally, vaginal dehydroepiandrosterone has been used for the treatment of VVA; its use is associated with lower levels of systemic estrogen and testosterone, but its long-term safety profile is unknown [47].

The role of testosterone therapy for the treatment of female sexual dysfunction is even more controversial. Although it is not FDA approved for this indication, it is frequently prescribed off label. Testosterone has been shown to improve sexual satisfaction, general well-being, and mood [48]; however, safety concerns such as potential development of breast cancer and negative effects on cardiovascular health have limited its use [35].

Bupropion is a mild dopamine and norepinephrine reuptake inhibitor/nicotinic acetylcholine receptor antagonist that is used as an antidepressant and smoking cessation aid. Prior studies have shown that it is also useful in treated low desire in women [49], including those with SSRI-induced low desire [50, 51], and women receiving adjuvant hormonal therapy for breast cancer [52]. Flibanserin is a 5-HT1A receptor agonist/5-HT2 receptor antagonist that was recently approved by the FDA for the treatment of premenopausal women with hypoactive sexual desire disorder (HSDD) [53, 54]. However, there are no data on its use in cancer survivors.

There are multiple sexual enhancement products that are available over the counter. While most have not been rigorously tested for efficacy and safety, many women with a history of cancer express interest in their use [55]. Most pharmacologic interventions for the treatment of sexual dysfunction have not been tested in cancer survivors [56], highlighting the importance of more research in this area.

When to Refer

Complex cases warrant referral to professionals who have specialized training in sexual health and medicine. Organizations such as the International Society for the Study of Women's Sexual Health (www.ISSWSH.org); the American Association of Sexuality Educators, Counselors and Therapists (www.AASECT.org); and the Society for Sex Therapy and Research (www.SSTARNET.Org) have online tools that can assist with locating healthcare providers that specialize in sexual health issues.

Conclusion

Healthy sexual functioning is important for girls and women who have/have had cancer. The ability to function sexually and experience sexual satisfaction significantly contributes to overall quality of life and can have implications for a woman's ability to develop and sustain intimate relationships [56]. Survivors of childhood, adolescent, and young adult cancers are at risk for sexual problems as a result of their cancer experience.

It is imperative that providers are proactive about addressing sexual concerns in this population. There are a range of treatments that can be used to optimize sexual health and function of survivors. Engaging girls and women in conversations about how cancer and cancer treatment might affect their sexual well-being at baseline can empower them to seek care for these problems if and when they develop.

References

1. Davison SL, Bell RJ, LaChina M, Holden SL, Davis SR. The relationship between self-reported sexual satisfaction and general well-being in women. J Sex Med. 2009;6(10):2690–7. Epub 2009/10/13. eng.
2. Field N, Mercer CH, Sonnenberg P, Tanton C, Clifton S, Mitchell KR, et al. Associations between health and sexual lifestyles in Britain: findings from the third National Survey of Sexual Attitudes and Lifestyles (Natsal-3). Lancet (London, England). 2013;382(9907):1830–44. Pubmed Central PMCID: PMC3898988. Epub 2013/11/30. eng.
3. Kornblith AB, Ligibel J. Psychosocial and sexual functioning of survivors of breast cancer. Semin Oncol. 2003;30(6):799–813. Epub 2003/12/10. eng.
4. Robison LL, Hudson MM. Survivors of childhood and adolescent cancer: life-long risks and responsibilities. Nat Rev Cancer. 2014;14(1):61–70. Epub 2013/12/07. eng.
5. DeSimone M, Spriggs E, Gass JS, Carson SA, Krychman ML, Dizon DS. Sexual dysfunction in female cancer survivors. Am J Clin Oncol. 2014;37(1):101–6. Epub 2012/05/31.eng.
6. Cantrell MA, Conte T, Hudson M, Shad A, Ruble K, Herth K, et al. Recruitment and retention of older adolescent and young adult female survivors of childhood cancer in longitudinal research. Oncol Nurs Forum. 2012;39(5):483–90. Pubmed Central PMCID: PMC3927146, Epub 2012/09/04. eng.

7. Rechis R, Boerner L, Nutt S, Shaw K, Berno D, Duchover Y. How cancer has affected post-treatment survivors: a LIVESTRONG report. 2010. http://imageslivestrongorg/downloads/flatfiles/what-we-do/our-approach/reports/how-cancer/LSSurvivorSurveyReportpdf.
8. Zebrack BJ, Foley S, Wittmann D, Leonard M. Sexual functioning in young adult survivors of childhood cancer. Psychooncology. 2010;19(8):814–22. Pubmed Central PMCID: PMC2888926, Epub 2009/10/29. eng.
9. Ford JS, Kawashima T, Whitton J, Leisenring W, Laverdiere C, Stovall M, et al. Psychosexual functioning among adult female survivors of childhood cancer: a report from the childhood cancer survivor study. J Clin Oncol Off J Am Soc Clin Oncol. 2014;32(28):3126–36. Pubmed Central PMCID: PMC4171357, Epub 2014/08/13. eng.
10. Bober SL, Zhou ES, Chen B, Manley PE, Kenney LB, Recklitis CJ. Sexual function in childhood cancer survivors: a report from Project REACH. J Sex Med. 2013;10(8):2084–93. Epub 2013/05/18. eng.
11. Murphy D, Klosky JL, Termuhlen A, Sawczyn KK, Quinn GP. The need for reproductive and sexual health discussions with adolescent and young adult cancer patients. Contraception. 2013;88(2):215–20. Epub 2012/10/09. eng.
12. Wiggins DL, Wood R, Granai CO, Dizon DS. Sex, intimacy, and the gynecologic oncologists: survey results of the New England Association of Gynecologic Oncologists (NEAGO). J Psychosoc Oncol. 2007;25(4):61–70. Epub 2007/11/23. eng.
13. D'Agostino NM, Penney A, Zebrack B. Providing developmentally appropriate psychosocial care to adolescent and young adult cancer survivors. Cancer. 2011;117(10 Suppl):2329–34. Epub 2011/05/20. eng.
14. van Dijk EM, van Dulmen-den Broeder E, Kaspers GJ, van Dam EW, Braam KI, Huisman J. Psychosexual functioning of childhood cancer survivors. Psychooncology. 2008;17(5):506–11. Epub 2007/10/16. eng.
15. Langeveld NE, Stam H, Grootenhuis MA, Last BF. Quality of life in young adult survivors of childhood cancer. Support Care Cancer Off J Multinatl Assoc Support Care Cancer. 2002;10(8):579–600. Epub 2002/11/19. eng.
16. Pui CH, Cheng C, Leung W, Rai SN, Rivera GK, Sandlund JT, et al. Extended follow-up of long-term survivors of childhood acute lymphoblastic leukemia. N Engl J Med. 2003;349(7):640–9. Epub 2003/08/15. eng.
17. Rauck AM, Green DM, Yasui Y, Mertens A, Robison LL. Marriage in the survivors of childhood cancer: a preliminary description from the Childhood Cancer Survivor Study. Med Pediatr Oncol. 1999;33(1):60–3. Epub 1999/07/13. eng.
18. Kokkonen J, Vainionpaa L, Winqvist S, Lanning M. Physical and psychosocial outcome for young adults with treated malignancy. Pediatr Hematol Oncol. 1997;14(3):223–32. Epub 1997/05/01. eng.
19. Puukko LR, Hirvonen E, Aalberg V, Hovi L, Rautonen J, Siimes MA. Sexuality of young women surviving leukaemia. Arch Dis Child. 1997;76(3):197–202. Pubmed Central PMCID: PMC1717091, Epub 1997/03/01. eng.
20. Schover LR, van der Kaaij M, van Dorst E, Creutzberg C, Huyghe E, Kiserud CE. Sexual dysfunction and infertility as late effects of cancer treatment. EJC Suppl EJC Off J EORTC Eur Org Res Treat Cancer. 2014;12(1):41–53. Pubmed Central PMCID: PMC4250536, Epub 2015/07/29. eng.
21. Spunt SL, Sweeney TA, Hudson MM, Billups CA, Krasin MJ, Hester AL. Late effects of pelvic rhabdomyosarcoma and its treatment in female survivors. J Clin Oncol Off J Am Soc Clin Oncol. 2005;23(28):7143–51. Epub 2005/09/30. eng.
22. Zantomio D, Grigg AP, MacGregor L, Panek-Hudson Y, Szer J, Ayton R. Female genital tract graft-versus-host disease: incidence, risk factors and recommendations for management. Bone Marrow Transplant. 2006;38(8):567–72. Epub 2006/09/06. eng.
23. Aerts L, Christiaens MR, Enzlin P, Neven P, Amant F. Sexual functioning in women after mastectomy versus breast conserving therapy for early-stage breast cancer: a prospective controlled study. Breast (Edinburgh, Scotland). 2014;23(5):629–36. Epub 2014/08/02. eng.
24. Sprangers MA, Taal BG, Aaronson NK, te Velde A. Quality of life in colorectal cancer. Stoma vs. nonstoma patients. Dis Colon Rectum. 1995;38(4):361–9. Epub 1995/04/01. eng.

25. Choi EK, Kim IR, Chang O, Kang D, Nam SJ, Lee JE, et al. Impact of chemotherapy-induced alopecia distress on body image, psychosocial well-being, and depression in breast cancer patients. Psychooncology. 2014;23(10):1103–10. Epub 2014/03/26. eng.
26. Lehmann V, Hagedoorn M, Gerhardt CA, Fults M, Olshefski RS, Sanderman R, et al. Body issues, sexual satisfaction, and relationship status satisfaction in long-term childhood cancer survivors and healthy controls. Psychooncology. 2015;25(2):210–6. Epub 2015/05/12. Eng.
27. American Psychiatric Association, American Psychiatric Association DSM-5 Task Force. Diagnostic and statistical manual of mental disorders: DSM-5. 5th ed. Washington, DC: American Psychiatric Association; 2013. xliv, 947.
28. Group CsO. Long-term follow-up guidelines for survivors of childhood, adolescent and young adult cancer 2013 [9/26/2015]. Version 4.0.
29. Metzger ML, Meacham LR, Patterson B, Casillas JS, Constine LS, Hijiya N, et al. Female reproductive health after childhood, adolescent, and young adult cancers: guidelines for the assessment and management of female reproductive complications. J Clin Oncol Off J Am Soc Clin Oncol. 2013;31(9):1239–47. Pubmed Central PMCID: PMC4500837, Epub 2013/02/06. eng.
30. Network NCC. NCCN Guidelines: Survivorship 2015 [cited 2015 9/01/2015]. Version 2.2015.
31. Baser RE, Li Y, Carter J. Psychometric validation of the Female Sexual Function Index (FSFI) in cancer survivors. Cancer. 2012;118(18):4606–18. Epub 2012/02/24. eng.
32. Flynn KE, Lin L, Cyranowski JM, Reeve BB, Reese JB, Jeffery DD, et al. Development of the NIH PROMIS (R) sexual function and Satisfaction measures in patients with cancer. J Sex Med. 2013;10 Suppl 1:43–52. Pubmed Central PMCID: PMC3729213, Epub 2013/03/21. eng.
33. Althof SE, Parish SJ. Clinical interviewing techniques and sexuality questionnaires for male and female cancer patients. J Sex Med. 2013;10 Suppl 1:35–42. Epub 2013/02/15. eng.
34. Clayton A, Ramamurthy S. The impact of physical illness on sexual dysfunction. Adv Psychosom Med. 2008;29:70–88. Epub 2008/04/09. eng.
35. Dizon DS, Suzin D, McIlvenna S. Sexual health as a survivorship issue for female cancer survivors. Oncologist. 2014;19(2):202–10. Pubmed Central PMCID: PMC3926787, Epub 2014/01/08. eng.
36. Gunzler C, Berner MM. Efficacy of psychosocial interventions in men and women with sexual dysfunctions – a systematic review of controlled clinical trials: part 2 – the efficacy of psychosocial interventions for female sexual dysfunction. J Sex Med. 2012;9(12):3108–25. Epub 2012/10/24. eng.
37. Kingsberg SA, Woodard T. Female sexual dysfunction: focus on low desire. Obstet Gynecol. 2015;125(2):477–86. Epub 2015/01/09. eng.
38. Riley AJ, Riley EJ. A controlled study to evaluate directed masturbation in the management of primary orgasmic failure in women. Br J Psychiatry J Ment Sci. 1978;133:404–9. Epub 1978/11/01. eng.
39. Reisinger JJ. Effects of erotic stimulation and masturbatory training upon situational orgasmic dysfunction. J Sex Marital Ther. 1978;4(3):177–85. Epub 1978/01/01. eng.
40. Andersen BL. A comparison of systematic desensitization and directed masturbation in the treatment of primary orgasmic dysfunction in females. J Consult Clin Psychol. 1981;49(4):568–70. Pubmed Central PMCID: PMC2719958, Epub 1981/08/01. eng.
41. Canada AL, Schover LR, Li Y. A pilot intervention to enhance psychosexual development in adolescents and young adults with cancer. Pediatr Blood Cancer. 2007;49(6):824–8. Epub 2007/01/18. eng.
42. Yang EJ, Lim JY, Rah UW, Kim YB. Effect of a pelvic floor muscle training program on gynecologic cancer survivors with pelvic floor dysfunction: a randomized controlled trial. Gynecol Oncol. 2012;125(3):705–11. Epub 2012/04/05. eng.
43. Bakker RM, ter Kuile MM, Vermeer WM, Nout RA, Mens JW, van Doorn LC, et al. Sexual rehabilitation after pelvic radiotherapy and vaginal dilator use: consensus using the Delphi method. Int J Fynecolog Cancer Off J Int Gynecol Cancer Soc. 2014;24(8):1499–506. Epub 2014/09/24. eng.

44. Miles T, Johnson N. Vaginal dilator therapy for women receiving pelvic radiotherapy. Cochrane Database Syst Rev. 2014;9:CD007291. Epub 2014/09/10. eng.
45. Law E, Kelvin JF, Thom B, Riedel E, Tom A, Carter J, et al. Prospective study of vaginal dilator use adherence and efficacy following radiotherapy. Radiother Oncol J Eur Soc Ther Radiol Oncol. 2015;116(1):149–55. Epub 2015/07/15. eng.
46. Portman DJ, Bachmann GA, Simon JA. Ospemifene, a novel selective estrogen receptor modulator for treating dyspareunia associated with postmenopausal vulvar and vaginal atrophy. Menopause (New York, NY). 2013;20(6):623–30. Epub 2013/01/31. eng.
47. Labrie F, Martel C, Berube R, Cote I, Labrie C, Cusan L, et al. Intravaginal prasterone (DHEA) provides local action without clinically significant changes in serum concentrations of estrogens or androgens. J Steroid Biochem Mol Biol. 2013;138:359–67. Epub 2013/08/21. eng.
48. Davis SR, Goldstat R, Papalia MA, Shah S, Kulkarni J, Donath S, et al. Effects of aromatase inhibition on sexual function and well-being in postmenopausal women treated with testosterone: a randomized, placebo-controlled trial. Menopause (New York, NY). 2006;13(1):37–45. Epub 2006/04/12. eng.
49. Segraves RT, Clayton A, Croft H, Wolf A, Warnock J. Bupropion sustained release for the treatment of hypoactive sexual desire disorder in premenopausal women. J Clin Psychopharmacol. 2004;24(3):339–42. Epub 2004/05/01. eng.
50. Safarinejad MR. Reversal of SSRI-induced female sexual dysfunction by adjunctive bupropion in menstruating women: a double-blind, placebo-controlled and randomized study. J Psychopharmacol (Oxford, England). 2011;25(3):370–8. Epub 2010/01/19. eng.
51. Pereira VM, Arias-Carrion O, Machado S, Nardi AE, Silva AC. Bupropion in the depression-related sexual dysfunction: a systematic review. CNS Neurol Disord Drug Targets. 2014;13(6):1079–88. Epub 2014/06/14. eng.
52. Mathias C, Cardeal Mendes CM, Ponde de Sena E, Dias de Moraes E, Bastos C, Braghiroli MI, et al. An open-label, fixed-dose study of bupropion effect on sexual function scores in women treated for breast cancer. Ann Oncol Off J Eur Soc Med Oncol/ESMO. 2006;17(12):1792–6. Epub 2006/09/19. eng.
53. Katz M, DeRogatis LR, Ackerman R, Hedges P, Lesko L, Garcia Jr M, et al. Efficacy of flibanserin in women with hypoactive sexual desire disorder: results from the BEGONIA trial. J Sex Med. 2013;10(7):1807–15. Epub 2013/05/16. eng.
54. Dhanuka I, Simon JA. Flibanserin for the treatment of hypoactive sexual desire disorder in premenopausal women. Expert Opin Pharmacother. 2015;22:1–7. Epub 2015/09/24. Eng.
55. Herbenick D, Reece M, Hollub A, Satinsky S, Dodge B. Young female breast cancer survivors: their sexual function and interest in sexual enhancement products and services. Cancer Nurs. 2008;31(6):417–25. Epub 2008/11/07. eng.
56. Lindau ST, Abramsohn EM, Matthews AC. A manifesto on the preservation of sexual function in women and girls with cancer. Am J Obstet Gynecol. 2015;213(2):166–74. Epub 2015/03/31. eng.

Chapter 6
Vitrification of Ovarian Tissue for Fertility Preservation

Alison Y. Ting, Steven F. Mullen, and Mary B. Zelinski

Introduction

Cryopreservation of embryos, oocytes, and ovarian tissue [16] is available to preserve fertility in female patients with cancer. Both embryo cryopreservation and oocyte cryopreservation are established methods, and ovarian tissue cryopreservation has emerged as a promising hope for future fertility for patients who are prepubertal, adolescent, lacking partners, or those who require immediate cancer therapy. Cryopreservation is also the only option for patients contraindicated for ovarian transplantation due to the risk of reintroducing malignant cells. Autografting of cryopreserved ovarian tissue to women restored ovarian endocrine function in almost every case reported [5]. Although there are 60 reported live births from transplantation of cryopreserved human ovarian tissue to date, this fertility preservation option is still considered experimental [6]. All but two of the reported human births have resulted from ovarian tissue cryopreserved using a slow-rate freezing protocol. The slower progress for clinical implementation of ovarian tissue

A.Y. Ting, PhD (✉)
Division of Reproductive & Developmental Sciences, Oregon National Primate Research Center, Oregon Health & Science University,
505 NW 185th Avenue, Beaverton, OR 97006, USA
e-mail: ting@ohsu.edu

S.F. Mullen, PhD
Cook Regentec, The Brown School Location,
500 W Simpson Chapel Road, Bloomington, IN 47404, USA

M.B. Zelinski, PhD
Division of Reproductive & Developmental Sciences, Oregon National Primate Research Center, Oregon Health & Science University,
505 NW 185th Avenue, Beaverton, OR 97006, USA

Department of Obstetrics & Gynecology, Oregon Health & Science University,
3181 SW Sam Jackson Park Road, Portland, OR 97239, USA

© Springer International Publishing Switzerland 2017
T.K. Woodruff, Y.C. Gosiengfiao (eds.), *Pediatric and Adolescent Oncofertility*,
DOI 10.1007/978-3-319-32973-4_6

vitrification is due to many factors. Two major limitations include the lack of a uniform vitrification protocol, in contrast to slow-rate freezing, that demonstrates consistent outcomes, that is exacerbated by few clinical attempts to use ovarian tissue vitrification followed by transplantation for fertility restoration in women. Recent advances in embryo and oocyte cryopreservation have driven clinical practice in the United States almost exclusively to vitrification, with the vast majority of infertility clinics no longer having access to programmable freezers in their embryology laboratories. Thus, there is a current demand for an ovarian tissue vitrification method that could extend the ability of clinics to offer this option for fertility preservation. This need is urgent because young patients make up the majority of those who survive their cancer and ultimately face the loss of their future fertility and for whom ovarian tissue cryopreservation is their only option for becoming a future parent.

Vitrification: Facts and Fallacies

Cryopreservation is a term used to describe procedures designed to preserve the viability of cells (either isolated or within the context of a tissue). As this term implies, very cold temperatures are paramount to achieving this goal. Extreme cold is useful for preservation because the rate of chemical reactions is directly proportional to the temperature, with reactions slowing markedly with a decrease in temperature. At true cryogenic temperatures, the motion of molecules has slowed to the point where translational movement ceases and only vibrational motion can occur [42]. Such a system can be thought of as being locked in place, and chemical reactions will not occur under such conditions.

Successfully preserving the viability of biological cells by moving them into a cryogenic environment is more difficult than it first may seem. This is, in large part, because the thermodynamically stable state of cytoplasmic water at such temperatures is in the crystalline (solid) phase, and this state is not conducive to living cells. However, cells can tolerate more concentrated (hypertonic) environments (both intracellularly and extracellularly) at lower temperatures and/or for short periods of time, and this is exploited to preserve the viability of cells by cryopreservation [24].

When ice forms inside of a living cell, it is almost always lethal [23]. As such, cryopreservation methods work by limiting the crystallization of intracellular water. This occurs in two fundamentally different ways, by the two major methods used to achieve cryopreservation, freezing and vitrification.

The first method is called freezing, and when performed properly, only the water on the outside of the cell freezes. It is fortunate that the cytoplasm of cells has the property of limiting the freezing of the intracellular water by depressing the ice nucleation temperature [39]. Additives to cryopreservation solutions, called cryoprotectants, increase the efficiency of ice nucleation suppression [31]. The result of this phenomenon provides a means by which the development of intracellular ice can be eliminated, and it works in the following way. Cells are cooled in a solution to the point where the extracellular water will freeze, yet the intracellular water will not. The change in phase of the extracellular water results in a chemical potential differential between the intracellular and extracellular water, causing water efflux from the cell. This effectively dehydrates the cell, and if the temperature decrease is slow enough, eventually the cytoplasm becomes too concentrated for ice to form [22]. When this occurs, the cells can safely be placed into long-term cryogenic storage without concern of damage due to intracellular ice.

Concentration of the cytoplasm is not healthy for cells, and they can perish due to excessive dehydration, even at reduced temperatures [23]. It is the optimal balance between minimizing these two sources of damage, intracellular ice formation and cellular dehydration, that results in successful freezing.

Unfortunately for tissue preservation, even extracellular ice formation can be damaging [30]. It is this problem that the second general method of cryopreservation, termed vitrification, is designed to overcome [7]. Vitrification methods attempt to preclude the formation of intracellular and extracellular ice by starting the system at a solute concentration that will not permit ice crystallization. This chapter focuses on recent developments in laboratory research that have the long-term goal of finding a successful method to vitrify primate ovarian tissue. We will describe the results of our research and summarize the progress made by others to provide an up-to-date summary of the state of the science as of today. Before we get to that, however, we will attempt to clarify some of the misconceptions about vitrification that make our approach counterintuitive to many in the field.

As mentioned above, freezing is a method that relies upon the formation of ice in the extracellular space to adequately dehydrate the cells or tissues to prevent intracellular ice formation and uses very slow cooling rates (usually less than or equal to 1° per minute after extracellular ice has formed) to facilitate safe dehydration. Vitrification, on the other hand, attempts to preclude all ice formation in the entire sample by the use of relatively high concentrations of solutes before cooling. Currently, most vitrification procedures used in the human embryology laboratory utilize very high rates of cooling and warming (between 10,000 and 100,000 °C per minute) in an attempt to vitrify the sample [40]. We use the word "attempt" here because many vitrification methods utilize solutions that are too dilute to prevent ice formation during the cryopreservation procedure despite the assumption to the contrary [13]. While it is beyond the scope of the current chapter to present a thorough review of the physical aspects of vitrification (please see excellent reviews such as [1, 8, 26, 29, 42]), it is sufficient to say that ice forms much more readily during warming than during cooling [13] as shown in Table 6.1. As a result, it is commonly assumed that a vitrification procedure is successful (i.e., prevents ice formation) when no ice can be seen to form during cooling. However, unless the solution is known to be stable during cooling and warming, ice is likely to form during warming.

Another common misconception is that the only way any solution can maintain a vitreous state is to cool and warm it at an extraordinary speed (on the order of 1500 °C per second). In fact, as demonstrated by the data in Fig. 6.1, the critical rates (rates necessary to prevent ice formation) are dependent upon both the solution composition and concentration. Some cryoprotectants (e.g., propylene glycol) are

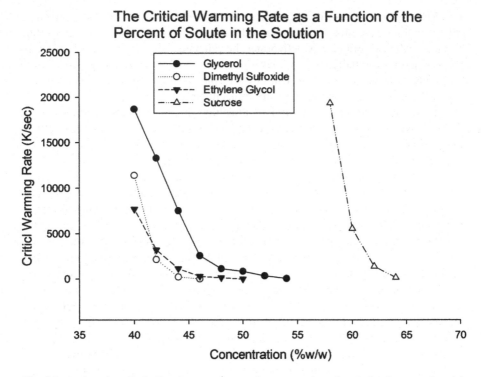

Fig. 6.1 As the solute (including the cryoprotectant) concentration of a solution increases (x axis), the cooling and warming rates (warming rates shown here on y axis) necessary to maintain an ice-free state decrease, and this decrease continues until no measurable ice forms in the solution and occurs at very low rates of temperature change (<1 °C per minute)

much better vitrifying agents than others. As the solute (including the cryoprotectant) concentration of a solution increases, the cooling and warming rates necessary to maintain an ice-free state decrease, and this decrease continues until no measurable ice forms in the solution at *very low rates of temperature change* (i.e., less than 1 °C per minute). A common criticism of the vitrification method developed in our lab is that the cooling and warming rates are far too slow. In fact, our vitrification solution was designed such that it maintained a vitreous state at the low cooling and warming rates applicable to our method.

Chemical and osmotic toxicity of cryoprotectant solutions are a far greater concern for vitrification procedures. This is because solutions used for freezing (versus vitrification) are much less concentrated at the temperature associated with initial cell and tissue exposure. The good news is that these problems can often be overcome. Adding and removing the cryoprotectants in several steps, and also using of osmotic buffers such as non-permeating sugars during cryoprotectant removal, can overcome excessive osmotic stress [29]. One caveat to using this approach is that the exposure time to the cryoprotectants will be longer and may exacerbate chemical toxicity. Adding and removing cryoprotectants at cold temperatures (i.e., 4 °C or lower), at least during the steps where higher concentrations are relevant, has the potential to reduce chemical toxicity. This approach may exacerbate osmotic stress, however, as the permeability of cryoprotectants to cells is usually much lower at these temperatures compared to water [25]. Another approach to reducing osmotic and chemical toxicity is to expose the cells to high values of these stresses for short periods of time. This approach is commonly utilized in current methods to vitrify oocytes and embryos, as the steps associated with exposure to the vitrification solution before cooling and during warming are very short (often less than 1 min). Such an approach will be more difficult for tissue, however, as the time necessary to concentrate the intracellular cryoprotectants sufficiently to maintain a stable vitreous state during the final step of cryoprotectant addition depends upon the size and geometry of the sample. This simply cannot be accomplished for tissue pieces on the same time scale as it is done for oocytes and embryos. As a result of these challenges inherent with tissue vitrification, thoughtful experiments must be designed and conducted in order to achieve effective vitrification.

A final challenge that we wish to discuss is that associated with the fracturing of a vitrified solution. The assumed need to cool and warm as fast as possible to successfully vitrify has led many investigators to plunge relatively large samples (e.g., cryostraws and cryovials) directly into liquid nitrogen to facilitate rapid cooling. While this approach does maximize the cooling rate, this approach can result in the generation of excessive thermomechanical stress within the vitrified sample, and fracturing of the vitrified glass is often seen, and occurs to relieve this stress [34]. The problem with glass fracturing is that the tissue is also prone to fracturing, and this can result in irreversible damage. One way to avoid the buildup of this stress is to slow down the cooling and warming of the sample. This apparent paradox leaves many confused. However, as we just described, rapid cooling and warming is not necessary to achieve and maintain a vitreous state if other variables in the system are properly designed.

As one can gather from the above discussion, vitrifying larger samples, such as tissue, becomes rather complicated due to the inherent limitations that the size of the material imposes on the system. However, it is our belief that with thoughtful experiments designed to understand the sensitivities of the material that one wishes to vitrify, it will be possible to engineer procedures that account for these sensitivities and result in a method that successfully preserves the viability of the biomaterial.

Development of Ovarian Tissue Vitrification Based on Cryobiological Principles

Vitrification has benefits independent from the ability to prevent lethal ice formation in a sample. From a practical standpoint, it is often a faster means to get samples into cryogenic storage. For isolated cells like oocytes, a procedure on one to two oocytes can be completed in approximately 12 min. On the contrary, because freezing cools the cells very slowly (i.e., 1 °C per minute between −5 and −35 °C), a freezing procedure usually takes more than an hour.

As with any multiparameter procedure, there are literally countless numbers of ways to vitrify biological material. The steps to vitrify a sample include incubating the biomaterial in a solution containing cryoprotectants, loading the sample into or onto a support system, cooling that system, holding the system in a long-term storage vessel, warming the sample, diluting the cryoprotectant solution, and then utilizing the sample in the intended way. Since each of these steps could be done in any one of a number of ways, the possible number of combinations of these parameters is theoretically infinite. This variety of combinations of parameters is reflected in the fact that more than 40 vitrification procedures have been developed and tested on human ovarian tissue throughout the years [1], the majority of protocols having been developed for oocyte or embryo vitrification, but not optimized for the complexity of cell types within ovarian cortical tissue that differ in cryoprotectant uptake and osmotic tolerance.

While it is likely that any number of methods could work equally effectively, it is also likely that more methods would fail than succeed. The difficulty, then, is to sort through all of the possible choices of parameters to find the right combination. We have approached this task in our efforts to vitrify nonhuman primate ovarian tissue by using some fundamental cryobiological principles to narrow the possible choices and, within that more limited sampling space, identified better choices based upon empirical testing.

One of the most important design restrictions upon which we imposed ourselves was that the sample had to be held inside of a truly closed system; closed in this context means that the sample is isolated from its environment during storage. We achieved this goal by using a straw that is large enough to hold small tissue pieces yet can be hermetically sealed. Using this vessel imposed restrictions on the other parameters, most noteworthy the achievable rates of temperature change during cooling and warming.

Since the straw we have chosen is much larger than the devices currently used to vitrify cells in embryology laboratories, we were limited to cooling and warming rates no greater than a few hundred °C per minute. As a result, this required us to develop vitrification solutions that would form stable glasses at such cooling and warming rates. As mentioned above, this is achievable, contrary to much of the current thinking.

Using a larger system does have some advantages, such as easier handling and labeling. The disadvantages include the use of higher concentrated solutions, with presumably higher toxicity, as discussed. However, we felt that, with enough effort, we would be able to overcome this challenge and develop a vitrification method that would form a stable glass and also have limited toxicity to primate ovarian tissue, allowing its use in a newly designed system.

Another advantage of having a larger system is that it is quite easy to observe ice formation during cooling and warming. We took advantage of this fact when designing our vitrification solutions and confirmed the absence of ice during cooling and warming by using a sensitive thermal analysis (differential scanning calorimetry).

Relatively few compounds have been identified that have cryoprotective properties and can be used as cryoprotectants. In the area of assisted reproduction, these include dimethyl sulfoxide (DMSO), ethylene glycol, propylene glycol, glycerol, and sucrose. All of these compounds except for sucrose fall into a class known as permeating cryoprotectants since they are able to diffuse across the cell membrane and enter the cytoplasm. In nearly all instances known, a cryopreservation solution must have at least one permeating cryoprotectant. Since vitrification solutions contain a relatively high concentration of cryoprotectants, a combination of two or more of these compounds are usually utilized, in an effort to reduce the specific toxicity of each single compound.

In one of our early experiments, we compared two vitrification solutions, one containing a combination of DMSO and ethylene glycol and the other containing a combination of glycerol and ethylene glycol. In order to determine the appropriate concentration of each of the compounds, we tested solutions containing an increasing concentration of the combination of each. Our goal was to have a solution with just enough of the solutes to form a stable glass in the straw system – too much would exacerbate chemical toxicity, and too little would facilitate ice formation. It was determined that with the combination of DMSO and ethylene glycol, a total concentration of 51 % by weight would suffice, and with the glycerol-ethylene glycol combination, 53 % was sufficient.

When testing these solutions, we witnessed a phenomenon that rarely occurs and goes against common assumptions. At these concentrations, while the solutions themselves remained vitreous during cooling and warming, the pieces of tissue actually froze during warming! It is often assumed that, because the cytoplasm of cells contains such a high concentration of proteins and other macromolecules, the cytoplasm is much more likely to vitrify than the surrounding solution. While this is probably true in a general sense, it is not an absolute fact, as we observed (also, see the discussion in [13]). We were able to overcome this problem by simply increasing the overall solute concentration by 1 % to a total of 54 % when using the glycerol and ethylene glycol combination. With the slightly higher concentration of solutes, both the solution and the tissue appeared to remain vitreous throughout both the cooling and warming process (Fig. 6.2).

We also tested the addition of synthetic polymers to the vitrification solutions, to determine their effect on the tissue after cooling and warming. The particular polymers were chosen for their ability to enhance vitrification at slow cooling and warming rates. Based upon the molecular configuration of these polymers, it is believed that they either directly interact with ice crystals, preventing their growth, or they interact with inherent nucleating agents that are often found in solutions, reducing the ability of ice crystals to form. Whatever their mechanism, we found that the addition of these polymers to the vitrification solution resulted in better preservation of the tissue. Because of their presumed mechanism of action, these polymers are only included in the vitrification solution (i.e., not the cryoprotectant loading or equilibration solutions) used in the last step prior to cooling of the tissue.

Fig. 6.2 *Top*:
Devitrification of macaque
ovarian tissue contained
inside a heat-sealed high
security plastic straw is
observed when the
concentration of
permeating cryoprotectants
(52 %) is not optimal.
Bottom: Successful
vitrification of macaque
ovarian tissue in a closed
system upon both cooling
and warming occurs with
optimal concentration of
permeating cryoprotectants
(54 %) (See Ting et al. [38]
for details)

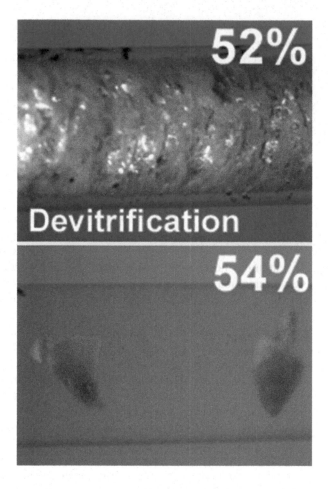

In each of the experiments that we conducted, we were able to identify levels of
parameters that resulted in improvements in the experimental outcomes. We pro-
gressed in an incremental fashion, choosing the best parameter levels to include in
future experiments, where other parameters were assessed. In the end, we have
developed a vitrification method that met our design criteria – having a closed system that is easy to use and insures that the sample remains vitreous throughout the
entire procedure. The good news is that the tissue, having been vitrified using this
system, maintains a high level of viability. The viability of the tissue remains
slightly less than the non-cryopreserved tissue, as measured by our experimental
endpoints, suggesting that further improvements might be achievable. Nevertheless,
we feel that, by applying good cryobiological principles and designing careful
experiments, we were able to make significant progress toward the development of
a very good vitrification method for nonhuman primate ovarian tissue that can eventually be applied to human tissue.

Endpoints of Vitrification Success

The gold standard and ultimate assessment for the success of a vitrification protocol for ovarian tissue preservation in cancer patients is live birth, which can take several years to achieve given that the patient has to be disease-free and healthy. Other endpoints, which are less time consuming, have been used frequently to evaluate the effectiveness of different vitrification methods for ovarian tissue. These endpoints include tissue morphology, follicle counts, protein markers for follicle health and function, as well as in vitro (tissue and isolated follicle culture) and in vivo follicle development (xenograft and autograft). The advantages and disadvantages of these endpoints are discussed here.

Tissue histology is the most common endpoint and provides an evaluation of the health of ovarian follicles and stroma based on morphology. Using tissue histology as an endpoint is simple and produces quick results. In addition, morphological change is often the first indicator of cryodamage such as abnormal cellular shrinkage and swelling resulting in lysed cells. The disadvantage of using tissue morphology as the sole endpoint is the lack of functional evaluation. Damage to intracellular organelles and intercellular contacts, which are important for follicle development and survival, can be triggered by cryoprotectant toxicity and the vitrification procedure without apparent histological changes.

Tissue morphology is often accompanied with follicle counts. Follicle counts provide an estimation of follicle numbers in fresh vs. vitrified tissues. However, one must take great caution in interpreting these results. In primate ovaries, the distribution of follicles is heterogeneous and follicular density can vary more than two orders of magnitude in cortical tissues within the same ovary [33]. Therefore, it is difficult, if not impossible, to compare numbers of follicles in different treatment groups. In addition, follicles that had been lysed would not be detected following counting, resulting in an overestimation of follicular survival. For these reasons, follicular quantification and tissue morphology, while providing a quick and general evaluation of tissue health, are much more useful when combined with analyses such as protein and functional endpoints in evaluation of vitrification protocols.

Protein markers are routinely used in examining tissue and follicle health prior to and following vitrification. Protein expression/localization is most frequently assessed using immunohistochemistry, and markers used are typically related to cellular growth/proliferation, apoptosis pathways, ovarian follicle-specific proteins, and vasculature. Classical markers of cellular proliferation include Ki-67 [2], proliferating cell nuclear antigen (PCNA; [27]), and phospho-histone H3 (PPH3; [37]). Apoptosis markers are often used to indicate follicle death/atresia and include active caspase-3 [44]; Fas, Fas ligand, Bcl-2, Bax, and p53 [14]; and TUNEL assay [21]. Follicle-specific markers are used to assess the health and developmental potential of the ovarian follicles, and these include growth differentiation factor 9 (GDF-9), anti-Müllerian hormone (AMH; [2]), activin, and phosphorylated Smad 2 (p-Smad 2; [17]). Both GDF-9 and AMH are members of the TGFβ family. GDF-9, expressed in the cytoplasm of the oocyte, plays an important role during early folliculogenesis

[28]. AMH is produced by granulosa cells of follicles from the primary to antral stage with its peak production in the small antral follicles [41]. Activin has been shown to be important for granulosa cell proliferation and follicle development, while Smad 2 is a downstream target of activin and is phosphorylated upon the activation of activin [12]. Finally, markers of vascularization are often used to assess the potential of the ovarian stroma to re-vascularize and support follicle survival and growth after transplantation. These markers include vascular endothelial growth factor (VEGF; [9]), a potent angiogenic factor that promotes growth of vascular endothelial cells, as well as CD31, also known as platelet endothelial cell adhesion molecule-1 (PECAM-1), an endothelial cell marker [21]. Endpoints such as tissue morphology and protein expression can give a rapid evaluation of the tested vitrification method; however, these endpoints do not reflect true ovarian function.

Other relatively short-term functional assays can be performed and are important for evaluating vitrification methods. Bromodeoxyuridine (BrdU) is incorporated into newly synthesized deoxyribonucleic acid (DNA) during the S phase of mitosis in dividing cells and can be used for the evaluation of tissue viability post-warming in culture. Vitrified ovarian tissues are cultured with BrdU for 48 h at 37 °C in 5 % CO_2 and subsequently fixed and immunostained for BrdU [20]. BrdU incorporation is mainly observed in granulosa cells of preantral follicles as well as stromal cells. BrdU incorporation may be a more accurate reflection of post-thaw viability as well as the ability of cells to recover from cryopreservation procedures.

Individual secondary follicles isolated from vitrified tissue have been encapsulated in alginate and cultured to evaluate follicle survival, growth, and ability to form an antrum and produce hormones (i.e., estradiol, progesterone, and AMH) as well as generate mature oocytes and live births (in rodent models only) [10, 38]. Vitrified ovarian tissue pieces have also been cultured in vitro; however, the current tissue culture system is still suboptimal and does not support long-term tissue viability; increased atretic follicles are observed in pieces of ovarian cortex cultured for longer 5 days [43]. Nevertheless, in vitro culture of ovarian cortical tissue provides insights into tissue morphology as well as short-term functional endpoints such as hormone production [15], the ability of follicles to grow [38], and expression of protein markers mentioned above [32].

Another option for examining the function of vitrified ovarian tissue is xeno-transplantation. A recent review by Dittrich and colleagues [4] summarizes studies wherein prepubertal or adult human ovarian tissue cryopreserved by slow-rate freezing was transplanted into various sites (kidney capsule, intra-abdominal pockets, subcutaneous spaces, intramuscular pockets) of immunocompromised mice with resultant recovery of ovarian function and, in a few cases, development of antral follicles from which metaphase II oocytes were recovered. Xenotransplantation of cryopreserved human ovarian tissue provides several advances over other in vitro functional assays such as the ability to evaluate re-vascularization of the ovarian graft, as well as long-term (months) in vivo support of follicular development to the antral stage. However, daily injections of human follicle-stimulating hormone are required to support follicle survival and growth. While an additional and critical application of xenotransplantation of human ovarian tissue is to assess the risk of reintroducing malignant cells [4], the concept of maturing human oocytes within another species is not yet clinically acceptable to be used as a means of fertility restoration.

Autotransplantation of vitrified ovarian tissue can be performed in the nonhuman primate model and can provide crucial information regarding the viability and function of vitrified ovarian tissue. Several groups have used nonhuman primates to evaluate vitrification methods for ovarian tissue and these studies are discussed in the section below.

Nonhuman Primate Models of Ovarian Tissue Vitrification

While valuable, studies using human ovarian tissues suffer from the limited availability of human ovarian tissue for research. As a result, these studies often use pooled samples from different patients of various ages and reproductive backgrounds, resulting in a lack of systematic comparison. The nonhuman primate is an ideal animal model for obtaining ovarian tissue for vitrification studies, due to the vast similarities in reproductive physiology and anatomy, including ovarian structure and function, between nonhuman primates and women. In addition to our laboratory, two other groups have utilized the nonhuman primate model in efforts to optimize ovarian tissue vitrification techniques; the current results to date are discussed here.

Suzuki and colleagues [11] systemically examined two different vitrification solutions (VSED, ethylene glycol, dimethyl sulfoxide, and sucrose, vs. VSEGP, ethylene glycol, polyvinylpyrrolidone [PVP], serum supplement substitute [SSS], and sucrose) and three different equilibration times (5, 10, and 20 min) on the morphology of cynomolgus macaque ovarian tissue post-thaw. In this study, the authors utilized an open system that involved direct plunging of the tissue into liquid nitrogen. While resulting in a high cooling rate, direct contact between the tissue and liquid nitrogen poses a safety risk for possible contamination from direct contact of tissue with liquid nitrogen as well as cross contamination between specimens during storage [3]. The VSEGP vitrification solution preserved a higher proportion of morphologically normal follicles compared to VSED. Transmission electron microscopy of vitrified-thawed ovarian tissue revealed that vitrification caused vacuolated mitochondria, an elevated surface ratio of lysosomes per oocyte cytoplasm, as well as collapsed collagen bundles between follicles and stromal cells. However, of the two vitrification solutions tested, VSED caused increased cryodamage compared to VSEGP. In addition, a shorter exposure time (5 min) using the VSEGP vitrification solution preserved follicle morphology, normality of mitochondria, and lysosomes in preantral follicles, compared to longer exposure times (10 and 20 min). Using the optimal vitrification solution and exposure time combination, this group adapted a closed system (0.5 cc straws) for tissue safety and assessed long-term function of vitrified ovarian tissue following heterotopic transplantation in cynomolgus macaques [35]. The heterotopic sites included retroperitoneal iliac fossa, omentum, uterine serosa, and mesosalpinx. Recovery of ovarian cyclicity, based on circulating estradiol and progesterone levels, was confirmed in three of four monkeys between 78 and 207 days posttransplantation and was maintained for as long as 716 days. In animals with confirmed ovarian cycles, ovarian stimulation with exogenous gonadotropin treatment was performed, and oocytes were collected 40 h after human chorionic gonadotropin (hCG) administration. This was the first study in primates wherein oocytes ($n = 9$ total) were collected from preovulatory follicles derived from vitrified ovarian tissue transplanted to non-ovarian sties. Some of the oocytes underwent fertilization with subsequent early embryonic development (8- to 16-cell stages) in vitro, establishing the potential of ovarian tissue vitrification to yield healthy gametes and embryos. The authors also utilized contrast-enhanced computed tomography to monitor reestablishment of vascularization and blood flow to the ovarian grafts and found abundant vasculature in the greater omentum, suggesting this as an optimal site for heterotopic transplantation of vitrified-thawed ovarian tissue.

Amorim and colleagues vitrified baboon ovarian tissue with dimethyl sulfoxide, ethylene glycol, human serum albumin, PVP, and sucrose by directly plunging the tissue into liquid nitrogen using Cryopins [2]. After warming in sucrose, ovarian tissue was transplanted orthotopically and covered with Interceed, a fabric composed of oxidized, regenerated cellulose designed to reduce the formation of postsurgical adhesions. Endpoints in this study included tissue histology and fibrosis (assessed using Masson's trichrome), follicle density, and immunohistochemistry for Ki67, AMH, GDF-9, caspase-3, and CD31. Results from this study demonstrated that ovarian follicles in vitrified-warmed ovarian grafts can survive, grow to the antral stage, and form corpora lutea, with evidence of ovulation in vivo 5 months posttransplantation. Follicles in vitrified-warmed grafts appeared healthy as they exhibited similar morphology and expressed Ki-67, AMH, and GDF-9 immunostaining with minimal caspase-3 staining relative to non-cryopreserved ovarian tissue. In addition, vitrified-warmed grafts also expressed similar numbers of blood vessels as marked by CD31 staining and did not exhibit increased areas of fibrosis relative to tissue that was not vitrified. Oocyte collection was not attempted. This study demonstrated promising results in the survival and development of vitrified-warmed grafts. The authors credited some of this success to the rapid transplantation time following ovarian biopsy; orthotopic transplantation was performed 24 h after removal of the cortex for vitrification. Thus, the fresh graft site might result in less ischemic damage typically observed after longer intervals between thawing and orthotopic transplantation. Ischemia remains an important issue for follicle survival because cancer patients will return to the clinic many years, if not decades depending upon the age of the patient at the time of ovarian tissue vitrification, to undergo orthotopic transplantation for restoration of ovarian function and fertility.

Our group employed the rhesus macaque as a model for vitrification of human ovarian tissue and developed first an open system [37] and then moved to a closed system [38]. Using an open system and ethylene glycol and glycerol as cryoprotectants, we discovered the benefits of adding a combination of synthetic polymers to the final vitrification solution, including a copolymer of polyvinyl alcohol (PVA, super cool X-1000™), PVP K12, and polyglycerol (super cool Z-1000™), in preserving ovarian morphology as well as cellular proliferation as assessed by PPH3 localization and BrdU incorporation post-vitrification [37]. Preantral follicles from vitrified-warmed tissues were also isolated and cultured in a three-dimensional (3D) environment within alginate as a biomatrix to assess follicle survival, growth, and ability to form an antrum and produce steroid hormones such as estradiol and progesterone. Encapsulated 3D follicle culture provided functional evidence of follicle viability post-vitrification and further supported the benefit of using polymers during tissue vitrification. However, secondary follicles isolated from vitrified-thawed tissue grew slower than those from non-cryopreserved tissue, and to date, healthy oocytes have not been obtained after 3D follicle culture in vitro. Similar to the study performed by Hashimoto et al. [11], we found that a shorter exposure time of ovarian cortical tissue to the vitrification solution (3 min in comparison to 8 min) resulted in less cryodamage, possibly due to toxicity induced by cryoprotective agents during a longer incubation [30]. In addition, we observed that the presence of DMSO in the vitrification solution promoted higher cryodamage in comparison to the vitrification solution without DMSO (Fig. 6.3). While DMSO is a frequently used cryoprotant in embryo, oocyte, and ovarian tissue vitrification, its negative effect found in our study could be attributed to the slow cooling rate, and therefore, a longer interval of exposure before the tissue is vitrified. DMSO induces toxicity by causing irreversible disruption of the microtubular system in mouse oocytes [18].

We also carefully examined the thermodynamics of our vitrification solution using differential scanning calorimetry (Fig. 6.4) for successful vitrification without devitrification in a fixed volume and confirmed the concentration required to stably vitrify in a 2 ml high security straw leading to successful development of a closed system for the vitrification of macaque ovarian tissue [38]. We incorporated the use of a tissue slicer to prepare uniformly thin pieces of ovarian cortical tissue (0.5–1 mm). Since the tissue thickness is uniform (optimal for cryoprotectant loading), the length and width of the pieces can vary according to the need for transplantation. We examined each piece of tissue for the presence of preantral follicles prior to initiation of the vitrification procedure. We enhanced tissue loading with solutions by placing the petri dishes containing tissue and solutions on top of an orbital laboratory shaker so that tissue was constantly moving thus facilitating tissue saturation. Since we have now determined the limiting concentration for 1 ml of vitrification solution to vitrify in a sealed straw, theoretically, as long as the tissue is saturated with the vitrification solution (facilitated by uniform thickness and constant stirring during loading) and can fit into the same configuration (6×60 mm^2), regardless of its size, it will vitrify. Figure 6.5 depicts the final composition of our optimal cryoprotectant and vitrification solutions used in our closed system for vitrification of macaque ovarian cortical tissue [30]. Tissues were exposed to one-fourth, one-half, and 1X vitrification solution containing 54 % permeating cryoprotectants [27 % ethylene glycol (weight/weight) and 27 % glycerol (weight/

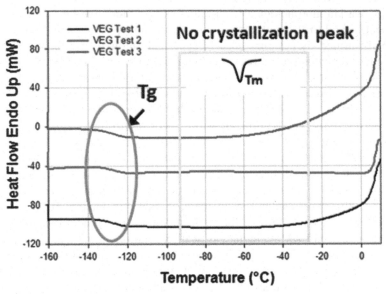

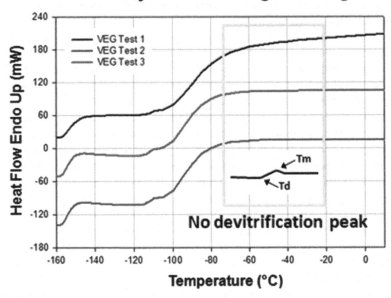

Fig. 6.3 Differential scanning calorimeter thermograms during cooling (*top*; temperature on the x axis decreasing from the left to the right) and warming (*bottom*; temperature on the x axis increasing from left to right) of vitrification solution containing ethylene glycol and glycerol (1:1). Glass transition temperature (Tg) was extrapolated as the midpoint of the thermal transition during cooling. The absence of phase transition peaks during cooling and warming validates the lack of crystallization during cooling as well as the lack of devitrification and melting during warming. *Arrows* indicate the onset of rapid warming at −110 °C, just above the temperature range of the glass transition (Adapted from Ting et al. [38])

Fig. 6.4 Morphology of vitrified-thawed macaque ovarian tissue (hematoxylin and eosin staining). *Top*: Ovarian tissue vitrified with 27% ethylene glycol (3.2 M) and 27% glycerol (4.7 M). *Bottom*: Ovarian tissue vitrified with 25.5% ethylene glycol (3 M) and 25.5% DMSO (4.5 M). The percentage of abnormal primordial and primary follicles as well as oocytes in secondary follicles was higher in tissue vitrified with DMSO. Cryodamage included shrunken and vacuolated oocytes, as well as abnormal space between the follicle and stroma. Granulosa cell morphology in secondary follicles and stromal integrity was similar in tissue vitrified with or without DMSO (Adapted from Ting et al. [38])

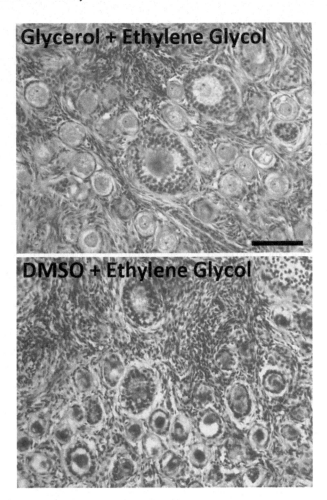

Fig. 6.5 Composition of our current working cryoprotectant and vitrification solutions for vitrification of macaque ovarian tissue in a closed system; see Ting et al. [38] for details

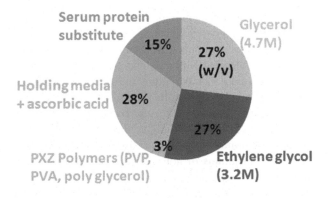

weight)] prepared in Sage holding medium containing ascorbic acid phosphate with the addition of 15 % synthetic serum protein supplement (SPS; v/v) for 5 min/step at 37 °C. In the last step, tissue is incubated for 1 min in vitrification solution containing non-permeating XYZ polymers (total of 1 %, v/v) and then loaded into the high security plastic straw, and the ends are heat sealed.

We also demonstrated that vitrification of ovarian tissue in 1 ml of vitrification solution requires a slower cooling rate (~35 °C/min; cooling was carried out in liquid nitrogen vapor as opposed to direct plunging into liquid nitrogen or super rapid cooling as described above) to avoid introducing fracture to the sample as discussed above [30]. Thus, we currently use a two-step cooling protocol wherein, after the last step of cryoprotectant loading, ovarian tissue is held in liquid nitrogen vapor at −150 °C to −180 °C for 10 min and then plunged into liquid nitrogen. Likewise, a two-step warming procedure is used to prevent devitrification of the tissue; closed straws containing ovarian tissue are held at 30 °C in the air for 1 min, followed by placement into a 40 °C water bath for 30 s. Thawed tissue is then exposed to decreasing concentrations of sucrose for removal of the vitrification solution [30].

When vitrified-thawed ovarian tissue was transplanted heterotopically to subcutaneous sites in the arm or abdomen, our preliminary results indicate restoration of ovarian cyclicity as well as development of preovulatory follicles that yielded mature oocytes capable of fertilization and early embryonic development [20]. Although the oocyte and embryo yield in our preliminary studies was also few, these results nonetheless lend credence to the effectiveness of our logical and systematic approach based on cryobiological principles for optimizing vitrification for ovarian cortical tissue. The "gold standard" endpoint of live offspring has not yet been achieved in nonhuman primate models but remains a major goal along with delineating the best sites for transplantation that will consistently yield competent oocytes for restoring fertility.

Successful Vitrification of Human Ovarian Tissue

The first documented attempts at transplantation of vitrified ovarian tissue in women were reported in two publications [19, 36]. In these pioneering studies, ovarian cortical tissue from patients with premature ovarian failure, not caused by cancer treatments, was vitrified with ethylene glycol and PVP and placed on a "Cryosupport" within a cryovial then into liquid nitrogen. Each of 20 patients with residual follicles present in their ovarian grafts prior to vitrification had 40–80 pieces of thawed ovarian tissue transplanted within a pocket of the mesosalpinx. The tissue was pretreated in vitro with drugs that stimulate the activity of Akt (protein kinase B) presumably to increase primordial follicle activation; unfortunately, there were no patients who received transplants of non-treated tissues to justify this conclusion. Nonetheless, nine patients resumed ovarian cyclicity, and 24 oocytes were retrieved from six patients. Three pregnancies ensued, with one miscarriage and two live births. These reports unequivocally demonstrate that vitrification can be an effective method of ovarian tissue cryopreservation that preserves ovarian function, including the fertile potential of this tissue, in women.

Conclusion

Collectively, studies in nonhuman primate models have provided a basis for consideration of ovarian tissue vitrification, in contrast to slow-rate freezing, for cryopreserving human ovarian tissue. Many parameters for optimization of ovarian tissue vitrification including tissue dimensions, cryoprotectant concentrations, cryoprotectant loading times and temperatures, cooling rates, warming rates, and cryoprotectant removal have been tested and validated in both open and closed systems in nonhuman primates. These studies also extended endpoint analysis beyond evaluation of static tissue morphology and follicle counts. Importantly, bona fide ovarian function in vivo was observed after transplantation of vitrified-thawed tissue which is required for moving toward the ultimate goal of restoring fertility and production of live offspring. The recent live births in women who underwent heterotopic transplantation with vitrified-thawed ovarian tissue can now provide some confidence that vitrification can move forward as an acceptable means of cryopreserving human tissue for restoring ovarian function and fertility. The necessity for ovarian tissue vitrification in the United States is evident from the fact that vitrification is now the accepted clinical method for cryopreserving oocytes and embryos. With this in mind, ovarian tissue vitrification using optimized protocols underscored by best manufacturing methods for vitrification solutions along with successful clinical practice for transplantation is also an immediate need for patients whose sole option for one day becoming parents is ovarian tissue cryopreservation.

Acknowledgments This work was supported by the Oncofertility Consortium NIH UL1 RR024926 (HD058293, HD058294, PL1-EB008542), U54-HD18185 (Eunice Kennedy Shriver Specialized Cooperative Centers Program in Reproduction and Infertility Research), and ONPRC 8P51OD011092.

References

1. Amorim CA, Curaba M, Van Langendonckt A, Dolmans MM, Donnez J. Vitrification as an alternative means of cryopreserving ovarian tissue. Reprod Biomed Online. 2011;23(2):160–86.
2. Amorim CA, Jacobs S, Devireddy RV, Van Langendonckt A, Vanacker J, Jaeger J, et al. Successful vitrification and autografting of baboon (Papio anubis) ovarian tissue. Hum Reprod. 2013;28(8):2146–56.
3. Bielanski A, Vajta G. Risk of contamination of germplasm during cryopreservation and cryobanking in IVF units. Hum Reprod. 2009;24(10):2457–67.
4. Dittrich R, Lotz L, Fehm T, Krussel J, von Wolff M, Toth B, et al. Xenotransplantation of cryopreserved human ovarian tissue – a systematic review of MII oocyte maturation and

discussion of it as a realistic option for restoring fertility after cancer treatment. Fertil Steril. 2015;103(6):1557–65.

5. Donnez J, Dolmans MM, Pellicer A, Diaz-Garcia C, Sanchez Serrano M, Schmidt KT, et al. Restoration of ovarian activity and pregnancy after transplantation of cryopreserved ovarian tissue: a review of 60 cases of reimplantation. Fertil Steril. 2013;99(6):1503–13.

6. Donnez J, Dolmans MM. Ovarian cortex transplantation: 60 reported live births brings the success and worldwide expansion of the technique towards routine clinical practice. J Assist Reprod Genet. 2015;32(8):1167–70.

7. Fahy GM, MacFarlane DR, Angell CA, Meryman HT. Vitrification as an approach to cryo-preservation. Cryobiology. 1984;21(4):407–26.

8. Fahy GM, Rall WF. Vitrification: an overview. In: Tucker MJ, Liebermann J, editors. Vitrification in assisted reproduction. London: Informa Healthcare; 2007. p. 1–20.

9. Grazul-Bilska AT, Banerjee J, Yazici I, Borowczyk E, Bilski JJ, Sharma RK, et al. Morphology and function of cryopreserved whole ovine ovaries after heterotopic autotransplantation. Reprod Biol Endocrinol. 2008;6:16.

10. Hasegawa A, Mochida N, Ogasawara T, Koyama K. Pup birth from mouse oocytes in preantral follicles derived from vitrified and warmed ovaries followed by in vitro growth, in vitro maturation, and in vitro fertilization. Fertil Steril. 2006;86(4 Suppl):1182–92.

11. Hashimoto S, Suzuki N, Yamanaka M, Hosoi Y, Ishizuka B, Morimoto Y. Effects of vitrification solutions and equilibration times on the morphology of cynomolgus ovarian tissues. Reprod Biomed Online. 2010;21(4):501–9.

12. Hogg K, Etherington SL, Young JM, McNeilly AS, Duncan WC. Inhibitor of differentiation (Id) genes are expressed in the steroidogenic cells of the ovine ovary and are differentially regulated by members of the transforming growth factor-beta family. Endocrinology. 2010;151(3):1247–56.

13. Hopkins JB, Badeau R, Warkentin M, Thorne RE. Effect of common cryoprotectants on critical warming rates and ice formation in aqueous solutions. Cryobiology. 2012;65(3):169–78.

14. Hussein MR, Bedaiwy MA, Falcone T. Analysis of apoptotic cell death, Bcl-2, and p53 protein expression in freshly fixed and cryopreserved ovarian tissue after exposure to warm ischemia. Fertil Steril. 2006;85 Suppl 1:1082–92.

15. Isachenko V, Lapidus I, Isachenko E, Krivokharchenko A, Kreienberg R, Woriedh M, et al. Human ovarian tissue vitrification versus conventional freezing: morphological, endocrinological, and molecular biological evaluation. Reproduction. 2009;138(2):319–27.

16. Jeruss JS, Woodruff TK. Preservation of fertility in patients with cancer. N Engl J Med. 2009;360(9):902–11.

17. Jin S, Lei L, Shea LD, Zelinski MB, Stouffer RL, Woodruff TK. Markers of growth and development in primate primordial follicles are preserved after slow cryopreservation. Fertil Steril. 2010;93(8):2627–32.

18. Johnson MH, Pickering SJ. The effect of dimethyl sulphoxide on the microtubular system of the mouse oocyte. Development. 1987;100(2):313–24.

19. Kawamura K, Cheng Y, Suzuki N, Deguchi M, Sato Y, Takae S, et al. Hippo signaling disruption and Akt stimulation of ovarian follicles for infertility treatment. Proc Natl Acad Sci U S A. 2013;110(43):17474–9.

20. Lee DM, Ting A, Thomas C, Bishop C, Xu F, Zelinski MB. Heterotopic transplants of vitrified ovarian tissue in macaques: assessment of follicular function, embryonic development and a novel microbubble assay for blood flow. Fertil Steril. 2012;98(3):S69.

21. Lee J, Kim SK, Youm HW, Kim HJ, Lee JR, Suh CS, et al. Effects of three different types of antifreeze proteins on mouse ovarian tissue cryopreservation and transplantation. PLoS One. 2015;10(5):e0126252.

22. Mazur P. Kinetics of water loss from cells at subzero temperatures and the likelihood of intracellular freezing. J Gen Physiol. 1963;47:47–69.

23. Mazur P, Leibo SP, Chu EH. A two-factor hypothesis of freezing injury. Evidence from Chinese hamster tissue-culture cells. Exp Cell Res. 1972;71(2):345–55.

24. Mazur P. Principles of cryobiology. In: Fuller BJ, Lane N, Benson EE, editors. Life in the frozen state. Boca Raton: CRC Press; 2004. p. 3–65.
25. Mullen SF, Li M, Li Y, Chen ZJ, Critser JK. Human oocyte vitrification: the permeability of metaphase II oocytes to water and ethylene glycol and the appliance toward vitrification. Fertil Steril. 2008;89(6):1812–25.
26. Mullen SF, Fahy GM. Fundamental aspects of vitrification as a method of reproductive cell, tissue, and organ cryopreservation. In: Donnez J, Kim SS, editors. Principles and practice of fertility preservation. Cambridge: Cambridge University Press; 2011. p. 145–63.
27. Onions VJ, Mitchell MR, Campbell BK, Webb R. Ovarian tissue viability following whole ovine ovary cryopreservation: assessing the effects of sphingosine-1-phosphate inclusion. Hum Reprod. 2008;23(3):606–18.
28. Otsuka F, McTavish KJ, Shimasaki S. Integral role of GDF-9 and BMP-15 in ovarian function. Mol Reprod Dev. 2011;78(1):9–21.
29. Pegg DE. The role of vitrification techniques of cryopreservation in reproductive medicine. Hum Fertil (Camb). 2005;8(4):231–9.
30. Pegg DE. The relevance of ice crystal formation for the cryopreservation of tissues and organs. Cryobiology. 2010;60(3 Suppl):S36–44.
31. Rall WF, Mazur P, McGrath JJ. Depression of the ice-nucleation temperature of rapidly cooled mouse embryos by glycerol and dimethyl sulfoxide. Biophys J. 1983;41(1):1–12.
32. Sadeu JC, Smitz J. Growth differentiation factor 9 and anti-Mullerian hormone expression in cultured human follicles from frozen-thawed ovarian tissue. Reprod Biomed Online. 2008;17(4):537–48.
33. Schmidt KL, Byskov AG, Nyboe Andersen A, Muller J, Yding Andersen C. Density and distribution of primordial follicles in single pieces of cortex from 21 patients and in individual pieces of cortex from three entire human ovaries. Hum Reprod. 2003;18(6):1158–64.
34. Steif PS, Palastro MC, Rabin Y. The effect of temperature gradients on stress development during cryopreservation via vitrification. Cell Preserv Technol. 2007;5(2):104–15.
35. Suzuki N, Hashimoto S, Igarashi S, Takae S, Yamanaka M, Yamochi T, et al. Assessment of long-term function of heterotopic transplants of vitrified ovarian tissue in cynomolgus monkeys. Hum Reprod. 2012;27(8):2420–9.
36. Suzuki N, Yoshioka N, Takae S, Sugishita Y, Tamura M, Hashimoto S, et al. Successful fertility preservation following ovarian tissue vitrification in patients with primary ovarian insufficiency. Hum Reprod. 2015;30(3):608–15.
37. Ting AY, Yeoman RR, Lawson MS, Zelinski MB. Synthetic polymers improve vitrification outcomes of macaque ovarian tissue as assessed by histological integrity and the in vitro development of secondary follicles. Cryobiology. 2012;65(1):1–11.
38. Ting AY, Yeoman RR, Campos JR, Lawson MS, Mullen SF, Fahy GM, et al. Morphological and functional preservation of pre-antral follicles after vitrification of macaque ovarian tissue in a closed system. Hum Reprod. 2013;28(5):1267–79.
39. Toner M, Cravalho EG, Karel M, Armant DR. Cryomicroscopic analysis of intracellular ice formation during freezing of mouse oocytes without cryoadditives. Cryobiology. 1991;28(1):55–71.
40. Vajta G, Nagy ZP. Are programmable freezers still needed in the embryo laboratory? Rev Vitrification Reprod Biomed Online. 2006;12(6):779–96.
41. Weenen C, Laven JS, Von Bergh AR, Cranfield M, Groome NP, Visser JA, et al. Anti-Mullerian hormone expression pattern in the human ovary: potential implications for initial and cyclic follicle recruitment. Mol Hum Reprod. 2004;10(2):77–83.
42. Wowk B. Thermodynamic aspects of vitrification. Cryobiology. 2010;60(1):11–22.
43. Wright CS, Hovatta O, Margara R, Trew G, Winston RM, Franks S, et al. Effects of follicle-stimulating hormone and serum substitution on the in-vitro growth of human ovarian follicles. Hum Reprod. 1999;14(6):1555–62.
44. Xiao Z, Wang Y, Li L, Li SW. Cryopreservation of the human ovarian tissue induces the expression of Fas system in morphologically normal primordial follicles. Cryo Letters. 2010;31(2):112–9.

Chapter 7
Opportunities for Enabling Puberty

Monica M. Laronda and Teresa K. Woodruff

Introduction

Puberty marks the transition from adolescence to adulthood and refers to physical and psychological changes as a result of the changes in male or female hormonal milieu during this critical point in development. Puberty establishes the hypothalamic-pituitary-gonadal axis, with the underlying goal of establishing reproductive maturity. Additionally, the transition through puberty solidifies development of hormone-responsive organ systems, such as neuronal, cardiovascular, and skeletal tissues. There are several ways in which this transition can be disrupted, including from naturally occurring mutations or from secondary effects of disease treatments that affect gonadal health or the health of other organs along this axis. This chapter will briefly describe the potential causes of delayed or failed puberty initiation and delve into the experimental paradigms undergoing investigation as a way to initiate puberty, restore fertility, and maintain endocrine support throughout a patient's adult life.

Normal Initiation of Puberty

Puberty is defined by a set of physiological, physical, and psychological changes that occur in the transition from an adolescent to a sexually mature being. These changes occur in girls between ages 10 and 14 and in boys between ages 12 and 16 [NIH.gov]. Puberty is initiated by gonadotropin-releasing hormone (GnRH)

M.M. Laronda • T.K. Woodruff (✉)
Obstetrics and Gynecology, Northwestern University, Feinberg School of Medicine, Chicago, IL, USA
e-mail: m-laronda@northwestern.edu; tkw@northwestern.edu

© Springer International Publishing Switzerland 2017
T.K. Woodruff, Y.C. Gosiengfiao (eds.), *Pediatric and Adolescent Oncofertility*,
DOI 10.1007/978-3-319-32973-4_7

neurons within the hypothalamus that triggers follicle-stimulating hormone (FSH) and luteinizing hormone (LH) release from the pituitary. These hormones act on the ovaries in females and testes in males to release estradiol and testosterone, respectively. The release of hormones from the gonads in response to the hypothalamus and pituitary sets up what is called the hypothalamic-pituitary-gonadal axis for continued cyclicity throughout a person's reproductively mature life. These sex hormones trigger several physical characteristics. Breast development is one of the earliest visible signs of a girl undergoing puberty. This is followed by hair growth in the pubic and armpit regions, and finally menstruation occurs. In boys, the first signs of puberty include enlargement of the penis and testicles, hair in the pubic region and armpits, followed by muscle growth, deepening of the voice, and facial hair growth.

The female reproductive tact is one of the most dynamic organ systems in the body and requires the pubertal transition to establish the cyclical response to pulsatile hormones. These active organs include the female gonads, ovaries, fallopian tubes, uterus, cervix, and vagina. Each of the lower reproductive tract organs responds to the main regulator of cyclicity and keeper of female fertility, the ovary, and is connected by a centralized luminal space.

The ovary is comprised of a primary functional unit, called the follicle, which houses, protects, and stimulates an oocyte, the female gamete. The follicle units exist within the ovary at different stages of differentiation, from the quiescent primordial follicle pool to the large antral follicle that has the potential to ovulate a mature egg and become fertilized. Follicle processes such as rest, activation, and atresia are highly regulated within the ovary, and this regulation is set up by the first wave of folliculogenesis. The first wave occurs prepubertally in a more rapid fashion and includes differentiation through the antral stage in the absence of hormonal stimulation [1, 2]. This wave can be visualized in unique transgenic mice with three developmentally unique oocyte-specific markers. First follicles to be activated were localized to the anterior-dorsal region. However the first follicles to undergo meiotic onset are located in the ventral region [3]. The controlled waves of folliculogenesis are also regulated by somatic cell support and the time and location from which these support cells are derived [2, 4, 5].

The two main support cells that surround a centralized oocyte and manufacture endocrine products are the granulosa and theca cells. Granulosa cells proliferate around the growing follicles as they produce increasing amounts of estradiol through aromatization of androgens secreted by the neighboring theca cells. Pulsatile FSH primes the granulosa cells of the growing follicles through the FSH receptor to develop an antrum, a fluid-filled sac that forms within the growing follicle, and respond to the immediate spike in LH. The granulosa cells are the primary source of inhibin A and release this peptide hormone to suppress FSH secretion from the pituitary [6]. Inhibins play an important role in this regulation as Inhibin A knockout mice produce granulosa cell tumors in females and the equivalent support cell tumors in males with 100 % penetrance [7]. The theca cells of the dominant follicle produce collagenase enzymes to break down the ovarian surface epithelium as the cumulus granulosa cells break away from the maturing oocyte and release it through ovulation. Progesterone receptors (PRs) have been localized to theca cells of small antral follicles and granulosa cells of preovulatory follicles in ovaries that have been exposed to LH in primates [8]. Once the egg is released, the ovary remodels and the follicular cells differentiate into a corpus luteum that responds less to FSH-stimulated estrogen production and becomes the primary source of progesterone production. This process is blocked at the level of the PR in isolated preovulatory granulosa cells by the antiprogestin RU486, also known as the "morning after pill" [9]. Circulating progesterone signals to the hypothalamus to reduce release of GnRH and also signals to the downstream reproductive tract to prepare for accepting the ovulated egg, potential fertilization, implantation, and embryo development.

The female reproductive tract undergoes dramatic changes through proliferation, differentiation, and extracellular matrix (ECM) remodeling. The mostly secretory and ciliated epithelial lining of the fallopian tube responds to the estradiol secretion from the ovary and facilitates the movement of the ovulated egg toward the uterus [10]. The frequency of muscle contractions of the fallopian tube increases to move the ovulated egg into the ampulla region where it can be fertilized in response to prostaglandin, progesterone, and LH [11]. Additionally, the oviductal-glycoprotein 1 (OVGP1) mucin is secreted by the fallopian tube in response to estrogen and facilitates fertilization if sperm is available during this ovulation window [12]. The uterus responds to estrogen produced by the growing ovarian follicles by generating a thickened uterine lining. The uterine lining prepares for implantation through estrogen-induced progesterone receptor action that induces glandular secretion and provides a nutrient-rich environment for implantation of a blastocyst [13–15]. Once the embryo embeds into the uterine wall, it releases human chorionic gonadotropin (hCG) that stimulates back to the ovary to maintain the progesterone-producing corpus luteum [16]. Otherwise, the corpus luteum degenerates and the uterine lining sheds through contractile movements; together this process is known as menstruation.

The cervix is the barrier between the uterus and vagina in the female reproductive tract. It protects the inner luminal space from pathogens by producing cloudy thick mucus during most of the reproductive cycle. Following implantation, the cervical glands remodel and produce a mucus plug in response to progesterone and to protect the developing embryo. During the proliferative phase of the menstrual cycle, estrogen promotes fluid-like alkaline mucus production from the cervix that supports the survival and passage of sperm through the vagina and into the internal luminal space [17, 18].

The male gonad, the testis, is like the female ovary as it houses both the production of sperm and the cells that produce sex hormones. The testis is organized into tubules and interstitial space. The tubules are comprised of a basement membrane, established by the peritubular myoid cells, that serves as a barrier function to protect the spermatogonial stem cells and the developing spermatozoa. Spermatogenesis occurs in a wave that begins with dividing spermatogonial stem cells (SSCs) that produce spermatogonia every 16 days, and the whole process of spermatogenesis in the human takes 72 days [19]. Spermatogonia mitotically amplify and differentiate in a manner highly controlled by positional location within the luminal space of the tubules and by the intimate tight junction cell contacts with the supporting Sertoli cell. Sertoli cells protect cells by establishing a blood-testis barrier and ensuring that only certain cells receive signals, such as the meiosis triggering molecules like retinoic acid [20, 21]. Cells further away from the basement membrane meiotically divide to produce 4 haploid cells, defined as round spermatids. Round spermatids begin to shed their cytoplasm and condense their nuclear contents, through tubulobulbar complexes with Sertoli cells, as they produce a single flagellum and develop into spermatozoa [22–24]. These cells are not yet mobile and require lots of fluid to be flushed from the luminal space and into the convoluted tubules of the epididymis. The caput epididymal cuboidal and ciliated epithelial cells resorb the excess fluid and concentrate the sperm, as they prepare the sperm for potential capacitation and fertilization. For example, epididymal human cysteine-rich secretory proteins (hCRISPs) associate with the head of the sperm in the epididymis and aid in the binding and penetration through the egg's zona pellucida to facilitate fertilization [25, 26]. The caudal epididymis provides an area where the highly concentrated sperm can be stored for 2–3 months. During ejaculation, the concentrated sperm is pushed, via peristaltic action, through the vas deferens, as it is diluted with fluids from the seminal vesicles and prostate.

During a male's peripubertal period, spermatogenesis occurs in an incomplete and accelerated manner. This process is similar to what happens in females and is also known as the first wave. It sets up the intracellular contacts and primes the testis to be receptive to hormonal cues. The interstitial compartments between the tubules contain Leydig cells, which produce testosterone in response to pulsatile LH and hCG secreted from the pituitary and peaking each morning. Leydig cells produce testosterone, which promote spermatogenesis through the AR receptors expressed in a cyclical manner on the Sertoli cells [27]. The Sertoli cells also express FSHR, and signaling through these receptors is required for establishing the testis tubules prior to puberty in mice [28] and maintains germ cell survival (reviewed in [29]).

Effects of Sex Hormone on Other Organ Systems

Male and female sex hormones regulate growth hormone (GH) secretion directly, at the hypothalamus and pituitary, and indirectly through modulating downstream tissue responses to GH, affecting height and body composition throughout a person's lifetime, but is exemplified during puberty. Three peptide hormones, GH-releasing hormone (GHRH), somatostatin (SS), and ghrelin, control GH secretion, while insulin-like growth factor I (IGF-I) provides negative feedback by acting on GHRH and SS neurons. Metabolic cues, including insulin, glucose, and adiposity, inhibit GH secretion. Pulsatile GH secretion increases 1.5- to 3 fold in both boys and girls during puberty [30]. GH secretion is positively regulated by testosterone and estrogen in prepubertal and transitioning boys and girls [31]. The response to testosterone in boys is due to the aromatization into estrogen and is mediated through the estrogen receptor. Adolescent boys with gynecomastia and treated with testosterone showed an increase in plasma GH and greater increase in height velocity over the group that was treated with non-aromatizing dihydrotestosterone (DHT), which showed a decrease in plasma GH [32, 33]. In addition to androgens and estrogens affecting GH levels, GH also seems to directly affect steroidogenesis. GH levels are higher in adult women, fluctuate during the menstrual cycle, and are strongly correlated with the serum estrogen levels, as GH decreases in postmenopausal women [34–36].

In addition to sex hormones' effect on growth through the regulation of GH during puberty, they also act directly on hormone-responsive chondrocytes at the epiphyseal plates, the region that contributes to the elongation of long bones. During the pubertal growth spurt, chondrocytes differentiate and proliferate; secrete extracellular matrix proteins (ECM), osteoblasts, and bone cell precursors; invade the growth plate; and differentiate (reviewed in [37]). Estrogen, progesterone, and androgen receptors (ER, PR, and AR) are all highly expressed in this group of cells in both males and females and contribute to the proliferative regulation [38]. Testosterone injected directly into this growth plate area increased the length of the tibia in rats, in comparison to the non-injected control [39]. A man with a mutation in ER alpha (ESR1) did not develop the normal epiphyseal plate closure [40]. There is mounting evidence, using rodent and cell culture models, that testosterone action works through aromatization into estrogen in the epiphyseal plate chondrocytes and is responsible for the proliferative response [41, 42]. This is most apparent in a sister and brother with a rare aromatase mutation that both had elevated serum testosterone levels with low levels of estrone and estradiol, with resulting osteoporosis and osteopenia [43]. Additionally, estrogen action has been shown to stimulate metabolic activity in rat metatarsal bones as well as human primary articular chondrocytes and immortalized cell lines from rib cartilage [44, 45]. While long bones are sealed at the epiphyseal plate following the pubertal transition, sex hormones continue to play a role in chondrocyte health. Increased bone resorption and impaired bone remodeling are accelerated during menopause, making women susceptible to developing osteoporosis, which is the loss of bone mass and strength [46, 47]. While the remaining lifetime risk for women to contract osteoporosis is 45–55 % at age 50, men also have a risk of 20–25 %, just as men with reduced testosterone have an increased chance of developing osteoporosis [48–51]. In addition, inhibin A increases bone mass and strength independent of sex steroids by stimulating osteoblast activity in mice with gonads disconnected or removed [52]. Inhibin from gonadal sources also modulates hemoglobin accumulation and erythropoiesis in human bone marrow cells [53, 54].

Sex hormones that drive the noticeable physical changes during puberty also establish other important physiological changes that are less apparent but are important for continued homeostasis throughout adulthood. Males develop a greater volume of white matter, the centralized inner portion of the brain that consists of myelin-coated axon bundles that facilitate communication between brain regions, which continues to outpace females in growth during puberty [55–58]. However, certain white matter tracts have been shown to be organized faster in adolescent girls than in boys [58]. Sex hormones in both boys and girls also significantly affect medial temporal lobe gray matter volumes, as these are regions with high density sex steroid receptors [59].

The timing of puberty transition is impressionable on resulting sexual behavior. Female mice exposed to stressors, such as shipment via crate or extended social isolation, during puberty responded less to estradiol- and progesterone-stimulated sexual behavior in comparison to mice that were exposed to stress during adulthood [60, 61].

Primary Hypogonadism from Natural Causes

The timing of puberty can be early or delayed for a number of reasons. Hypogonadism refers to the reduced or failed ability of the gonads, ovaries, or testes to produce sufficient hormones to initiate puberty and/or maintain systemic homeostasis. Endocrine disorders, such as hypogonadotropic hypogonadism, can occur as a result of decreased or absent release of GnRH and can be caused by injury to the pituitary, gene mutations as in Prader-Willis Syndrome, or excessive opioid or steroid use [62, 63]. Primary hypogonadism occurs as a result of gonadal dysfunction, while secondary hypogonadism occurs as a result of hypothalamus or pituitary dysfunction. Premature ovarian insufficiency (POI) or early menopause occurs in 1.1 % of women under 40 years old from all ethnicities with Japanese women having the lowest incidence at 0.1 % and African-American and Hispanic women having the highest incidence rate at 1.4 % [64]. POI is defined by 4–6 months of amenorrhea, elevated FSH levels, and low estrogen levels and could be caused by a number of factors including genetic and exogenous causes. Gene mutations that can cause POI include mutations on the X chromosome like fragile X mental retardation 1 gene (FMR1) [65], mutations in oocyte and granulosa communicating ligands like bone morphogenic factor 15 (BMP15) mutations [66], or mutations in gonadotropin receptors like FSHR and LHR [67, 68] or sex hormone receptors like PR [69]. Hypogonadism in males is defined by low testosterone levels. This syndrome can develop in many of the same ways that female hypogonadism develops through mutations in gonadotropin receptors [70] and sex hormone receptors like AR [71] but also through mutations in sex-determining region Y box 3 gene (SOX3) and Kallmann syndrome 1 gene (KAL1) [72].

Primary Hypogonadism from Gonadotoxic Reagents

Hypogonadism can also develop through nonnatural means, such as gonadotoxic chemotherapy and radiation treatment regimens. Approximately 10,400 children, under the age of 15, are diagnosed with cancer in the USA each year. The most common types of cancer in children include acute lymphocytic leukemia, central nervous system tumors, neuroblastomas, and non-Hodgkin's lymphoma. Approximately 5 % of childhood cancers result from an inherited mutation (NCI posted May 13, 2015; cancer.gov). Almost 380,000 adults had survived childhood or adolescent (0–19 years old) cancer in the USA in January 2010, when the National Cancer Institute took their last Surveillance, Epidemiology, and End Results (SEER) program survey [73]. Treatments that prolong the life of children with cancer often have off-target effects. This includes disruption of the endocrine cells within the ovary and testes that provide the spike of hormone release to initiate puberty and maintain systemic homeostasis of cardiovascular, neurological, and bone health throughout adult life. Males and females treated for lymphomas or bone marrow transplants for various malignancies with alkylating agents, such as mustine, pro-carbazine, or busulfan, have a high risk of azoospermia or early menopause [74, 75] (reviewed in [76, 77]). Additional diseases that require harsh treatments, such as lupus nephritis, also may result in secondary hypogonadism with reduced fertility and decreased endocrine support [78].

Current Practices for Restoring Endocrine Function

Puberty is triggered by the increasing pulsatile release of GnRH from the hypo-thalamus, which triggers the secretion of FSH and LH. In response, estrogens and androgens will be secreted from the ovaries and testes along with inhibins that sup-press further FSH release (see above for more details). Levels of FSH during early follicular phase are used as an indicator of growing follicles. Anti-Mullerian hor-mone (AMH), also expressed by granulosa cells, has been indicated as a potential indicator of follicle reserve [79]. However, there is also caution taken with these assessments as women using hormonal contraceptive pills have reduced AMH that is restored once the women ceased use of the pills [79, 80]. Additionally, a life-span study of AMH in males has determined that it may represent a good marker of Sertoli cell function in response to intratestosterone levels [81]. Alternatively, levels of inhibin A and B, produced by granulosa cells of growing and small follicles, respectively, were used to detect potential ovarian reserve in adolescent girls and young women with Turner's syndrome that did not have signs of spontaneous puberty [82]. However, whether or not this is an accurate test for ovarian reserve would be difficult to determine as it would require removal of the ovarian tissue. While it is difficult to determine late onset of puberty or inability to undergo natural puberty through testing of gonadotropins or other ovarian peptides, additional infor-mation of familial statistics and skeletal age can help to determine the potential of natural initiation of puberty.

If the need for endocrine replacement therapies is established to help with puber-tal transition, adolescent girls and boys have a limited number of options. GH replacement therapy at 55 μg/kg per day is considered standard for girls with Turner's syndrome and linear growth failure. These treatments may start as early as 9 months old as the average age to begin GH treatments is 9–10 years [83]. As a result of estrogens' role in accelerated bone maturation, Turner's syndrome girls taking GH postpone estrogen replacement therapy until they are 15–16 years old [83]. However in boys with known hypogonadotropic hypogonadism, pulsatile GH levels increased and further responded to endogenous GH-releasing hormone following testosterone treatments in three incremental doses over 4 weeks to mimic the onset of puberty [84]. Most girls with Turner's syndrome require hormone replacement therapy for the development of secondary sex characteristics, like breast development, uterine growth, and bone health, in addition to treating short stature. These studies provide a good indication of how adolescent girls with treatment-induced hypogonadism may respond to hormone replacement therapies. Generally estradiol replacement begins as a low-dose monotherapy, and progesterone therapy is added 1–2 years later or upon the girl's first menses [85]. Transdermal estrogens are often preferred in this population as the oral estrogens increase the amount of circulating estrones because of the first-pass metabolism of the oral administration through the liver. Additionally, the transdermal administration of estradiol resulted in a more physiological breakdown of estradiol, estrone, and bioestrogen concentrations, along with a greater suppression of LH and FSH [86]. The most appropriate progesterone regimens are more difficult to deduce. A study with early POF patients that displayed estrogen-primed endometrium showed a more effective "inphase" induction of secretory endometrium with progesterone administered vaginally than orally [87].

While there are many advantages to replacing the endocrine support that fails to initiate puberty or maintain homeostasis in adult tissues, there can be adverse effects to these replacement therapies. For example, oral administration of estradiol impairs the metabolic action of GH that is not seen with transdermal injections in postmenopausal women [88]. Additionally, a study with postmenopausal women identified that IGF-1 decreases and C-reactive protein, the strongest predictor of myocardial infarction and cardiovascular mortality in healthy women, increases with oral estrogen replacement therapies, but not transdermal therapies [89]. However, large doses of oral estradiol administration, and not transdermal estradiol, promote endothelium-dependent vasodilation and antiatherogenic changes to promote vascular health in healthy postmenopausal women [90].

Additionally, the amount of sex hormones administered as a therapy could affect the response. There are an increasing number of reproductive age men in the USA taking testosterone replacement drugs, around 75.7 per 10,000 per year in 2011 [91]. Exogenous testosterone has the potential to suppress the hypothalamic-pituitary-gonadal axis and reduce FSH and LH causing a reduction in intratesticular testosterone and reduced spermatogenesis in patients. In fact, increasing exogenous testosterone levels in normal patients is being tested as a male contraceptive [92].

Summary: While hormone replacement therapies function to adequately initiate the adolescent to adulthood physical and psychological changes that occur at puberty and alleviate many of the morbidities of premature hormone loss, they fail to account for the peptide hormones, gonadal inhibins and activins, and other endocrines that the gonads secrete, respond to, or regulate to maintain whole body homeostasis. Additionally, those patients treated for decades with these therapies needed regular assessments to determine the physiological response to these treatments and to avoid additional side effects as a result of treatment metabolites.

Current Practices of Fertility Preservation and Restoration in Females

The American Society for Reproductive Medicine published guidelines for physicians treating cancer patients to discuss fertility preservation options. Egg banking, embryo banking, and sperm banking are the only nonexperimental options for women and men who want to preserve their fertility [93]. If treatment can be delayed and the woman has undergone puberty, then eggs can be retrieved for egg or embryo banking. This procedure requires approximately 1 month of gonadotropin injections to stimulate selected follicles to grow larger and mature. Oocytes or eggs are retrieved through vaginal aspiration. The resulting healthy and matured eggs can be cryopreserved or fertilized through in vitro fertilization (IVF) with donor's or partner's sperm. When the patient desires a pregnancy, a woman will undergo another round of gonadotropin injections to prime the uterine lining for receipt of the embryos, and the cryopreserved embryos can be retrieved and administered to the receptive womb. These procedures can only be performed in postpubertal women who do not have gonadotropin-responsive tumors, are willing to postpone potentially lifesaving treatments, and can produce mature eggs. However, cryopreservation of oocytes or ovarian tissue for girls and testicular tissue for boys was mentioned by the ASRM as an option that could be offered to patients at an equipped research institution [93].

Experimental Practices for Fertility and Endocrine Restoration in Females

The field of oncofertility aims to explore and expand the options for restoring and preserving fertility in males and females detrimentally affected by gonadotoxic treatments [94]. The National Physicians Cooperative, within the Oncofertility Consortium, strives to expand fertility preservation and the options for restoring reproductive and endocrine health. Recently, research from this cooperative was performed on ovarian cortical tissue that can be easily removed through laparoscopy prior to chemotherapy or radiation treatment to retrieve primordial follicles, the quiescent follicle reserve. They found that ovarian tissue from each patient observed (up to 18 years old) contained primordial follicles, irrespective of previous treatment, transported or fresh or disease profile [95]. Additionally, alginate encapsulation and culture of these primordial follicle-containing cortical tissues resulted in growing preantral and antral follicles [96]. These studies support the argument to cryopreserve ovarian tissue for fertility restoration in patient cohorts where egg banking is not an option.

An experimental technique currently being explored as an option to restore endocrine function and fertility in girls with gonadotoxic diseases or treatments also involves the isolation and utilization of ovarian cortical strips. For this technique, four to five cortical strips (1 cm×0.5 mm×1.5 mm) from an adult, or one ovary from a child, are laparoscopically isolated prior to gonadotoxic therapies and cryopreserved. The strips are then thawed following cancer remission and fixed onto the remaining portion of the ovary or inserted underneath the cortical capsule [97, 98]. A pocket can be created within the peritoneal space for cortical strips if the ovaries are absent or have been removed [99, 100]. Alternatively, cortical strips have been inserted under the skin of the forearm to restore some endocrine function and to stimulate mature eggs for IVF [101, 102]. There have been 60 reported live births from these ovarian cortical tissue transplants (summarized [103]). There are varying degrees of success with these transplants. For example, one patient has had two successful deliveries with one transplant, and the graft is still functioning (suppresses FSH) after 5 years, while another patient has undergone two cortical strip surgeries and successfully delivered one baby with an egg donation [103]. The second scenario demonstrates ovarian tissue burnout and brings to light one limiting factor of utilizing this technique [104]. The varying success could be attributed to the type or degree of gonadotoxic treatment endured, the amount of ovary that remains prior to transplant, and the number of follicles transplanted within the cortical strips to restore function and fertility. Because these tissue strips are generally isolated prior to gonadotoxic and cancer-killing treatments, there should be extreme caution prior to transplanting these potentially cancer-containing tissues back into women who have just beat their cancer. Cancer cells have been identified in many of the ovarian cortical tissues, especially in blood-based cancers like acute lymphoblastic leukemia [105]. A cancer marker was detected within the ovarian tissue isolated from a patient with advanced-stage breast cancer by PCR analysis [106]. A review of this literature and assessment of risk was published by Bastings et al. [107].

The success of these cortical strip transplants provides some hope in the underlying technique, that a strip of tissue with follicles could promote ovarian function, including endocrine restoration and fertility. However, considering the pitfalls of the technique including tissue "burnout" and especially the real risk of cancer transmission, alternative approaches need to be studied. To minimize this risk, experimentation with small animal models is ongoing. One example of endocrine restoration to initiate puberty in a mouse model utilized the decellularized matrix of an ovary and isolated ovarian cells [105]. This technique describes use of the biologically active, ovary-specific ECM in which to seed safely isolated cells and follicles. Another example is the use of a bioengineered artificial ovary consisting of mouse ovarian follicles seeded within a 3D printed scaffold modeled from the ovarian extracellular matrix composition and architecture to create a 3D printed follicle niche (3DP-FN), for follicles to reside and grow (unpublished data). Both of these experimental paradigms rely on development of the follicle niche to provide the appropriate biochemical and biophysical cues to result in viable and functioning follicle units. Potential cell sources include follicles, containing both endocrine support and potential gametes that could be fertilized, from the patient herself. However, this

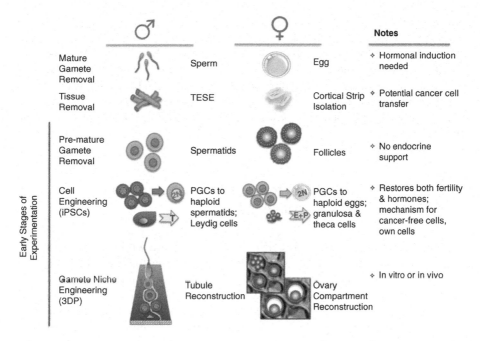

Fig. 7.1 Experimental and existing technologies useful to the restoration of fertility in males and females.

source, as described above, is limiting. Induced pluripotent stem cells derived from the patient could provide a source of endocrine cells, or even oocytes in the future, as human ESCs have been differentiated into both populations [108, 109]. These techniques would provide a theoretically unlimited source of patient-specific cells and could result in the complete restoration of the ovary (Fig. 7.1).

Current Practices of Fertility Preservation in Males

Adult male cancer patients, who wish to preserve their fertility, have options to cryopreserve sperm through semen samples to be used for future-assisted reproductive techniques, including intrauterine insemination (IUI), in vitro fertilization (IVF), and intracytoplasmic sperm injection (ICSI). Additionally, percutaneous epididymal sperm aspiration (PESA), testicular sperm extraction (TESE), testicular sperm aspiration (TESA), and microsurgical epididymal sperm aspiration (MESA) can be used to collect sperm or haploid gametes in patients with azoospermia or oligospermia. IVF and ICSI could then be performed with as little as a single haploid gamete. Assisted reproductive technologies (ART) have been widely used in the USA since 1981, in over 440 fertility clinics nationwide [110]. Unfortunately, prepubertal boys are unable to provide sperm samples, as they have not undergone the hormonal changes necessary to undergo complete spermatogenesis. There are currently no regular procedures for preserving gametes from prepubertal boys. An experimental procedure where testicular tissue is cryopreserved is recommended as a potential fertility-saving option by the American Society for Reproductive Medicine for prepubertal patients undergoing gonadotoxic cancer treatments [93]. These techniques are performed throughout the world in the hopes of one day utilizing advanced technologies to grow or transplant spermatogonial stem cells (SSCs) for future use in ART technologies or to restore fertility in cancer survivors in the future [111–116].

Experimental Procedures for Fertility Preservation and Endocrine Restoration in Males

Patients undergoing potentially sterilizing techniques are willing to participate in studies that may promote the availability of their tissue for later use [112], and retrieval of tissue biopsies as part of a treatment regimen for prepubertal or peripubertal boys has been shown to be safe and effective [111, 112]. Cryopreservation was accepted by 93.5 % of patients asked, and all cryopreserved patient tissue contained visible spermatogonia [111]. Experimental procedures to obtain mature sperm can occur as a transplantation of SSCs into depleted tubules or transplantation of testicular tissue. SSCs are stem cells that produce sperm continuously throughout the adult male's life and exist as mitotically active cells within even prepubertal boys. SSCs are susceptible to chemotherapy and radiation therapy, especially in prepubertal boys where they are more mitotically active as they populate the tubules in preparation for the initiation of spermatogenesis at puberty, called spermarche. First attempts to grow and differentiate human SSCs in small animal hosts demonstrated some survival and potential proliferation. SSCs were isolated from human tissue biopsies from adult patients with a variety of diagnosed azoospermia or oligospermia causes. They were then transplanted into the seminiferous tubules of immunocompromised mouse testes, who had undergone germ cell ablation. Human germ cells were most abundant 1 month after transplantation and almost absent by 6 months post transplant [117]. Analysis of xenotransplant of SSCs into mouse recipients may indicate that the somatic cell compartment or stem cell niche may be the limiting factor for activation of meiosis and spermatocyte differentiation. Testis biopsies that maintain the SSC and somatic cell niche from neonatal mice, pigs, goats, and rhesus monkeys were grafted into immunocompromised mice [118]. These grafts produced complete spermatogenesis with viable sperm that were then used for ICSI into rhesus monkey eggs, for example [118, 119].

As in the experimental ovarian tissue transplant techniques performed for women, there are legitimate concerns about the safety of transferring cells retrieved prior to cancer treatment, especially for leukemia patients [120]. Therefore, sorting methods for enriching the SSC population, while eliminating the cancer cells, needs to be standardized and transplants need to be handled with caution. Additional methods for growing SSCs in vitro and utilizing ART techniques that utilize haploid male gametes in vitro could surpass the concern for transferring cancer into recipients. Testis biopsies isolated prior to gonadotoxic therapies could preserve the chance of restoring fertility later in life through SSC transplant or through in vitro or in situ differentiation of SSCs into haploid gametes. The xenotransplant successes described above maintain that mitotically active SSC supported within the appropriate niche could provide a source of donor-specific haploid cells that could be used in ART to produce offspring. Transplantation of these niches into the patient could additionally provide the necessary endocrine restoration as well.

Summary

Puberty is an important physiological, psychological, and physical transition from adolescence to adulthood. It lays the groundwork for adult reproductive capacity and further differentiation of organ systems that respond to the increased hormonal milieu, including neurons, chondrocytes, and cells within the reproductive tract. In the absence of puberty, individuals would not establish normal neuronal growth and connectivity, normal height, or reproductive maturity. The current options for fertility and hormone restoration for prepubertal cancer survivors are inadequate. Some experimental paradigms utilizing tissue extraction that would house the follicle reserve in females and the SSCs in males are promising. Isolated follicles and haploid spermatogonia could provide a potential gamete and, therefore, the option for biological offspring following ART procedures. However, this does not address the need to restore natural hormone cyclicity. Some promising results from ovarian cortical tissue transplants ensure that a surgical procedure with ovarian cells could restore limited hormone cyclicity and fertility. However, these tissues could also reinoculate the patient with cancer cells, as they are taken and preserved prior to treatment. A collaborative effort between reproductive biologists, endocrinologists, regenerative medicine scientists, clinicians, and engineers is necessary to develop a transplant that could provide long-term endocrine function and fertility in patients with hypogonadism or premature gonadal failure.

References

1. McGee EA, Hsu SY, Kaipia A, Hsueh AJ. Cell death and survival during ovarian follicle development. Mol Cell Endocrinol. 1998;140:15–8.
2. Zheng W, Zhang H, Gorre N, Risal S, Shen Y, Liu K. Two classes of ovarian primordial follicles exhibit distinct developmental dynamics and physiological functions. Hum Mol Genet. 2014;23:920–8. doi:10.1093/hmg/ddt486.
3. Cordeiro MH, Kim S-Y, Ebbert K, Duncan FE, Ramalho-Santos J, Woodruff TK. Geography of follicle formation in the embryonic mouse ovary impacts activation pattern during the first wave of folliculogenesis. Biol Reprod. 2015:1–19. doi:10.1095/biolreprod.115.131227.

4. Mork L, Maatouk DM, McMahon JA, Guo JJ, Zhang P, McMahon AP, et al. Temporal differences in granulosa cell specification in the ovary reflect distinct follicle fates in mice. Biol Reprod. 2012;86:37. doi:10.1095/biolreprod.111.095208.
5. Harikae K, Miura K, Shinomura M, Matoba S, Hiramatsu R, Tsunekawa N, et al. Heterogeneity in sexual bipotentiality and plasticity of granulosa cells in developing mouse ovaries. J Cell Sci. 2013;126:2834–44. doi:10.1242/jcs.122663. The Company of Biologists Ltd.
6. Muttukrishna S, Child T, Lockwood GM, Groome NP, Barlow DH, Ledger WL. Serum concentrations of dimeric inhibins, activin A, gonadotrophins and ovarian steroids during the menstrual cycle in older women. Hum Reprod. 2000;15:549–56.
7. Matzuk MM, Finegold MJ, Su JG, Hsueh AJ, Bradley A. Alpha-inhibin is a tumour-suppressor gene with gonadal specificity in mice. Nature (Nature Publishing Group). 1992;360:313–9. doi:10.1038/360313a0.
8. Hild-Petito S, Stouffer RL, Brenner RM. Immunocytochemical localization of estradiol and progesterone receptors in the monkey ovary throughout the menstrual cycle*. Endocrinology (The Endocrine Society). 1988;123:2896–905. doi:10.1210/endo-123-6-2896.
9. Natraj U, Richards JS. Hormonal regulation, localization, and functional activity of the progesterone receptor in granulosa cells of rat preovulatory follicles. Endocrinology. 1993;133:761–9. doi:10.1210/endo.133.2.8344215.
10. Mahmood T, Saridogan E, Smutna S, Habib AM, Djahanbakhch O. The effect of ovarian steroids on epithelial ciliary beat frequency in the human Fallopian tube. Hum Reprod. 1998;13:2991–4.
11. Wanggren K, Stavreus-Evers A, Olsson C, Andersson E, Gemzell-Danielsson K. Regulation of muscular contractions in the human Fallopian tube through prostaglandins and progestagens. Hum Reprod. 2008;23:2359–68. doi:10.1093/humrep/den260.
12. Verhage HG, Fazleabas AT, Mavrogianis PA, O'Day-Bowman MB, Donnelly KM, Arias EB, et al. The baboon oviduct: characteristics of an oestradiol-dependent oviduct-specific glycoprotein. Hum Reprod Update. 1997;3:541–52.
13. Lydon JP, Demayo FJ, Funk CR, Mani SK, Hughes AR, Montgomery CA, et al. Mice lacking progesterone receptor exhibit pleiotropic reproductive abnormalities. Genes Dev (Cold Spring Harbor Lab). 1995;9:2266–78. doi:10.1101/gad.9.18.2266.
14. Cha J, Sun X, Dey SK. Mechanisms of implantation: strategies for successful pregnancy. Nat Med. 2012;18:1754–67. doi:10.1038/nm.3012.
15. Kastner P, Krust A, Turcotte B, Stropp U, Tora L, Gronemeyer H, et al. Two distinct estrogen-regulated promoters generate transcripts encoding the two functionally different human progesterone receptor forms A and B. EMBO J Eur Mol Biol Organ. 1990;9:1603–14.
16. Hay DL. Placental histology and the production of human choriogonadotrophin and its subunits in pregnancy. Br J Obstet Gynaecol. 1988;95:1268–75.
17. Gorodeski GI, Hopfer U, Liu CC, Margles E. Estrogen acidifies vaginal pH by up-regulation of proton secretion via the apical membrane of vaginal-ectocervical epithelial cells. Endocrinology. 2005;146:816–24. doi:10.1210/en.2004-1153.
18. Gorodeski GI. Estrogen increases the permeability of the cultured human cervical epithelium by modulating cell deformability. Am J Physiol. 1998;275:C888–99.
19. Heller CG, Clermont Y. Spermatogenesis in man: an estimate of its duration. Science. 1963;140:184–6.
20. Hasegawa K, Saga Y. Retinoic acid signaling in Sertoli cells regulates organization of the blood-testis barrier through cyclical changes in gene expression. Development. 2012;139:4347–55. doi:10.1242/dev.080119.
21. Russell LD. The blood-testis barrier and its formation relative to spermatocyte maturation in the adult rat: a lanthanum tracer study. Anat Rec. 1978;190:99–111. doi:10.1002/ar.1091900109.
22. Russell LD, Malone JP. A study of Sertoli-spermatid tubulobulbar complexes in selected mammals. Tissue Cell. 1980;12:263–85.
23. Russell LD, Lee IP, Ettlin R, Peterson RN. Development of the acrosome and alignment, elongation and entrenchment of spermatids in procarbazine-treated rats. Tissue Cell. 1983;15:615–26.

24. Sprando RL, Russell LD. Comparative study of cytoplasmic elimination in spermatids of selected mammalian species. Am J Anat. 1987;178:72–80. doi:10.1002/aja.1001780109.
25. Hayashi M, Fujimoto S, Takano H, Ushiki T, Abe K, Ishikura H, et al. Characterization of a human glycoprotein with a potential role in sperm-egg fusion: cDNA cloning, immunohisto-chemical localization, and chromosomal assignment of the gene (AEGL1). Genomics. 1996;32:367–74. doi:10.1006/geno.1996.0131.
26. Maldera JA, Weigel Munoz M, Chirinos M, Busso D, GE Raffo F, Battistone MA, et al. Human fertilization: epididymal hCRISP1 mediates sperm-zona pellucida binding through its interaction with ZP3. Mol Hum Reprod (Oxford University Press). 2014;20:341–9. doi:10.1093/molehr/gat092.
27. Bremner WJ, Millar MR, Sharpe RM, Saunders PT. Immunohistochemical localization of androgen receptors in the rat testis: evidence for stage-dependent expression and regulation by androgens. Endocrinology. 1994;135:1227–34. doi:10.1210/endo.135.3.8070367.
28. O'Shaughnessy PJ, Monteiro A, Abel M. Testicular development in mice lacking receptors for follicle stimulating hormone and androgen. Lobaccaro J-MA, editor. PLoS ONE. 2012;7:e35136–9. doi:10.1371/journal.pone.0035136.
29. George JW, Dille EA, Heckert LL. Current concepts of follicle-stimulating hormone receptor gene regulation. Biol Reprod (Society for the Study of Reproduction). 2011;84:7–17. doi:10.1095/biolreprod.110.085043.
30. Juul A, Bang P, Hertel NT, Main K, Dalgaard P, Jørgensen K, et al. Serum insulin-like growth factor-I in 1030 healthy children, adolescents, and adults: relation to age, sex, stage of puberty, testicular size, and body mass index. J Clin Endocrinol Metab. 1994;78:744–52. doi:10.1210/jcem.78.3.8126152.
31. Veldhuis JD, Roemmich JN, Rogol AD. Gender and sexual maturation-dependent contrasts in the neuroregulation of growth hormone secretion in prepubertal and late adolescent males and females – a general clinical research center-based study. J Clin Endocrinol Metab. 2000;85:2385–94. doi:10.1210/jcem.85.7.6697.
32. Keenan BS, Richards GE, Ponder SW, Dallas JS, Nagamani M, Smith ER. Androgen-stimulated pubertal growth: the effects of testosterone and dihydrotestosterone on growth hormone and insulin-like growth factor-I in the treatment of short stature and delayed puberty. J Clin Endocrinol Metab. 1993;76:996–1001. doi:10.1210/jcem.76.4.8473416.
33. Veldhuis JD, Metzger DL, Martha PM, Mauras N, Kerrigan JR, Keenan B, et al. Estrogen and testosterone, but not a nonaromatizable androgen, direct network integration of the hypothalamo somatotrope (growth hormone)-insulin-like growth factor I axis in the human: evidence from pubertal pathophysiology and sex-steroid hormone replacement. J Clin Endocrinol Metab. 1997;82:3414–20. doi:10.1210/jcem.82.10.4317.
34. Ho KY, Evans WS, Blizzard RM, Veldhuis JD, Merriam GR, Samojlik E, et al. Effects of sex and age on the 24-hour profile of growth hormone secretion in man: importance of endoge-nous estradiol concentrations*. J Clin Endocrinol Metab (The Endocrine Society). 1987;64:51–8. doi:10.1210/jcem-64-1-51.
35. van den Berg G, Veldhuis JD, Frolich M, Roelfsema F. An amplitude-specific divergence in the pulsatile mode of growth hormone (GH) secretion underlies the gender difference in mean GH concentrations in men and premenopausal women. J Clin Endocrinol Metab. 1996;81:2460–7. doi:10.1210/jcem.81.7.8675561.
36. Faria ACS, Bekenstein LW, Booth RA, Vaccaro VA, Asplin CM, Veldhuis JD, et al. Pulsatile growth hormone release in normal women during the menstrual cycle. Clin Endocrinol (Blackwell Publishing Ltd). 1992;36:591–6. doi:10.1111/j.1365-2265.1992.tb02270.x.
37. Nilsson O, Marino R, De Luca F, Phillip M, Baron J. Endocrine regulation of the growth plate. Horm Res (Karger Publishers). 2005;64:157–65. doi:10.1159/000088791.
38. Ben-Hur H, Thole HH, Mashiah A, Insler V, Berman V, Shezen E, et al. Estrogen, progester-one and testosterone receptors in human fetal cartilaginous tissue: immunohistochemical studies. Calcif Tissue Int. 1997;60:520–6.
39. Ren SG, Malozowski S, Sanchez P, Sweet DE, Loriaux DL, Cassorla F. Direct administration of testosterone increases rat tibial epiphyseal growth plate width. Acta Endocrinol (European Society of Endocrinology). 1989;121:401–5. doi:10.1530/acta.0.1210401.

40. Smith EP, Boyd J, Frank GR, Takahashi H, Cohen RM, Specker B, et al. Estrogen resistance caused by a mutation in the estrogen-receptor gene in a man. N Engl J Med. 1994;331: 1056–61. doi:10.1056/NEJM199410203311604.
41. Sun H, Zang W, Zhou B, Xu L, Wu S. DHEA suppresses longitudinal bone growth by acting directly at growth plate through estrogen receptors. Endocrinology. 2011;152:1423–33. doi:10.1210/en.2010-0920.
42. Chagin AS, Karimian E, Sundstrom K, Eriksson E, Savendahl L. Catch-up growth after dexamethasone withdrawal occurs in cultured postnatal rat metatarsal bones. J Endocrinol. 2009;204:21–9. doi:10.1677/JOE-09-0307.
43. Morishima A, Grumbach MM, Simpson ER, Fisher C, Qin K. Aromatase deficiency in male and female siblings caused by a novel mutation and the physiological role of estrogens. J Clin Endocrinol Metab. 2013;80:3689–98. doi:10.1210/jcem.80.12.8530621.
44. Schicht M, Ernst J, Nielitz A, Fester L, Tsokos M, Guddat SS, et al. Articular cartilage chondrocytes express aromatase and use enzymes involved in estrogen metabolism. Arthritis Res Ther. 2014;16:1–9. doi:10.1186/ar4539.
45. Chagin AS. Locally produced estrogen promotes fetal rat metatarsal bone growth; an effect mediated through increased chondrocyte proliferation and decreased apoptosis. J Endocrinol. 2006;188:193–203. doi:10.1677/joe.1.06364.
46. Ebeling PR, Atley LM, Guthrie JR, Burger HG, Dennerstein L, Hopper JL, et al. Bone turnover markers and bone density across the menopausal transition. J Clin Endocrinol Metab. 1996;81:3366–71. doi:10.1210/jcem.81.9.8784098.
47. Finkelstein JS, Brockwell SE, Mehta V, Greendale GA, Sowers MR, Ettinger B, et al. Bone mineral density changes during the menopause transition in a multiethnic cohort of women. J Clin Endocrinol Metab. 2008;93:861–8. doi:10.1210/jc.2007-1876.
48. Laurent M, Gielen E, Claessens F, Boonen S, Vanderschueren D. Osteoporosis in older men: recent advances in pathophysiology and treatment. Best Pract Res Clin Endocrinol Metab (Elsevier Ltd). 2013;27:527–39. doi:10.1016/j.beem.2013.04.010.
49. Melton LJ, Chrischilles EA, Cooper C, Lane AW, Riggs BL. Perspective. How many women have osteoporosis? J Bone Miner Res (John Wiley and Sons and The American Society for Bone and Mineral Research (ASBMR)). 1992;7:1005–10. doi:10.1002/jbmr.5650070902.
50. Laurent M, Sinnesael M, Vanderschueren D, Antonio L, Classens F, Dubois V, et al. Androgens and estrogens in skeletal sexual dimorphism. Asian J Androl. 2014;16:213–10. doi:10.4103/1008-682X.122356.
51. Finkelstein JS, Klibanski A, Neer RM, Greenspan SL, Rosenthal DI, Crowley WF. Osteoporosis in men with idiopathic hypogonadotropic hypogonadism. Ann Intern Med (American College of Physicians). 1987;106:354–61. doi:10.7326/0003-4819-106-3.
52. Perrien DS, Akel NS, Edwards PK, Carver AA, Bendre MS, Swain FL, et al. Inhibin A is an endocrine stimulator of bone mass and strength. Endocrinology. 2007;148:1654–65. doi:10.1210/en.2006-0848.
53. Meunier H, Rivier C, Evans RM, Vale W. Gonadal and extragonadal expression of inhibin alpha, beta A, and beta B subunits in various tissues predicts diverse functions. Proc Natl Acad Sci U S A (National Academy of Sciences). 1988;85:247–51.
54. Yu J, Shao L-E, Lemas V, Yu AL, Vaughan J, Rivier J, et al. Importance of FSH-releasing protein and inhibin in erythrodifferentiation. Published online: 31 December 1987; doi:101038/330765a0. Nature. Nature Publishing Group; 1987;330:765–7. doi:10.1038/330765a0.
55. Perrin JS, Herve PY, Leonard G, Perron M, Pike GB, Pitiot A, et al. Growth of white matter in the adolescent brain: role of testosterone and androgen receptor. J Neurosci. 2008;28:9519–24. doi:10.1523/JNEUROSCI.1212-08.2008.
56. Giedd JN, Blumenthal J, Jeffries NO, Castellanos FX, Liu H, Zijdenbos A, et al. Brain development during childhood and adolescence: a longitudinal MRI study. Nat Neurosci. 1999;2:861–3. doi:10.1038/13158.
57. Paus T. Growth of white matter in the adolescent brain: myelin or axon? Brain Cogn (Elsevier Inc). 2010;72:26–35. doi:10.1016/j.bandc.2009.06.002.

58. Ladouceur CD, Peper JS, Crone EA, Dahl RE. White matter development in adolescence: the influence of puberty and implications for affective disorders. Dev Cogn Neurosci. 2012;2:36–54. doi:10.1016/j.dcn.2011.06.002.

59. Bramen JE, Hranilovich JA, Dahl RE, Forbes EE, Chen J, Toga AW, et al. Puberty influences medial temporal lobe and cortical gray matter maturation differently in boys than girls matched for sexual maturity. Cereb Cortex. 2011;21:636–46. doi:10.1093/cercor/bhq137.

60. Laroche J, Gasbarro L, Herman JP, Blaustein JD. Reduced behavioral response to gonadal hormones in mice shipped during the peripubertal/adolescent period. Endocrinology. 2009;150:2351–8. doi:10.1210/en.2008-1595.

61. Kercmar J, Tobet SA, Majdic G. Social isolation during puberty affects female sexual behavior in mice. Front Behav Neurosci (Frontiers). 2014;8:337. doi:10.3389/fnbeh.2014.00337.

62. Bruni JF, Van Vugt D, Marshall S, Meites J. Effects of naloxone, morphine and methionine enkephalin on serum prolactin, luteinizing hormone, follicle stimulating hormone, thyroid stimulating hormone and growth hormone. Life Sci. 1977;21:461–6.

63. Miller NLG, Wevrick R, Mellon PL. Necdin, a Prader-Willi syndrome candidate gene, regulates gonadotropin-releasing hormone neurons during development. Hum Mol Genet. 2008;18:248–60. doi:10.1093/hmg/ddn344.

64. Luborsky JL, Meyer P, Sowers MF, Gold EB, Santoro N. Premature menopause in a multi-ethnic population study of the menopause transition. Hum Reprod. 2003;18:199–206. doi:10.1093/humrep/deg005.

65. Allen EG, Sullivan AK, Marcus M, Small C, Dominguez C, Epstein MP, et al. Examination of reproductive aging milestones among women who carry the FMR1 premutation. Hum Reprod. 2007;22:2142–52. doi:10.1093/humrep/dem148.

66. Di Pasquale E, Rossetti R, Marozzi A, Bodega B, Borgato S, Cavallo L, et al. Identification of new variants of human BMP15 gene in a large cohort of women with premature ovarian failure. J Clin Endocrinol Metab. 2006;91:1976–9. doi:10.1210/jc.2005-2650.

67. Prakash GJ, Kanth VVR, Shelling AN, Rozati R, Sujatha M. Absence of 566C>T mutation in exon 7 of the FSHR gene in Indian women with premature ovarian failure. Int J Gynaecol Obstet (Elsevier). 2009;105:265–6. doi:10.1016/j.ijgo.2009.01.023.

68. Latronico AC, Anasti J, Arnhold IJ, Rapaport R, Mendonca BB, Bloise W, et al. Brief report: testicular and ovarian resistance to luteinizing hormone caused by inactivating mutations of the luteinizing hormone-receptor gene. N Engl J Med. 1996;334:507–12. doi:10.1056/NEJM199602223340805.

69. Mansouri MR, Schuster J, Badhai J, Stattin EL, Losel R, Wehling M, et al. Alterations in the expression, structure and function of progesterone receptor membrane component-1 (PGRMC1) in premature ovarian failure. Hum Mol Genet. 2008;17:3776–83. doi:10.1093/hmg/ddn274.

70. Sinha SK, Bhangoo A, Ten S, Gromoll J. Leydig cell hypoplasia due to inactivating luteinizing hormone/chorionic gonadotropin receptor gene mutation presenting as a 46, XY DSD. Adv Exp Med Biol (New York NY: Springer New York). 2011;707:147–8. doi:10.1007/978-1-4419-8002-1_32.

71. Tordjman KM, Yaron M, Berkovitz A, Botchan A, Sultan C, Lumbroso S. Fertility after high-dose testosterone and intracytoplasmic sperm injection in a patient with androgen insensitivity syndrome with a previously unreported androgen receptor mutation. Andrologia. 2014;46:703–6. doi:10.1111/and.12126.

72. Izumi Y, Suzuki E, Kanzaki S, Yatsuga S, Kinjo S, Igarashi M, et al. Genome-wide copy number analysis and systematic mutation screening in 58 patients with hypogonadotropic hypogonadism. Fertil Steril. 2014;102:1130–6.e3. doi:10.1016/j.fertnstert.2014.06.017.

73. Ward E, DeSantis C, Robbins A, Kohler B, Jemal A. Childhood and adolescent cancer statistics. CA Cancer J Clin. 2014;64:83–103. doi:10.3322/caac.21219.

74. Whitehead E, Shalet SM, Blackledge G, Todd I, Crowther D, Beardwell CG. The effects of Hodgkin's disease and combination chemotherapy on gonadal function in the adult male. Cancer. 1982;49:418–22.

75. Thomas-Teinturier C, El Fayech C, Oberlin O, Pacquement H, Haddy N, Labbé M, et al. Age at menopause and its influencing factors in a cohort of survivors of childhood cancer: earlier but rarely premature. Hum Reprod (Oxford University Press). 2013;28:488–95. doi:10.1093/humrep/des391.

76. Howell SJ, Shalet SM. Testicular function following chemotherapy. Hum Reprod Update. 2001;7:363–9.

77. Torino F, Barnabei A, De Vecchis L, Sini V, Schittulli F, Marchetti P, et al. Chemotherapy-induced ovarian toxicity in patients affected by endocrine-responsive early breast cancer. Crit Rev Oncol Hematol (Elsevier Ireland Ltd). 2014;89:27–42. doi:10.1016/j.critrevonc.2013.07.007.

78. Park M-C, Park YB, Jung SY, Chung IH, Choi KH, Lee S-K. Risk of ovarian failure and pregnancy outcome in patients with lupus nephritis treated with intravenous cyclophosphamide pulse therapy. Lupus. 2004;13:569–74. doi:10.1191/0961203304lu1063oa.

79. Birch Petersen K, Hvidman HW, Forman JL, Pinborg A, Larsen EC, Macklon KT, et al. Ovarian reserve assessment in users of oral contraception seeking fertility advice on their reproductive lifespan. Hum Reprod. 2015;30:2364–75. doi:10.1093/humrep/dev197.

80. Lambalk CB. Anti-Müllerian hormone, the holy grail for fertility counselling in the general population? Hum Reprod. 2015;30:2257–8. doi:10.1093/humrep/dev199.

81. Aksglaede L, Sorensen K, Boas M, Mouritsen A, Hagen CP, Jensen RB, et al. Changes in Anti-Müllerian Hormone (AMH) throughout the life span: a population-based study of 1027 healthy males from birth (cord blood) to the age of 69 years. J Clin Endocrinol Metab. 2010;95:5357–64. doi:10.1210/jc.2010-1207.

82. Gravholt CH, Naeraa RW, Andersson A-M, Christiansen JS, Skakkebaek NE. Inhibin A and B in adolescents and young adults with Turner's syndrome and no sign of spontaneous puberty. Hum Reprod. 2002;17:2049–53. doi:10.1093/humrep/17.8.2049.

83. Davenport ML. Moving toward an understanding of hormone replacement therapy in adolescent girls. Ann N Y Acad Sci. 2008;1135:126–37. doi:10.1196/annals.1429.031.

84. Giustina A, Scalvini T, Tassi C, Desenzani P, Poiesi C, Wehrenberg WB, et al. Maturation of the regulation of growth hormone secretion in young males with hypogonadotropic hypogonadism pharmacologically exposed to progressive increments in serum testosterone. J Clin Endocrinol Metab. 1997;82:1210–9. doi:10.1210/jcem.82.4.3871.

85. Gonzalez L, Witchel SF. The patient with Turner syndrome: puberty and medical management concerns. Fertil Steril. 2012;98:780–6. doi:10.1016/j.fertnstert.2012.07.1104.

86. Taboada M, Santen R, Lima J, Hossain J, Singh R, Klein KO, et al. Pharmacokinetics and pharmacodynamics of oral and transdermal 17β estradiol in girls with turner syndrome. J Clin Endocrinol Metab. 2011;96:3502–10. doi:10.1210/jc.2011-1449.

87. Fatemi HM, Bourgain C, Donoso P, Blockeel C, Papanikolaou EG, Popovic-Todorovic B, et al. Effect of oral administration of dydrogestrone versus vaginal administration of natural micronized progesterone on the secretory transformation of endometrium and luteal endocrine profile in patients with premature ovarian failure: a proof of concept. Hum Reprod. 2007;22:1260–3. doi:10.1093/humrep/del520.

88. O'Sullivan AJ, Crampton LJ, Freund J, Ho KK. The route of estrogen replacement therapy confers divergent effects on substrate oxidation and body composition in postmenopausal women. J Clin Invest (American Society for Clinical Investigation). 1998;102:1035–40. doi:10.1172/JCI2773.

89. Vongpatanasin W, Tuncel M, Wang Z, Arbique D, Mehrad B, Jialal I. Differential effects of oral versus transdermal estrogen replacement therapy on C-reactive protein in postmenopausal women. J Am Coll Cardiol. 2003;41:1358–63. doi:10.1016/S0735-1097(03)00156-6.

90. Vehkavaara S, Hakala-Ala-Pietilä T, Virkamäki A, Bergholm R, Ehnholm C, Hovatta O, et al. Differential effects of oral and transdermal estrogen replacement therapy on endothelial function in postmenopausal women. Circulation. 2000;102:2687–93.

91. Layton JB, Li D, Meier CR, Sharpless J, Stürmer T, Jick SS, et al. Testosterone lab testing and initiation in the United Kingdom and the United States, 2000–2011. J Clin Endocrinol Metab. 2013:jc.2013-3570–8. doi:10.1210/jc.2013-3570.

92. Gonzalo ITG, Swerdloff RS, Nelson AL, Clevenger B, Garcia R, Berman N, et al. Levonorgestrel implants (Norplant II) for male contraception clinical trials: combination with transdermal and injectable testosterone. J Clin Endocrinol Metab. 2002;87:3562–72. doi:10.1210/jcem.87.8.8710.

93. The Practice Committee of the American Society for Reproductive Medicine. Fertility preservation in patients undergoing gonadotoxic therapy or gonadectomy: a committee opinion. Fertil Steril (American Society for Reproductive Medicine). 2013;100:1214–23. doi:10.1016/j.fertnstert.2013.08.012.

94. Woodruff TK. The emergence of a new interdiscipline: oncofertility. In: Woodruff TK, Snyder KA, editors. Oncofertility fertility preservation for cancer survivors. Springer US; 2007. p. 3–11. doi:10.1007/978-0-387-72293-1.

95. Duncan FE, Pavone ME, Gunn AH, Badawy S, Gracia C, Ginsberg JP, et al. Pediatric and teen ovarian tissue removed for cryopreservation contains follicles irrespective of age, disease diagnosis, treatment history, and specimen processing methods. J Adolesc Young Adult Oncol. 2015:150908124647009–10. doi:10.1089/jayao.2015.0032.

96. Laronda MM, Duncan FE, Hornick JE, Xu M, Pahnke JE, Whelan KA, et al. Alginate encapsulation supports the growth and differentiation of human primordial follicles within ovarian cortical tissue. J Assist Reprod Genet (Springer US). 2014;31:1013–28. doi:10.1007/s10815-014-0252-x.

97. Donnez J, Dolmans M M. Fertility preservation in women. Nat Rev Endocrinol (Nature Publishing Group). 2013;9:735–49. doi:10.1038/nrendo.2013.205.

98. Silber S, Kagawa N, Kuwayama M, Gosden R. Duration of fertility after fresh and frozen ovary transplantation. Fertil Steril (Elsevier Ltd). 2010;94:2191–6. doi:10.1016/j.fertnstert.2009.12.073.

99. Donnez JJ, Dolmans M-M, Demylle DD, Jadoul PP, Pirard CC, Squifflet JJ, et al. Livebirth after orthotopic transplantation of cryopreserved ovarian tissue. Lancet. 2004;364:1405–10. doi:10.1016/S0140-6736(04)17222-X.

100. Donnez J, Jadoul P, Pirard C, Hutchings G, Demylle D, Squifflet J, et al. Live birth after transplantation of frozen-thawed ovarian tissue oophorectomy for benign disease. Fertil Steril (Elsevier Inc). 2012;98:720–5. doi:10.1016/j.fertnstert.2012.05.017.

101. Oktay K, Economos K, Kan M, Rucinski J, Veeck L, Rosenwaks Z. Endocrine function and oocyte retrieval after autologous transplantation of ovarian cortical strips to the forearm. JAMA (American Medical Association). 2001;286:1490–3.

102. Oktay KK, Buyuk EE, Rosenwaks ZZ, Rucinski JJ. A technique for transplantation of ovarian cortical strips to the forearm. Fertil Steril. 2003;80:193–8. doi:10.1016/S0015-0282(03)00568-5.

103. Donnez J, Dolmans M-M. Ovarian cortex transplantation: 60 reported live births brings the success and worldwide expansion of the technique towards routine clinical practice. J Assist Reprod Genet (Springer US). 2015;32:1167–70. doi:10.1007/s10815-015-0544-9.

104. Gavish Z, Peer G, Hadassa R, Yoram C, Meirow D. Follicle activation and "burn-out" contribute to post-transplantation follicle loss in ovarian tissue grafts: the effect of graft thickness. Hum Reprod. 2014;29:989–96. doi:10.1093/humrep/deu015.

105. Laronda MM, Jakus AE, Whelan KA, Wertheim JA, Shah RN, Woodruff TK. Initiation of puberty in mice following decellularized ovary transplant. Biomaterials (Elsevier Ltd). 2015;50:20–9. doi:10.1016/j.biomaterials.2015.01.051.

106. Luyckx V, Durant JF, Camboni A, Gilliaux S, Amorim CA, Langendonckt A, et al. Is transplantation of cryopreserved ovarian tissue from patients with advanced-stage breast cancer safe? A pilot study. J Assist Reprod Genet. 2013. doi:10.1007/s10815-013-0065-3.

107. Bastings L, Beerendonk CCM, Westphal JR, Massuger LFAG, Kaal SEJ, van Leeuwen FE, et al. Autotransplantation of cryopreserved ovarian tissue in cancer survivors and the risk of reintroducing malignancy: a systematic review. Hum Reprod Update. 2013;19:483–506. doi:10.1093/humupd/dmt020.

108. Sasaki K, Yokobayashi S, Nakamura T, Okamoto I, Yabuta Y, Kurimoto K, et al. Robust in vitro induction of human germ cell fate from pluripotent stem cells. Stem Cell (Elsevier Inc). 2015;17:178–94. doi:10.1016/j.stem.2015.06.014.

109. Lan C-W, Chen M-J, Jan P-S, Chen H-F, Ho H-N. Differentiation of human embryonic stem cells into functional ovarian granulosa-like cells. J Clin Endocrinol Metab. 2013;98:3713–23. doi:10.1210/jc.2012-4302.
110. US Department of Health and Human Services Centers for Disease Control and Prevention. 2012 Assisted reproductive technology national summary report. 2014, p. 1–82.
111. Wyns C, Curaba M, Petit S, Vanabelle B, Laurent P, Wese JFX, et al. Management of fertility preservation in prepubertal patients: 5 years' experience at the Catholic University of Louvain. Hum Reprod (Oxford University Press). 2011;26:737–47. doi:10.1093/humrep/deq387.
112. Ginsberg JP, Carlson CA, Lin K, Hobbie WL, Wigo E, Wu X, et al. An experimental protocol for fertility preservation in prepubertal boys recently diagnosed with cancer: a report of acceptability and safety. Hum Reprod (Oxford University Press). 2010;25:37–41. doi:10.1093/humrep/dep371.
113. Sadri-Ardekani H. Propagation of human spermatogonial stem cells in vitro. JAMA. 2009;302:2127–12. doi:10.1001/jama.2009.1689.
114. Keros V, Hultenby K, Borgström B, Fridström M, Jahnukainen K, Hovatta O. Methods of cryopreservation of testicular tissue with viable spermatogonia in pre-pubertal boys undergoing gonadotoxic cancer treatment. Hum Reprod (Oxford University Press). 2007;22:1384–95. doi:10.1093/humrep/del508.
115. Goossens E, Van Saen D, Tournaye H. Spermatogonial stem cell preservation and transplantation: from research to clinic. Hum Reprod (Oxford University Press). 2013;28:897–907. doi:10.1093/humrep/det039.
116. Payne CJ. The next frontier: the promise of in vitro spermatogenesis coupled with intracytoplasmic sperm injection. Andrology-Open Access. 2012. doi:10.4172/2167-0420.1000191.
117. Nagano M, Patrizio P, Brinster RL. Long-term survival of human spermatogonial stem cells in mouse testes. Fertil Steril. 2002;78:1225–33.
118. Honaramooz A, Li M-W, Penedo MCT, Meyers S, Dobrinski I. Accelerated maturation of primate testis by xenografting into mice. Biol Reprod (Society for the Study of Reproduction). 2004;70:1500–3. doi:10.1095/biolreprod.103.025536.
119. Honaramooz A, Snedaker A, Boiani M, Schöler H, Dobrinski I, Schlatt S. Sperm from neonatal mammalian testes grafted in mice. Nature. 2002;418:778–81. doi:10.1038/nature00918.
120. Kim TH, Hargreaves HK, Brynes RK, Hawkins HK, Lui VK, Woodard J, et al. Pretreatment testicular biopsy in childhood acute lymphocytic leukaemia. Lancet. 1981;2:657–8.

Chapter 8
Male Fertility Preservation: Current Options and Advances in Research

Kathrin Gassei, Peter H. Shaw, Glenn M. Cannon, Lillian R. Meacham, and Kyle E. Orwig

Introduction

Improvements in cancer therapies have resulted in improved 5-year survival rates [1] and an increasing focus on the quality of life after cure. Cancer survivors report that parenthood is important to them and distress over infertility has long-term psychological and relationship implications [2]. Therefore, the American Society for Clinical Oncology [3, 4] and the American Society for Reproductive Medicine [5, 6] recommend that patients be educated about the reproductive risks associated with their therapy as well as options for preserving fertility.

K. Gassei
Department of Obstetrics, Gynecology and Reproductive Sciences, Magee-Womens Research Institute, University of Pittsburgh School of Medicine, Pittsburgh, PA, USA

P.H. Shaw
Department of Pediatrics, University of Pittsburgh School of Medicine, Pittsburgh, PA, USA

Children's Hospital of Pittsburgh, University of Pittsburgh Medical Center, Pittsburgh, PA, USA

G.M. Cannon
Children's Hospital of Pittsburgh, University of Pittsburgh Medical Center, Pittsburgh, PA, USA

Department of Urology, University of Pittsburgh School of Medicine, Pittsburgh, PA, USA

L.R. Meacham
Department of Pediatrics, Emory University School of Medicine, Atlanta, GA, USA

Aflac Cancer Center/Children's Healthcare of Atlanta, Atlanta, GA, USA

K.E. Orwig, PhD (✉)
Department of Obstetrics, Gynecology and Reproductive Sciences, Magee-Womens Research Institute, University of Pittsburgh School of Medicine, Pittsburgh, PA, USA

Magee-Womens Research Institute, Rm B711, 204 Craft Avenue, Pittsburgh, PA 15213, USA
e-mail: orwigke@upmc.edu

© Springer International Publishing Switzerland 2017
T.K. Woodruff, Y.C. Gosiengfiao (eds.), *Pediatric and Adolescent Oncofertility*,
DOI 10.1007/978-3-319-32973-4_8

Whole body radiation; radiation to the hypothalamus, pituitary or gonads; and alkylating chemotherapies are particularly toxic to male fertility [7–10]. This is an important public health concern because nearly 25,000 males under the age of 44 will be diagnosed with cancer each year in the USA. Epidemiological data [10–12] indicate that most of these patients will survive their cancer, but many will receive treatments that put them at high risk for infertility. The Childhood Cancer Survivor Study (CCSS) has shown that male survivors of childhood cancer are half as likely to achieve a pregnancy with their partner compared to their male siblings [10]. When rates of infertility were studied in the CCSS, 46 % of survivors compared to 18 % of siblings reported experiencing infertility [13].

Patients and families with children facing a cancer diagnosis and planning for treatment may be ill prepared to discuss, think about, or take action to preserve their future fertility before initiating treatment. Unfortunately, while healthcare professionals in general acknowledge the need to discuss fertility preservation with their patients, fertility counseling is not consistently implemented [14, 15]. Consequently, many families are poorly informed of the risk of infertility [14] and the options they have to preserve their child's fertility [16]. Insufficient training for medical staff to counsel patients on this sensitive topic has been identified as an important factor, along with patient factors such as degree of disease, age, and cultural/religious concerns [17]. Both parents and adolescent cancer patients identify fertility as an important life goal after cancer [18].

Spermatogonial stem cells (SSCs) are at the foundation of spermatogenesis and maintain continuous sperm production throughout the postpubertal life of men [19–22]. Spermatogenesis is an extraordinarily productive process that generates more than 100 million sperm each day from the testes of adult men [23]. Because spermatogenesis is such a productive system, it can sometimes become an unintended target of cancer therapies that are toxic to rapidly dividing cells. Therapies that deplete the stem cell pool and/or damage the somatic niche can cause temporary or permanent infertility. Infertility in cancer survivors is due to impaired spermatogenesis, which can be characterized as oligospermia (<15 million sperm/ml of semen) or azoospermia (no sperm in the semen). High-dose alkylating agents (e.g., cyclophosphamide, busulfan, melphalan, chlorambucil), bleomycin, testicular radiation >400 cGy, or genitourinary surgery are associated with the highest risk of developing azoospermia [7–9, 13, 24, 25]. In contrast to spermatogenesis, the steroidogenic function of the testes appears to be less affected by cancer therapy, and the testosterone-producing Leydig cells appear to be fairly resistant to damage by cancer treatments [26].

Sperm Banking: The Gold Standard Procedure for Male Fertility Preservation

Postpubertal boys and adult men have the option to cryopreserve a semen sample containing sperm before initiating treatment, which can be thawed at a later date to achieve pregnancy by intrauterine insemination [27], in vitro fertilization (IVF [28]), or IVF with intracytoplasmic sperm injection (ICSI [29]). Unfortunately, only about 24 % of adult men freeze a semen sample before initiating their therapy [30]. Some males as young as 12 or 13 years of age are capable of producing a semen sample. Semen is produced via masturbation, but other methods such as vibratory stimulation [31] or electroejaculation [32, 33] have been used. Ideally patients should provide two specimens obtained 2–3 days apart. Standard semen analysis would be performed by the andrology laboratory and results will be available within 1 day to confirm whether the semen specimens contained sperm.

Testicular Sperm Extraction (TESE)

For patients who did not preserve a semen sample and have persistent azoospermia after cancer therapy, there is the option to retrieve rare sperm directly from the testis during a surgical procedure called testicular sperm extraction (TESE). This is possible because a few SSCs may survive the gonadotoxic therapy and produce focal areas of spermatogenesis in the seminiferous tubules. Hsiao and colleagues recently described their experience with 73 patients with post-chemotherapy azoospermia [34]. They reported that sperm were successfully retrieved from 37 % of patients on initial attempt with an overall success rate of 42.9 %. Fertilization rate with the retrieved sperm was 57 %; the pregnancy rate was 50 % and the live birth rate was 42 %. Success retrieving sperm was treatment dependent in that study with the lowest sperm recovery success rates (21 %) in patients receiving alkylating chemotherapy [34]. Picton and colleagues surveyed results from a total of five centers (including the Hsiao et al. study) and reported an overall sperm recovery rate of 44 % in azoospermic patients undergoing TESE after chemotherapy [35].

TESE for Men and Adolescent Boys with Klinefelter Syndrome

TESE is also used effectively for Klinefelter syndrome (KS) patients who typically have a 46, XXY karyotype and azoospermia, often characterized as a Sertoli cell-only phenotype. However, germ cells are sometimes present in the testes of KS patients, which produce focal areas of spermatogenesis in the testes. Success rates retrieving sperm by TESE from the testes of KS patients are consistently above 50 % (50–72 %) [36–41] and are similar to the success rates reported for TESE in azoospermic patients without Klinefelter syndrome. Most importantly, pregnancy rates and live birth rates after ICSI are similar in couples with or without KS, and children fathered by KS patients have a normal karyotype [36, 38, 39]. The infertility phenotype of KS patients is considered progressive, with rapid declines in spermatogenesis during the teenage years [42–44]. Previous studies in adult KS patients reported that sperm recovery rates were significantly lower after the age of 35 [39–41]. Therefore, early intervention may be important to preserve the fertility of Klinefelter patients. In fact, some centers have protocols to retrieve sperm by TESE from adolescent boys with KS based on the understanding that the likelihood of retrieving sperm in later years will be reduced [42, 45]. Other groups, however, did not find that performing TESE at a younger age increased the chances of successful sperm retrieval [43, 46], and there is considerable debate about the benefit of early fertility intervention for KS patients [45, 47].

Typically, pubertal development is determined by Tanner Staging of pubic hair and genitalia development, testicular size, and hormone levels. In normal boys, the median age of spermatogenesis onset is 13–14 years, correlating to a Tanner Stage II or III. In KS patients that present with developmental delays and altered developmental patterns, these parameters may not be useful to determine if spermatogenesis is present. It is currently unknown when spermatogenesis starts in boys with KS. While it seems to be commonly accepted that there is a progressive depletion of germ cells in the testes of KS patients after the onset of puberty, the data to support this notion are equivocal with small patient populations, lack of controls, and no longitudinal data. In addition, the standard therapy for boys with KS is testosterone replacement therapy in order to trigger entry and progression of puberty, secondary sexual characteristics, bone development, and longitudinal growth. However, testosterone supplementation also suppresses spermatogenesis (if present) even further through negative feedback on the hypothalamus-pituitary-gonadal axis. Some argue that any intervention to preserve fertility for KS patients should ideally precede hormone replacement therapy [48], although in one study it was proposed that topical testosterone therapy might not negatively affect spermatogenesis in adolescent KS patients [42]. The risks of invasive surgical procedures like TESE for boys have to be carefully weighed against the possible benefits for this unique patient population. Systematic, longitudinal studies are needed to characterize spermatogenic decline in KS patients.

There are currently no standard options to treat the infertility of adult patients who did not cryopreserve a semen sample and were not successful with the TESE/ICSI procedure. Adoption and third-party reproduction are family building options for these patients, but most cancer survivors prefer to have their own biological children [3]. Therefore, sperm banking should also be discussed with all pubertal, adolescent, and adult males who are able to produce a semen sample.

Gonadal Shielding

Gonadal shielding can be used to protect the testes from scatter radiation using lead shielding. The proper shielding technique should be carefully evaluated on a case by case basis depending on total radiation dose, fractionation, and the specific mode of delivery of the external beam therapy [49–51]. However, when the testicular tissue requires radiation therapy as a part of cancer treatment, shielding cannot be used. At other times, the proximity of the testes to the target of radiation results in scatter radiation to the testes which can also result in impaired spermatogenesis.

Testicular Tissue Banking: An Experimental Procedure for Fertility Preservation

There are currently no standard of care options to preserve the future fertility of prepubertal boys who are not yet producing sperm. This is an important human health concern because, with improved therapies, the event-free survival rate of children with cancer is 85 % [12, and these survivors can look forward to a full and productive life after cure. We estimate that each year in the USA more than 2000 boys will receive gonadotoxic treatments for cancer or other conditions (e.g., mye-loablative conditioning prior to bone marrow transplantation) that put them at high risk for infertility [52]. Prepubertal boys are not producing sperm, but they do have spermatogonial stem cells (SSCs) in their testes that are poised to initiate sperm production at the time of puberty [53]. There are several methods in the research pipeline, including SSC transplantation, testicular tissue grafting or xenografting, testicular tissue organ culture, and de novo testicular morphogenesis, that might be used to restore spermatogenesis or fertility from cryopreserved SSCs and/or testicular tissue. Induced pluripotent stem cell (iPSC) technologies may also be a fertility option for cancer survivors in the future. These methods are reviewed in this chapter.

Anticipating that new therapies will be available in the future; many centers in the USA and abroad have determined that it is reasonable to preserve testicular tissue for young patients who are at high risk for infertility and have no other options to preserve their fertility [35, 54–60]. Testicular tissue-based fertility preservation methods for children are considered experimental and should be performed with Institutional Review Board (IRB) oversight and approval. Although no pregnancies from cryopreserved testicular tissues have been reported in humans to date, two centers reported that the majority of parents consented to fertility preservation procedures on behalf of their children [55, 61, 62].

Considerations for Testicular Tissue Collection, Processing, and Freezing

Testicular tissue for cryopreservation is obtained via needle biopsy, wedge biopsy, or orchiectomy, ideally before the initiation of gonadotoxic treatment (surgery, chemotherapy, radiation). There is insufficient experience or evidence to recommend a particular surgical approach or orchiectomy, and each center will make those decisions based on individual and/or institutional biases about what is in the best interest of the patient in the short term and long term. Needle biopsy may be the least invasive but has an increased risk of unmitigated bleeding and recovers the least amount of tissue for downstream fertility applications. Wedge resection is more invasive than needle biopsy but may allow recovery of more testicular tissue (depending on surgeon preference), and bleeding can be controlled during surgery. Orchiectomy (removal of an entire testis) is the most invasive but allows for the greatest recovery of testicular tissue for downstream fertility applications, and bleeding can be controlled during surgery. Collection of more tissue at the time of surgery should correlate with increased recovery of SSCs and greater flexibility for future fertility applications. However, limited tissue should not be a deterrent to enrollment in a testicular tissue cryopreservation protocol. There are several experimental cell-based and tissue-based options under development with different requirements for the amount of cells/tissue that will be needed.

There are no established "best practices" for processing and freezing testicular tissue or cells. Two labs examined the post-thaw recovery of spermatogonia from cryopreserved human testis cell suspensions versus intact pieces of testicular tissue. Yango and colleagues reported that the recovery of SSEA4+ spermatogonia from cryopreserved fetal testicular tissue was similar to cryopreserved testicular cells, but recovery of SSEA4+ cells from cryopreserved adult testicular cells was greater than cryopreserved testicular tissue [63]. Pacchiarotti and coworkers reported that cryopreservation of testicular tissue was comparable in most aspects to cryopreservation of a cell suspension. However, while the viability of total cells from the cryopreserved tissue was higher than the cryopreserved cell suspension, the recovery of SSEA4+ and VASA+ germ cells from cryopreserved tissue pieces tended to be greater than cryopreserved cell suspensions. These differences were not significant [64].

For fertility preservation, most centers are freezing intact pieces of testicular tissue for patients because this preserves the option for both tissue-based and cell-based therapies in the future [35, 55, 56, 59, 60, 65]. Biopsied testicular tissues are typically cut into small pieces (1–9 mm^3), suspended in a DMSO-based freezing medium, and frozen at a controlled slow rate using a programmable freezing machine (Fig. 8.1) [35, 54–56, 59, 65–67]. Some centers have reported using an ethylene glycol-based freezing medium instead of DMSO [68–70], and some centers have reported that viability of vitrified testicular tissue is similar to tissue frozen at a controlled slow rate [71–74]. This may improve access to testicular tissue-freezing technology in centers that do not have programmable freezing machines. The experimental endpoints that have been used to evaluate freezing protocols have been varied and include cell viability; immunocytochemistry for spermatogonial markers; ultrastructural, histological, and/or immunohistochemical examination of cultured or grafted tissue; and hormone production (reviewed in Table 8.1). Systematic studies on prepubertal human testicular tissues with evaluation of both cell-based and tissue-based endpoints are needed. It is possible that the optimal freezing condition depends on the intended use of the tissue or cells.

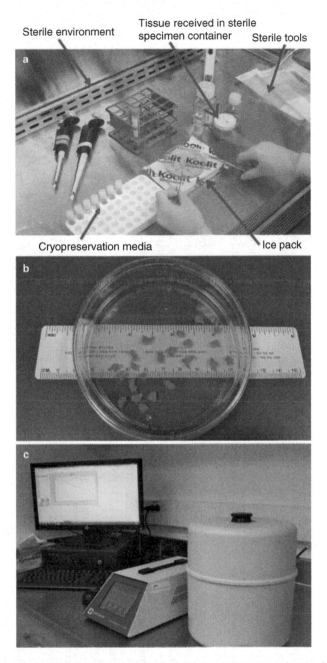

Fig. 8.1 Testicular tissue cryopreservation. Testicular tissues are transported on ice from the operating room to the andrology lab in a sterile specimen container containing medium. (**a**) Tissue is kept cool and processed in a sterile environment with sterile tools. (**b**) Most centers cut the testicular tissue into small pieces (2–9 mm³) and deposit in cryovials with DMSO-based freezing medium. (**c**) Controlled slow rate using a freezing machine

Table 8.1 Cryopreservation of human testicular tissue and cells

Tissue or cells	Freezing method	Freezing conditions	Endpoints	References
Cells	Controlled slow freezing	10% HSA, 10% DMSO, 1% dextran	Viability, Fc – SSEA4, LHR, VASA	[64]
Tissue	Controlled slow freezing	0.7 M DMSO, 0.1 M sucrose	Xenografting, IHC – MAGE-A4, Ki67, 3p-HSD	[73]
Tissue	Vitrification	Eq. sol. – 7.5% EG, 7.5% DMSO, 0.25 M sucrose. Vitr. Sol. 15% EG, 15% DMSO, 0.5 M sucrose		
Tissue	Controlled slow freezing	0.7 M DMSO, 5% HSA	IHC – MAGE-A4, TEM, organ culture	[67]
Tissue	Controlled slow freezing	0.7 M DMSO, 0.1 M sucrose, 10 mg/ml HSA	IHC – MAGE-A4 and Ki67	[72]
Tissue	Vitrification	?		
Tissue	Controlled slow freezing	1.5 M EG, 0.1 M sucrose, 10% HSA	Morphology, IHC – KIT	[68]
Tissue	Controlled slow freezing	0–2.5 M DMSO or EG or glycerol with 0.1% ITS and 20% FBS	Viability, seminiferous tubule culture	[70]
Tissue	Controlled slow freezing	5% DMSO, 5% HSA	IHC – MAGE-A4, vimentin, CD34. TEM. Tissue culture	[59]
Tissue	Controlled slow freezing	(1) 0.7 M or 1.5 M DMSO and 5% HSA (2) 0.7 M DMSO, 0.1 M sucrose, 10% HSA	IHC – TUNEL, PCNA, UCHL1. TEM	[71]
	Uncontrolled slow freezing	0.7 M or 1.5 M DMSO, 0.15 M sucrose, 10% HSA		
	Solid-surface vitrification	Eq. sol. – 1.35 M EG, 1.05 M DMSO. Vitr. Sol. 2.7 M EG, 2.1 M DMSO, 20% HSA		
	Direct cover vitrification			
Cells	Controlled slow freezing	1.28 M DMSO, 25% FBS	Fc – CD45, THY1, SSEA4	[63]
Tissue				
Cells	Controlled slow freezing	2% HSA, 1.4 M DMSO	Cell recovery, viability	[74]
	Uncontrolled slow freezing	2% HSA, 0.7 M DMSO		
	Vitrification	Eq. sol. – 2% HSA, 1.1 M DMSO, 1.34 M EG. Vitr. Sol. – 2% HSA, 0.67 M sucrose, 2.3 M DMSO, 1.34 M EG		
Cells	Controlled slow freezing	4% FBS, 1.5 M DMSO or EG or glycerol or 1,2-propanediol	Viability	[69]

HSA human serum albumin, *DMSO* dimethyl sulfoxide, *Fc* flow cytometry, *EG* ethylene glycol, *IHC* immunohistochemistry, *TEM* transmission electron microscopy, *FBS* fetal bovine serum

Table 8.1 is reproduced from Valli et al., 2015 [65], with permission of Springer

Testicular Cell-Based Methods to Preserve and Restore Male Fertility

Spermatogonial Stem Cell Transplantation

Spermatogonial stem cell transplantation was first described by Ralph Brinster and colleagues in 1994, who demonstrated that SSCs could be isolated and transplanted to regenerate spermatogenesis in infertile recipient mice [75, 76]. SSC transplantation has now been reported in mice, rats, pigs, goats, bulls, sheep, dogs, and monkeys, and donor-derived progeny has been produced by natural breeding in mice, rats, goats, and sheep [77–88]. SSCs from donors of all ages, newborn to adult, are competent to regenerate spermatogenesis [78, 89], and SSCs can be cryopreserved and retain spermatogenic function upon thawing and transplantation [85, 90, 91]. Thus, it appears feasible that a testicular tissue biopsy (containing SSCs) could be obtained from a prepubertal boy prior to gonadotoxic therapy, frozen, thawed at a later date, and transplanted back into his testes to regenerate spermatogenesis. If spermatogenesis from transplanted cells is robust, this approach may restore natural fertility, allowing survivors to achieve pregnancy with their partner by natural intercourse and have biological children.

Radford and colleagues already reported cryopreserving testicular cells for 11 adult non-Hodgkin's lymphoma patients in 1999 and subsequently reported transplanting autologous frozen and thawed testis cells back into the testes of seven survivors [92, 93]. The fertility outcomes for patients in that study have not been reported, and even if the men fathered children, it would not be possible to ascertain whether the sperm arose from transplanted stem cells or surviving endogenous stem cells. This uncertainty will always plague the interpretation of human SSC transplant studies where it is not ethically possible to genetically mark the transplanted cells because the genetic modification would be transmitted to progeny. Therefore, large epidemiological datasets generated over decades will be required to prove the fertility benefit of SSC transplantation. Nonetheless, this study demonstrates that patients are willing to pursue experimental stem cell-based options even when there is no guarantee of a fertile outcome. There are no published reports of SSC transplantation in humans since Radford's follow-up report of his non-Hodgkin's lymphoma patients in 2003 [93].

Translating Spermatogonial Stem Cell Transplantation into the Clinic: Challenges and Opportunities

Considering the progress in several animal models and the fact that testicular tissues have already been cryopreserved for hundreds of human patients worldwide [54–60, 92, 93], it seem reasonable to expect that SSC transplantation and/or other stem cell technologies will impact the fertility clinic in the next decade. However, there are several safety and feasibility issues that must be considered.

Spermatogonial Stem Cell Culture

Based on our experiences at the Fertility Preservation Program in Pittsburgh [54] and published reports [56, 59], it is reasonable to expect that 50–500 mg of testicular tissue can be obtained by wedge biopsy or needle biopsy from a single testis of a prepubertal boy. This is a small amount of tissue relative to size of adult human testes that can range from 11 to 26 g in size [94]. It is widely believed that the number of stem cells in biopsies from prepubertal boys will be small and that SSCs will have to be expanded in culture prior to transplant. Conditions for maintaining and expanding rodent SSCs in culture are well established and SSCs maintained in long-term culture remain competent to regenerate spermatogenesis and restore fertility [95–100].

If cultured human SSCs function similar to cultured rodent SSCs, it should be feasible to expand a few stem cells obtained from the testis biopsy of a prepubertal boy to a number sufficient to produce robust spermatogenesis upon transplantation back into his testes when he is an adult. Several studies have reported culturing human SSCs [57, 58, 101–109], including two studies in which cultures were established from the testes of prepubertal patients [58, 101]. Human SSC cultures have been evaluated by quantitative PCR or immunocytochemistry for spermatogonial markers or xenotransplantation into mouse testes. Strategies to isolate and culture human spermatogonia have been unique to each study, and to date no approach has been independently replicated in another laboratory. Also, the field is frustrated by the lack of a functional assay to test the full spermatogenic potential of cultured human cells.

Malignant Contamination

A testicular biopsy obtained from a cancer patient could harbor malignant cells, especially for patients with leukemia. Kim and colleagues [110] reported that 20 % of boys with acute lymphocytic anemia had malignant cells in their testicular tissue prior to the initiation of oncologic treatment. Jahnukainen and colleagues [111] reported the transmission of leukemia after transplantation of testis cells from terminally ill leukemic rats into the testes of non-leukemic recipients. The same group further demonstrated that transplantation of as few as 20 leukemic cells was sufficient for disease transmission, leading to terminal leukemia within 3 weeks.

Because infertility is not life threatening and fertility treatments are elective, it is essential that risk of cancer recurrence after transplant be reduced to zero. Fluorescence-activated cell sorting (FACS) and magnetic-activated cell sorting (MACS) strategies to isolate and enrich therapeutic spermatogonia while removing malignant contamination have been explored with mixed results. To date, transplantable human spermatogonia have been recovered in the Ep-CAM^{lo}, THY-1^{lo}, CD49f$^+$, SSEA4$^+$, GPR125$^+$, and CD9$^+$ fractions of human testis cells [94, 102, 105, 112–114].

Fujita and coworkers isolated germ cells from the testes of leukemic mice in the forward scatter high and side scatter low fraction (positive selection), which was then further divided into fractions that were CD45/MHC class I antigens (H-2K^b/H-2D^b) double positive and CD45/MHC class I double negative cells. All recipient males injected with the CD45$^+$/MHC class I$^+$ cells developed terminal leukemia within 40 days. All mice injected with CD45$^-$/MHC class I$^-$ cells survived for 300 days without onset of leukemia and produced donor-derived offspring [115]. In a subsequent study, the same group reported that seven out of eight human leukemic cell lines expressed the cell surface antigens CD45 and MHC class I [116]. In a rat model of Roser's T-cell leukemia, Hou and colleagues concluded that single parameter selection using either leukemic (CD4 and MHC Class I) or SSC (Ep-CAM) markers was not sufficient to eliminate malignant contamination [117], but malignant contamination was successfully removed using a combination of leukemia and SSC markers (plus/minus selection) [114, 118]. Using similar positive/negative selection strategies, Hermann and colleagues isolated VASA+ germ cells in the THY-1$^+$/ CD45$^-$ fraction of leukemia-contaminated prepubertal nonhuman primate testis cells [118], and this fraction did not produce tumors in mice. Dovey and colleagues contaminated human testis cells with MOLT-4 acute lymphoblastic leukemia cells and demonstrated by xenotransplantation that the Ep-CAM^{lo}/ HLA-ABC$^-$/CD49e$^-$ fraction was enriched 12-fold for transplantable human SSCs and was devoid of malignant contamination [114]. Collectively, these results are encouraging, but caution is still warranted as Geens and colleagues concluded, using EL-4 lymphoma contaminated mouse and human testis cells, that FACS- and MACS-based methods were insufficient to remove malignant contamination [119].

It will not be possible to perform comprehensive in vivo testing on patient samples because this would limit the amount of sample available for fertility therapy. More sensitive PCR-based methods have been described for detection of minimal residual disease (MRD), and this approach has identified malignant contamination in many ovarian tissue samples that were preserved for leukemia patients, even after negative histology and immunocytochemistry examination [120, 121]. However, in one of those studies, Dolmans and colleagues obtained disparate results from histology, qRT-PCR, and xenografting of ovarian tissues from leukemia patients. Quantitative RT-PCR to detect MRD revealed the possibility of malignant contamination in 9 of the 16 samples that was not detected by histological examination. However, when those ovarian tissues were grafted into recipient mice, only five of the nine samples with positive MRD had evidence of leukemic cells 3 months after transplantation [120]. Were the MRD results in the other four cases nefarious, or were they accurate and the leukemic cells simply failed to survive freezing, thawing, and grafting? In the absence of a definitive and practical test of malignant contamination, alternatives to autologous transplantation are needed for patients with hematogenous cancers, testis cancers, or cancers that metastasize to the testes.

De Novo Testicular Morphogenesis

Testicular cells (including germ cells, Sertoli cells, peritubular myoid cells, and Leydig cells) have the remarkable ability to reorganize to form normal looking seminiferous tubules when grafted under the skin of recipient mice [122–126]. Ina Dobrinski and colleagues disaggregated neonatal pig and sheep testis cells, pelleted them by centrifugation, and grafted them under the skin of immune-deficient mice. When grafts were recovered between 16 and 41 weeks after transplant, cells had reorganized to form seminiferous tubules with complete spermatogenesis [125, 126]. In a remarkable extension of this approach, Kita and colleagues [124] mixed fetal or neonatal testis cells from mice or rats with GFP+-cultured mouse germline stem cells and growth factor-reduced Matrigel and grafted under the skin of immune-deficient mice. Seven to 10 weeks after grafting, seminiferous tubules with complete spermatogenesis originating from both intrinsic germ cells and cultured (GFP+) germ cells were observed. Tubules were dissected and GFP+ round spermatids were recovered, injected into mouse oocytes. The resulting embryos were transferred to recipient females and gave rise to ten mouse pups, including four with the GFP transgene. It may be feasible to build a human testis from disaggregated human testis cells, but this has not been reported to our knowledge. The human experiment may be complicated by limited availability of fetal, neonatal, or prepubertal human testis cells. It does not appear that anyone has tried to "build a testis" from disaggregated adult testis cells for any species. One day it may be possible to "build a testis," in vitro or in vivo, on the scaffold of a decellularized human testis [127].

Testicular Tissue-Based Methods to Preserve and Restore Male Fertility

Testicular Tissue Grafting and Xenografting

Testicular tissue grafting may provide an alternative approach for generating fertilization-competent sperm from small testicular biopsies. In contrast to the SSC transplantation method in which SSCs are removed from their cognate niches and transplanted into recipient seminiferous tubules, grafting involves transplantation of the intact SSC/niche unit in pieces of testicular tissue. Honaramooz and colleagues reported that grafted testicular tissue from newborn mice, rats, pigs, and goats, in which spermatogenesis was not yet established, could mature and produce complete spermatogenesis when xenografted into nude mice [128]. The same group later reported the production of live offspring from sperm obtained from mouse testicular tissue grafts [129]. Fertilization-competent sperm was also produced from xenografts of prepubertal nonhuman primate testicular tissue transplanted into mice [130]. These results suggest that it may be possible to obtain fertilization-competent sperm by xenografting small pieces of testicular tissue from a prepubertal cancer patient under the skin of mice or other animal recipients such as pigs that are already an established source for human food consumption, replacement heart valves [131, 132], and potentially other organs [133]. Xenografting would also circumvent the issue of malignant contamination. However, the xenografting approach raises concerns about xenobiotics because viruses from mice, pigs, and other species can be transmitted to human cells [134, 135]. There is no evidence to date that xenografted human testicular tissue can produce spermatogenesis or sperm in mice [136–141]. However, there is reason for optimism because Sato and colleagues observed primary spermatocytes 1 year after xenografting testicular tissue from a 3-month-old boy that clearly did not have spermatocytes at the time of transplantation [140]. Xenografting of human testicular tissue to species other than mice has not been tested to our knowledge.

If malignant contamination of the testicular tissue is not a concern, autologous testicular tissue grafting can be considered. Luetjens and colleagues demonstrated that fresh autologous testicular tissue grafts from prepubertal marmosets could produce complete spermatogenesis when transplanted into the scrotum but not under the skin [142]. Frozen and thawed grafts did not produce complete spermatogenesis in that study, but those grafts were only transplanted under the skin. Therefore, additional experimentation is merited. Testicular tissue grafting will not restore natural fertility but could generate haploid sperm that can be used to fertilize oocytes by ICSI.

Testicular Tissue Organ Culture

Sato and colleagues reported that intact testicular tissues from newborn mice (2.5–3.5 days old) could be maintained in organ culture and mature to produce spermatogenesis, including the production of fertilization-competent haploid germ cells [143, 144]. Testicular tissues from neonatal mice were minced into pieces (1–3 mm^3) and placed in culture at the gas/liquid interface on a slab of agarose that was soaked in medium. Haploid round spermatids and sperm were recovered from the tissue after 3–6 weeks in culture and used to fertilize mouse eggs by ICSI. The resulting embryos were transferred to pseudopregnant females and gave rise to healthy offspring that matured to adulthood and were fertile. If testicular tissue organ culture can be translated to humans, it will provide an alternative to autologous SSC transplantation, autologous grafting, and xenografting in cases where there is concern about malignant contamination of the testicular tissue. The same authors were also successful to produce haploid germ cells in organ culture of frozen and thawed testicular tissues, which is particularly relevant to the cancer survivor paradigm. However, the fertilization potential of those sperm was not tested [143].

Induced Pluripotent Stem Cell-Based Methods to Preserve and Restore Male Fertility

Several groups have now reported that it is possible to produce germ cells from pluripotent embryonic stem cells (ESCs) or induced pluripotent stem cells (iPSCs) [145–158]. Hayashi and coworkers reported that it is possible to differentiate ESCs or iPSCs into epiblast-like cells (EpiLCs) that then give rise to primordial germ cell-like cells (PGCLCs) when cultured in the presence of BMP4 [145]. The resulting germ cells were transplanted into the seminiferous tubules of infertile recipient mice where they regenerated spermatogenesis and produced haploid gametes that were used to fertilize mouse oocytes by ICSI. The embryos were transferred to recipient females and gave rise to live offspring. However, some of the offspring developed tumors in the neck area and died prematurely, suggesting that further optimization of the culture and differentiation protocols will be required [145]. Two groups recently reported the differentiation of human pluripotent stem cells into putative hPGCLCs exhibiting gene expression patterns similar to bona fide human PGCs [146, 147]. Of course, functional validation by generation of progeny is not possible in studies with human cells.

An important implication of the iPSC to germ cell differentiation technology, if responsibly developed, is that it will no longer be necessary to preserve fertility before the initiation of gonadotoxic treatments. An adult survivor of a childhood cancer who desires to start his family and discovers that he is infertile can theoretically produce sperm and biological offspring from his own skin, blood, or other somatic cell type. This scenario applies not only to childhood cancer survivors but all survivors who did not preserve semen or testicular tissue prior to gonadotoxic therapy. Nonhuman primate and human pluripotent stem cells have also been differentiated to the germ lineage, producing putative transplantable germ cells and even rare cells that appear to be haploid [148–155, 157–159]. The challenge with the human studies is that it is not possible to test the spermatogenic potential or fertilization potential of putative germ cells, which are the gold standards in animal studies. Thus, the burden of proof required of human studies is much lower than animal studies. Spermatogenic lineage development and testicular anatomy in nonhuman primates is similar to humans [22], and this may serve as a platform for safety and feasibility studies in which putative germ cells can be tested by transplantation, and the resulting gametes can be tested by fertilization [85], embryo transfer, and production of live offspring. Perhaps 1 day it will be possible to build a human testis in vitro or in vivo on a decellularized human testis scaffold, and this will provide the ultimate platform to test the spermatogenic potential of experimentally derived human germ cells.

Conclusions

Many centers worldwide are actively preserving testicular tissue or testicular cells for cancer patients in anticipation that those samples can be used in the future for reproductive purposes. Therefore, it is incumbent on the medical and research communities to responsibly develop the technologies that will allow patients to use their samples to achieve their family building goals. This is important because cancer survivors report that fertility has a significant impact on their quality of life after cure. It seems reasonable to assume that similar quality of life issues are relevant to men who are infertile due to genetic (e.g., Klinefelter), surgical, age-related, accidental, or other causes. The first, best, and proven approach for fertility preservation in males is to freeze sperm that can be obtained in a semen sample or extracted from the testis. With IVF and IVF with ICSI, only a relatively small number of sperm are required to achieve fertilization and pregnancy. Unfortunately, sperm banking is not an option for all patients, including prepubertal boys who are not yet producing sperm.

There are several testicular cell- and tissue-based technologies in the research pipeline that may have application for patients who cannot preserve sperm. All of the technologies described in this chapter are dependent on stem cells (SSCs or iPSCs) with the potential to generate or regenerate autologous spermatogenesis. Spermatogonial stem cell transplantation, de novo testicular morphogenesis, testicular tissue organ culture, testicular tissue grafting/xenografting, and iPSC-derived germ cells have all produced spermatogenesis with sperm that are competent to fertilize oocytes and give rise to viable offspring in mice. Several of these methods have also been translated to larger animal models, including nonhuman primates, indicating a potential for application in the human fertility clinic.

The greatest challenge in the development of stem cell technologies for treatment of human male infertility is the lack of experimental tools for testing the spermatogenic and fertile potential of human cells. This means that human studies cannot be held to the same standard for burden of proof that is required of animal studies. While it is not realistic or possible to demonstrate the fertilization potential of human stem cell-derived gametes, it may be possible to develop systems to test the spermatogenic potential of human cells, such as de novo testicular morphogenesis or engraftment of a decellularized testis. Progress along these lines will provide powerful tools to ensure responsible development and validation of stem cell technologies before they are translated to the male fertility clinic.

Acknowledgments The authors would like to thank the Scaife Foundation, the Richard King Mellon Foundation, the Magee-Womens Research Institute and Foundation, the Children's Hospital of Pittsburgh Foundation, and the University of Pittsburgh Departments of Obstetrics, Gynecology & Reproductive Sciences and Urology, which have generously provided funds to support the Fertility Preservation Program in Pittsburgh (http://www.mwrif.org/220). It is in this context that we have had the opportunity to meet the infertile patients that fuel our passion for fertility research. The Orwig lab is supported by the Magee-Womens Research Institute and Foundation, the *Eunice Kennedy Shriver* National Institute of Child Health and Human Development grants HD075795 and HD076412, the USA-Israel Binational Science Foundation, and gift funds from Montana State University, Sylvia Bernassoli, and Julie and Michael McMullen.

References

1. Surviving Childhood Cancer. http://www.cancer.org/cancer/cancerinchildren/detailedguide/cancer-in-children-treating-survival-rates: American Cancer Society; 2015. Available from: http://www.cancer.org/cancer/cancerinchildren/detailedguide/cancer-in-children-treating-survival-rates.
2. Schover LR. Patient attitudes toward fertility preservation. Pediatr Blood Cancer. 2009;53(2):281–4.

3. Lee SJ, Schover LR, Partridge AH, Patrizio P, Wallace WH, Hagerty K, Beck LN, Brennan LV, Oktay K. American Society of Clinical Oncology recommendations on fertility preservation in cancer patients. J Clin Oncol Off J Am Soc Clin Oncol. 2006;24(18):2917–31.

4. Loren AW, Mangu PB, Beck LN, Brennan L, Magdalinski AJ, Partridge AH, Quinn G, Wallace WH, Oktay K, American Society of Clinical Oncology. Fertility preservation for patients with cancer: American Society of Clinical Oncology clinical practice guideline update. J Clin Oncol Off J Am Soc Clin Oncol. 2013;31(19):2500–10.

5. Ethics Committee of the American Society for Reproductive Medicine. Fertility preservation and reproduction in cancer patients. Fertil Steril. 2005;83(6):1622–28.

6. Practice Committee of American Society for Reproductive Medicine. Fertility preservation in patients undergoing gonadotoxic therapy or gonadectomy: a committee opinion. Fertil Steril. 2013;100(5):1214–23.

7. Wallace WH, Anderson RA, Irvine DS. Fertility preservation for young patients with cancer: who is at risk and what can be offered? Lancet Oncol. 2005;6(4):209–18.

8. Meistrich ML. Male gonadal toxicity. Pediatr Blood Cancer. 2009;53(2):261–6.

9. Levine J, Canada A, Stern CJ. Fertility preservation in adolescents and young adults with cancer. J Clin Oncol Off J Am Soc Clin Oncol. 2010;28(32):4831–41.

10. Green DM, Kawashima T, Stovall M, Leisenring W, Sklar CA, Mertens AC, Donaldson SS, Byrne J, Robison LL. Fertility of male survivors of childhood cancer: a report from the Childhood Cancer Survivor Study. J Clin Oncol Off J Am Soc Clin Oncol. 2010;28(2):332–9.

11. Meistrich ML, Vassilopoulou-Sellin R, Lipshultz LI. Adverse effects of treatment: gonadal dysfunction. In: DeVita VT, Hellman S, Rosenberg SA, editors. Principles and practice of oncology. 7th ed. Philadelphia: Lippincott Williams & Wilkins; 2004. p. 2560–74.

12. Howlader N, Noone AM, Krapcho M, Neyman N, Aminou R, Waldron W, Altekruse SF, Kosary CL, Ruhl J, Tatalovich Z, Cho H, Mariotto A, Eisner MP, Lewis DR, Chen HS, Feuer EJ, Cronin KA, Edwards BK. SEER cancer statistic review 1975–2008. Bethesda: National Cancer Institute; 2010. [cited 2011], Available from: http://seer.cancer.gov/csr/1975_2008/.

13. Wasilewski-Masker K, Seidel KD, Leisenring W, Mertens AC, Shnorhavorian M, Ritenour CW, Stovall M, Green DM, Sklar CA, Armstrong GT, Robison LL, Meacham LR. Male infertility in long-term survivors of pediatric cancer: a report from the childhood cancer survivor study. J Cancer Surviv. 2014;8(3):437–47.

14. Schover LR, Brey K, Lichtin A, Lipshultz LI, Jeha S. Knowledge and experience regarding cancer, infertility, and sperm banking in younger male survivors. J Clin Oncol Off J Am Soc Clin Oncol. 2002;20(7):1880–9.

15. Schover LR, Brey K, Lichtin A, Lipshultz LI, Jeha S. Oncologists' attitudes and practices regarding banking sperm before cancer treatment. J Clin Oncol Off J Am Soc Clin Oncol. 2002;20(7):1890–7.

16. Sadri-Ardekani H, Akhondi MM, Vossough P, Maleki H, Sedighnejad S, Kamali K, Ghorbani B, van Wely M, van der Veen F, Repping S. Parental attitudes toward fertility preservation in boys with cancer: context of different risk levels of infertility and success rates of fertility restoration. Fertil Steril. 2013;99(3):796–802.

17. Gilbert E, Adams A, Mehanna H, Harrison B, Hartshorne GM. Who should be offered sperm banking for fertility preservation? A survey of UK oncologists and haematologists. Ann Oncol Off J Eur Soc Med Oncol/ESMO. 2011;22(5):1209–14.

18. Klosky JL, Simmons JL, Russell KM, Foster RH, Sabbatini GM, Canavera KE, Hodges JR, Schover LR, McDermott MJ. Fertility as a priority among at-risk adolescent males newly diagnosed with cancer and their parents. Support Care Cancer Off J Multinatl Assoc Support Care Cancer. 2015;23(2):333–41.

19. Tegelenbosch RA, de Rooij DG. A quantitative study of spermatogonial multiplication and stem cell renewal in the C3H/101 F1 hybrid mouse. Mutat Res. 1993;290(2):193–200.

20. de Rooij DG, Grootegoed JA. Spermatogonial stem cells. Curr Opin Cell Biol. 1998;10(6):694–701.

21. Phillips BT, Gassei K, Orwig KE. Spermatogonial stem cell regulation and spermatogenesis. Philos Trans R Soc Lond B Biol Sci. 2010;365(1546):1663–78.

22. Valli H, Phillips BT, Gassei K, Nagano MC, Orwig KE. Spermatogonial stem cells and spermatogenesis. In: Plant TM, Zeleznik AJ, editors. Knobil and Neill's physiology of reproduction, vol. 1. 4th ed. San Diego: Elsevier; 2015. p. 595–635.
23. Sharpe RM. Regulation of spermatogenesis. In: Knobil E, Neill JD, editors. The physiology of reproduction. New York: Raven Press, Ltd.; 1994. p. 1363–434.
24. Bucci LR, Meistrich ML. Effects of busulfan on murine spermatogenesis: cytotoxicity, sterility, sperm abnormalities, and dominant lethal mutations. Mutat Res. 1987;176(2):259–68.
25. Meistrich ML, Wilson G, Brown BW, da Cunha MF, Lipshultz LI. Impact of cyclophosphamide on long-term reduction in sperm count in men treated with combination chemotherapy for Ewing and soft tissue sarcomas. Cancer. 1992;70(11):2703–12.
26. Chemaitilly W, Sklar CA. Endocrine complications in long-term survivors of childhood cancers. Endocr Relat Cancer. 2010;17(3):R141–59.
27. Agarwal A, Allamaneni SR. Artificial insemination. In: Falcone T, Hurd W, editors. Clinical reproductive medicine and surgery. Philadelphia: Elsevier; 2007. p. 539–48.
28. Steptoe PC, Edwards RG. Birth after the reimplantation of a human embryo. Lancet. 1978;2(8085):366.
29. Palermo G, Joris H, Devroey P, Van Steirteghem AC. Pregnancies after intracytoplasmic injection of single spermatozoon into an oocyte. Lancet. 1992;340(8810):17–8.
30. Schover LR, Brey K, Lichtin A, Lipshultz LI, Jeha S. Knowledge and experience regarding cancer, infertility, and sperm banking in younger male survivors. J Clin Oncol. 2002;20(7):1880–9.
31. Schmiegelow ML, Sommer P, Carlsen E, Sønksen JOR, Schmiegelow K, Muller JR. Penile vibratory stimulation and electroejaculation before anticancer therapy in two pubertal boys. J Pediatr Hematol Oncol. 1998;20(5):429–30.
32. Adank MC, van Dorp W, Smit M, van Casteren NJ, Laven JSE, Pieters R, van den Heuvel-Eibrink MM. Electroejaculation as a method of fertility preservation in boys diagnosed with cancer: a single-center experience and review of the literature. Fertil Steril. 2014;102(1):199–205.e191.
33. Gat I, Toren A, Hourvitz A, Raviv G, Band G, Baum M, Lerner-Geva L, Inbar R, Madgar I. Sperm preservation by electroejaculation in adolescent cancer patients. Pediatr Blood Cancer. 2014;61(2):286–90.
34. Hsiao W, Stahl PJ, Osterberg EC, Nejat E, Palermo GD, Rosenwaks Z, Schlegel PN. Successful treatment of postchemotherapy azoospermia with microsurgical testicular sperm extraction: the Weill Cornell experience. J Clin Oncol. 2011;29(12):1607–11.
35. Picton HM, Wyns C, Anderson RA, Goossens E, Jahnukainen K, Kliesch S, Mitchell RT, Pennings G, Rives N, Tournaye H, van Pelt AM, Eichenlaub-Ritter U, Schlatt S. A European perspective on testicular tissue cryopreservation for fertility preservation in prepubertal and adolescent boysdagger. Hum Reprod. 2015;30(11):2463–75.
36. Schiff JD, Palermo GD, Veeck LL, Goldstein M, Rosenwaks Z, Schlegel PN. Success of testicular sperm extraction [corrected] and intracytoplasmic sperm injection in men with Klinefelter syndrome. J Clin Endocrinol Metab. 2005;90(11):6263–7.
37. Koga M, Tsujimura A, Takeyama M, Kiuchi H, Takao T, Miyagawa Y, Takada S, Matsumiya K, Fujioka H, Okamoto Y, Nonomura N, Okuyama A. Clinical comparison of successful and failed microdissection testicular sperm extraction in patients with nonmosaic Klinefelter syndrome. Urology. 2007;70(2):341–5.
38. Yarali H, Polat M, Bozdag G, Gunel M, Alpas I, Esinler I, Dogan U, Tiras B. TESE-ICSI in patients with non-mosaic Klinefelter syndrome: a comparative study. Reprod Biomed Online. 2009;18(6):756–60.
39. Bakircioglu ME, Ulug U, Erden HF, Tosun S, Bayram A, Ciray N, Bahceci M. Klinefelter syndrome: does it confer a bad prognosis in treatment of nonobstructive azoospermia? Fertil Steril. 2011;95(5):1696–9.
40. Ramasamy R, Ricci JA, Palermo GD, Gosden LV, Rosenwaks Z, Schlegel PN. Successful fertility treatment for Klinefelter's syndrome. J Urol. 2009;182(3):1108–13.
41. Okada H, Goda K, Yamamoto Y, Sofikitis N, Miyagawa I, Mio Y, Koshida M, Horie S. Age as a limiting factor for successful sperm retrieval in patients with nonmosaic Klinefelter's syndrome. Fertil Steril. 2005;84(6):1662–4.

42. Mehta A, Paduch DA, Schlegel PN. Successful testicular sperm retrieval in adolescents with Klinefelter syndrome treated with at least 1 year of topical testosterone and aromatase inhibitor. Fertil Steril. 2013;100(4):e27.
43. Wikstrom AM, Raivio T, Hadziselimovic F, Wikstrom S, Tuuri T, Dunkel L. Klinefelter syndrome in adolescence: onset of puberty is associated with accelerated germ cell depletion. J Clin Endocrinol Metab. 2004;89(5):2263–70.
44. Aksglaede L, Wikstrom AM, Rajpert-De Meyts E, Dunkel L, Skakkebaek NE, Juul A. Natural history of seminiferous tubule degeneration in Klinefelter syndrome. Hum Reprod Update. 2006;12(1):39–48.
45. Oates RD. Sperm retrieval in adolescents with Klinefelter syndrome. Fertil Steril. 2013;100(4):943–4.
46. Plotton I, Giscard d'Estaing S, Cuzin B, Brosse A, Benchaib M, Lornage J, Ecochard R, Dijoud F, Lejeune H. Preliminary results of a prospective study of testicular sperm extraction in young versus adult patients with nonmosaic 47, XXY Klinefelter syndrome. J Clin Endocrinol Metab. 2015;100(3):961–7.
47. Rives N, Milazzo JP, Perdrix A, Castanet M, Joly-Helas G, Sibert L, Bironneau A, Way A, Mace B. The feasibility of fertility preservation in adolescents with Klinefelter syndrome. Hum Reprod. 2013;28(6):1468–79.
48. Verit FF, Verit A. Klinefelter syndrome: an argument for early aggressive hormonal and fertility management. Fertil Steril. 2012;98(5):e25. author reply e26.
49. Fraass BA, Kinsella TJ, Harrington FS, Glatstein E. Peripheral dose to the testes: the design and clinical use of a practical and effective gonadal shield. Int J Radiat Oncol Biol Phys. 1985;11(3):609–15.
50. Yadav P, Kozak K, Tolakanahalli R, Ramasubramanian V, Paliwal BR, Welsh JS, Rong Y. Adaptive planning using megavoltage fan-beam CT for radiation therapy with testicular shielding. Med Dosim. 2012;37(2):157–62.
51. Sanghvi PR, Kaurin DG, McDonald TL, Holland JM. Testicular shielding in low-dose total body irradiation. Bone Marrow Transplant. 2007;39(4):247–8.
52. Valli H, Phillips BT, Shetty G, Byrne JA, Clark AT, Meistrich ML, Orwig KE. Germline stem cells: toward the regeneration of spermatogenesis. Fertil Steril. 2014;101(1):3–13.
53. Paniagua R, Nistal M. Morphological and histometric study of human spermatogonia from birth to the onset of puberty. J Anat. 1984;139(Pt 3):535–52.
54. Orwig KE, Shaw PH, Sanfilippo JS, Kauma SW, Nayak S, Cannon GM. Fertility preservation program of Magee-Womens Hospital in Pittsburgh. http://www.mwrif.org/220. Available from: http://www.mwrif.org/220.
55. Wyns C, Curaba M, Petit S, Vanabelle B, Laurent P, Wese JF, Donnez J. Management of fertility preservation in prepubertal patients: 5 years' experience at the Catholic University of Louvain. Hum Reprod. 2011;26(4):737–47.
56. Ginsberg JP, Carlson CA, Lin K, Hobbie WL, Wigo E, Wu X, Brinster RL, Kolon TF. An experimental protocol for fertility preservation in prepubertal boys recently diagnosed with cancer: a report of acceptability and safety. Hum Reprod. 2010;25(1):37–41.
57. Sadri-Ardekani H, Mizrak SC, van Daalen SK, Korver CM, Roepers-Gajadien HL, Koruji M, Hovingh S, de Reijke TM, de la Rosette JJ, van der Veen F, de Rooij DG, Repping S, van Pelt AM. Propagation of human spermatogonial stem cells in vitro. J Am Med Assoc. 2009;302(19):2127–34.
58. Sadri-Ardekani H, Akhondi MA, van der Veen F, Repping S, van Pelt AM. In vitro propagation of human prepubertal spermatogonial stem cells. J Am Med Assoc. 2011;305(23):2416–8.
59. Keros V, Hultenby K, Borgstrom B, Fridstrom M, Jahnukainen K, Hovatta O. Methods of cryopreservation of testicular tissue with viable spermatogonia in pre-pubertal boys undergoing gonadotoxic cancer treatment. Hum Reprod. 2007;22(5):1384–95.
60. Goossens E, Van Saen D, Tournaye H. Spermatogonial stem cell preservation and transplantation: from research to clinic. Hum Reprod. 2013;28(4):897–907.

61. Ginsberg JP. New advances in fertility preservation for pediatric cancer patients. Curr Opin Pediatr. 2011;23(1):9–13.
62. Wyns C, Collienne C, Shenfield F, Robert A, Laurent P, Roegiers L, Brichard B. Fertility preservation in the male pediatric population: factors influencing the decision of parents and children. Hum Reprod. 2015;30:2022–30.
63. Yango P, Altman E, Smith JF, Klatsky PC, Tran ND. Optimizing cryopreservation of human spermatogonial stem cells: comparing the effectiveness of testicular tissue and single cell suspension cryopreservation. Fertil Steril. 2014;102(5):1491–8. e1491.
64. Pacchiarotti J, Ramos T, Howerton K, Greilach S, Zaragoza K, Olmstead M, Izadyar F. Developing a clinical-grade cryopreservation protocol for human testicular tissue and cells. BioMed Res Int. 2013;2013:10.
65. Valli H, Gassei K, Orwig KE. Stem cell therapies for male infertility: where are we now and where are we going? In: Carrell DT, Schlegel PN, Racowsky C, Gianaroli L, editors. Biennial review of infertility, vol. 4. Switzerland: Springer International Publishing; 2015. p. 17–39.
66. Wyns C, Curaba M, Martinez-Madrid B, Van Langendonckt A, Francois-Xavier W, Donnez J. Spermatogonial survival after cryopreservation and short-term orthotopic immature human cryptorchid testicular tissue grafting to immunodeficient mice. Hum Reprod. 2007;22(6):1603–11.
67. Keros V, Rosenlund B, Hultenby K, Aghajanova L, Levkov L, Hovatta O. Optimizing cryopreservation of human testicular tissue: comparison of protocols with glycerol, propanediol and dimethylsulphoxide as cryoprotectants. Hum Reprod. 2005;20(6):1676–87.
68. Kvist K, Thorup J, Byskov AG, Hoyer PE, Mollgard K, Yding AC. Cryopreservation of intact testicular tissue from boys with cryptorchidism. Hum Reprod. 2006;21(2):484–91.
69. Brook PF, Radford JA, Shalet SM, Joyce AD, Gosden RG. Isolation of germ cells from human testicular tissue for low temperature storage and autotransplantation. Fertil Steril. 2001;75(2):269–74.
70. Unni S, Kasiviswanathan S, D'Souza S, Khavale S, Mukherjee S, Patwardhan S, Bhartiya D. Efficient cryopreservation of testicular tissue: effect of age, sample state, and concentration of cryoprotectant. Fertil Steril. 2012;97(1):200–8. e201.
71. Baert Y, Van Saen D, Haentjens P, In't Veld P, Tournaye H, Goossens E. What is the best cryopreservation protocol for human testicular tissue banking? Hum Reprod. 2013;28:1816–26.
72. Curaba M, Poels J, van Langendonckt A, Donnez J, Wyns C. Can prepubertal human testicular tissue be cryopreserved by vitrification? Fertil Steril. 2011;95(6):2123.e2129–12.
73. Poels J, Van Langendonckt A, Many MC, Wese FX, Wyns C. Vitrification preserves proliferation capacity in human spermatogonia. Hum Reprod. 2013;28(3):578–89.
74. Sa R, Cremades N, Malheiro I, Sousa M. Cryopreservation of human testicular diploid germ cell suspensions. Andrologia. 2012;44(6):366–72.
75. Brinster RL, Zimmermann JW. Spermatogenesis following male germ-cell transplantation. Proc Natl Acad Sci U S A. 1994;91(24):11298–302.
76. Brinster RL, Avarbock MR. Germline transmission of donor haplotype following spermatogonial transplantation. Proc Natl Acad Sci U S A. 1994;91(24):11303–7.
77. Ogawa T, Dobrinski I, Avarbock MR, Brinster RL. Transplantation of male germ line stem cells restores fertility in infertile mice. Nat Med. 2000;6(1):29–34.
78. Shinohara T, Orwig KE, Avarbock MR, Brinster RL. Remodeling of the postnatal mouse testis is accompanied by dramatic changes in stem cell number and niche accessibility. Proc Natl Acad Sci U S A. 2001;98(11):6186–91.
79. Nagano M, Brinster CJ, Orwig KE, Ryu BY, Avarbock MR, Brinster RL. Transgenic mice produced by retroviral transduction of male germ-line stem cells. Proc Natl Acad Sci U S A. 2001;98(23):13090–5.
80. Brinster CJ, Ryu BY, Avarbock MR, Karagenc L, Brinster RL, Orwig KE. Restoration of fertility by germ cell transplantation requires effective recipient preparation. Biol Reprod. 2003;69(2):412–20.

81. Honaramooz A, Behboodi E, Megee SO, Overton SA, Galantino-Homer H, Echelard Y, Dobrinski I. Fertility and germline transmission of donor haplotype following germ cell transplantation in immunocompetent goats. Biol Reprod. 2003;69(4):1260–4.
82. Mikkola M, Sironen A, Kopp C, Taponen J, Sukura A, Vilkki J, Katila T, Andersson M. Transplantation of normal boar testicular cells resulted in complete focal spermatogenesis in a boar affected by the immotile short-tail sperm defect. Reprod Domest Anim (Zuchthygiene). 2006;41(2):124–8.
83. Kim Y, Turner D, Nelson J, Dobrinski I, McEntee M, Travis AJ. Production of donor-derived sperm after spermatogonial stem cell transplantation in the dog. Reproduction. 2008;136(6):823–31.
84. Herrid M, Olejnik J, Jackson M, Suchowerska N, Stockwell S, Davey R, Hutton K, Hope S, Hill JR. Irradiation enhances the efficiency of testicular germ cell transplantation in sheep. Biol Reprod. 2009;81(5):898–905.
85. Hermann BP, Sukhwani M, Winkler F, Pascarella JN, Peters KA, Sheng Y, Valli H, Rodriguez M, Ezzelarab M, Dargo G, Peterson K, Masterson K, Ramsey C, Ward T, Lienesch M, Volk A, Cooper DK, Thomson AW, Kiss JE, Penedo MC, Schatten GP, Mitalipov S, Orwig KE. Spermatogonial stem cell transplantation into rhesus testes regenerates spermatogenesis producing functional sperm. Cell Stem Cell. 2012;11(5):715–26.
86. Izadyar F, Den Ouden K, Stout TA, Stout J, Coret J, Lankveld DP, Spoormakers TJ, Colenbrander B, Oldenbroek JK, Van der Ploeg KD, Woelders H, Kal HB, De Rooij DG. Autologous and homologous transplantation of bovine spermatogonial stem cells. Reproduction. 2003;126(6):765–74.
87. Schlatt S, Foppiani L, Rolf C, Weinbauer GF, Nieschlag E. Germ cell transplantation into X-irradiated monkey testes. Hum Reprod. 2002;17(1):55–62.
88. Jahnukainen K, Ehmcke J, Quader MA, Saiful Huq M, Epperly MW, Hergenrother S, Nurmio M, Schlatt S. Testicular recovery after irradiation differs in prepubertal and pubertal non-human primates, and can be enhanced by autologous germ cell transplantation. Hum Reprod. 2011;26(8):1945–54.
89. Ryu BY, Orwig KE, Avarbock MR, Brinster RL. Stem cell and niche development in the postnatal rat testis. Dev Biol. 2003;263(2):253–63.
90. Dobrinski I, Avarbock MR, Brinster RL. Transplantation of germ cells from rabbits and dogs into mouse testes. Biol Reprod. 1999;61(5):1331–9.
91. Dobrinski I, Avarbock MR, Brinster RL. Germ cell transplantation from large domestic animals into mouse testes. Mol Reprod Dev. 2000;57(3):270–9.
92. Radford JA, Shalet SM, Lieberman BA. Fertility after treatment for cancer. BMJ. 1999;319(7215):935–6.
93. Radford J. Restoration of fertility after treatment for cancer. Horm Res. 2003;59 Suppl 1:21–3.
94. Valli H, Sukhwani M, Dovey SL, Peters KA, Donohue J, Castro CA, Chu T, Marshall GR, Orwig KE. Fluorescence- and magnetic-activated cell sorting strategies to isolate and enrich human spermatogonial stem cells. Fertil Steril. 2014;102(2):566–80.
95. Hamra FK, Chapman KM, Nguyen DM, Williams-Stephens AA, Hammer RE, Garbers DL. Self renewal, expansion, and transfection of rat spermatogonial stem cells in culture. Proc Natl Acad Sci U S A. 2005;102(48):17430–5.
96. Richardson TE, Chapman KM, Tenenhaus Dann C, Hammer RE, Hamra FK. Sterile testis complementation with spermatogonial lines restores fertility to DAZL-deficient rats and maximizes donor germline transmission. PLoS ONE. 2009;4(7):e6308.
97. Ryu BY, Kubota H, Avarbock MR, Brinster RL. Conservation of spermatogonial stem cell self-renewal signaling between mouse and rat. Proc Natl Acad Sci U S A. 2005;102(40):14302–7.
98. Kanatsu-Shinohara M, Ogonuki N, Inoue K, Miki H, Ogura A, Toyokuni S, Shinohara T. Long-term proliferation in culture and germline transmission of mouse male germline stem cells. Biol Reprod. 2003;69(2):612–6.
99. Kubota H, Avarbock MR, Brinster RL. Growth factors essential for self-renewal and expansion of mouse spermatogonial stem cells. Proc Natl Acad Sci U S A. 2004;101(47):16489–94.

100. Kanatsu-Shinohara M, Muneto T, Lee J, Takenaka M, Chuma S, Nakatsuji N, Horiuchi T, Shinohara T. Long-term culture of male germline stem cells from hamster testes. Biol Reprod. 2008;78(4):611–7.

101. Wu X, Schmidt JA, Avarbock MR, Tobias JW, Carlson CA, Kolon TF, Ginsberg JP, Brinster RL. Prepubertal human spermatogonia and mouse gonocytes share conserved gene expression of germline stem cell regulatory molecules. Proc Natl Acad Sci U S A. 2009;106(51):21672–7.

102. He Z, Kokkinaki M, Jiang J, Dobrinski I, Dym M. Isolation, characterization, and culture of human spermatogonia. Biol Reprod. 2010;82(2):363–72.

103. Mirzapour T, Movahedin M, Tengku Ibrahim TA, Koruji M, Haron AW, Nowroozi MR, Rafieian SH. Effects of basic fibroblast growth factor and leukaemia inhibitory factor on proliferation and short-term culture of human spermatogonial stem cells. Andrologia. 2012;44:41–55.

104. Chen B, Wang YB, Zhang ZL, Xia WL, Wang HX, Xiang ZQ, Hu K, Han YF, Wang YX, Huang YR, Wang Z. Xeno-free culture of human spermatogonial stem cells supported by human embryonic stem cell-derived fibroblast-like cells. Asian J Androl. 2009;11(5):557–65.

105. Kokkinaki M, Djourabtchi A, Golestaneh N. Long-term culture of human SSEA-4 positive spermatogonial stem cells (SSCs). J Stem Cell Res Ther. 2011;2(2):pii: 2488.

106. Liu S, Tang Z, Xiong T, Tang W. Isolation and characterization of human spermatogonial stem cells. Reprod Biol Endocrinol RB&E. 2011;9:141.

107. Smith JF, Yango P, Altman E, Choudhry S, Poelzl A, Zamah AM, Rosen M, Klatsky PC, Tran ND. Testicular niche required for human spermatogonial stem cell expansion. Stem Cells Transl Med. 2014;3(9):1043–54.

108. Nowroozi MR, Ahmadi H, Rafiian S, Mirzapour T, Movahedin M. In vitro colonization of human spermatogonia stem cells: effect of patient's clinical characteristics and testicular histologic findings. Urology. 2011;78(5):1075–81.

109. Piravar Z, Jeddi-Tehrani M, Sadeghi MR, Mohazzab A, Eidi A, Akhondi MM. In vitro culture of human testicular stem cells on feeder-free condition. J Reprod Infertility. 2013;14(1):17–22.

110. Kim TH, Hargreaves HK, Brynes RK, Hawkins HK, Lui VK, Woodard J, Ragab AH. Pretreatment testicular biopsy in childhood acute lymphocytic leukaemia. Lancet. 1981;2(8248):657–8.

111. Jahnukainen K, Hou M, Petersen C, Setchell B, Soder O. Intratesticular transplantation of testicular cells from leukemic rats causes transmission of leukemia. Cancer Res. 2001;61(2):706–10.

112. Izadyar F, Wong J, Maki C, Pacchiarotti J, Ramos T, Howerton K, Yuen C, Greilach S, Zhao HH, Chow M, Chow YC, Rao J, Barritt J, Bar-Chama N, Copperman A. Identification and characterization of repopulating spermatogonial stem cells from the adult human testis. Hum Reprod. 2011;26(6):1296–306.

113. Zohni K, Zhang X, Tan SL, Chan P, Nagano M. CD9 is expressed on human male germ cells that have a long-term repopulation potential after transplantation into mouse testes. Biol Reprod. 2012;87(2):27.

114. Dovey SL, Valli H, Hermann BP, Sukhwani M, Donohue J, Castro CA, Chu T, Sanfilippo JS, Orwig KE. Eliminating malignant contamination from therapeutic human spermatogonial stem cells. J Clin Invest. 2013;123(4):1833–43.

115. Fujita K, Ohta H, Tsujimura A, Takao T, Miyagawa Y, Takada S, Matsumiya K, Wakayama T, Okuyama A. Transplantation of spermatogonial stem cells isolated from leukemic mice restores fertility without inducing leukemia. J Clin Investig. 2005;115(7):1855–61.

116. Fujita K, Tsujimura A, Miyagawa Y, Kiuchi H, Matsuoka Y, Takao T, Takada S, Nonomura N, Okuyama A. Isolation of germ cells from leukemia and lymphoma cells in a human in vitro model: potential clinical application for restoring human fertility after anticancer therapy. Cancer Res. 2006;66(23):11166–71.

117. Hou M, Andersson M, Zheng C, Sundblad A, Soder O, Jahnukainen K. Decontamination of leukemic cells and enrichment of germ cells from testicular samples from rats with Roser's T-cell leukemia by flow cytometric sorting. Reproduction. 2007;134(6):767–79.

118. Hermann BP, Sukhwani M, Salati J, Sheng Y, Chu T, Orwig KE. Separating spermatogonia from cancer cells in contaminated prepubertal primate testis cell suspensions. Hum Reprod. 2011;26(12):3222–31.

119. Geens M, Van de Velde H, De Block G, Goossens E, Van Steirteghem A, Tournaye H. The efficiency of magnetic-activated cell sorting and fluorescence-activated cell sorting in the decontamination of testicular cell suspensions in cancer patients. Hum Reprod. 2007;22(3):733–42.

120. Dolmans MM, Marinescu C, Saussoy P, Van Langendonckt A, Amorim C, Donnez J. Reimplantation of cryopreserved ovarian tissue from patients with acute lymphoblastic leukemia is potentially unsafe. Blood. 2010;116(16):2908–14.

121. Rosendahl M, Andersen MT, Ralfkiaer E, Kjeldsen L, Andersen MK, Andersen CY. Evidence of residual disease in cryopreserved ovarian cortex from female patients with leukemia. Fertil Steril. 2010;94(6):2186–90.

122. Dufour JM, Rajotte RV, Korbutt GS. Development of an in vivo model to study testicular morphogenesis. J Androl. 2002;23(5):635–44.

123. Gassei K, Schlatt S, Ehmcke J. De novo morphogenesis of seminiferous tubules from dissociated immature rat testicular cells in xenografts. J Androl. 2006;27(4):611–8.

124. Kita K, Watanabe T, Ohsaka K, Hayashi H, Kubota Y, Nagashima Y, Aoki I, Taniguchi H, Noce T, Inoue K, Miki H, Ogonuki N, Tanaka H, Ogura A, Ogawa T. Production of functional spermatids from mouse germline stem cells in ectopically reconstituted seminiferous tubules. Biol Reprod. 2007;76(2):211–7.

125. Honaramooz A, Megee SO, Rathi R, Dobrinski I. Building a testis: formation of functional testis tissue after transplantation of isolated porcine (Sus scrofa) testis cells. Biol Reprod. 2007;76(1):43–7.

126. Arregui L, Rathi R, Megee SO, Honaramooz A, Gomendio M, Roldan ER, Dobrinski I. Xenografting of sheep testis tissue and isolated cells as a model for preservation of genetic material from endangered ungulates. Reproduction. 2008;136(1):85–93.

127. Baert Y, Stukenborg JB, Landreh M, De Kock J, Jornvall H, Soder O, Goossens E. Derivation and characterization of a cytocompatible scaffold from human testis. Hum Reprod. 2015;30(2):256–67.

128. Honaramooz A, Snedaker A, Boiani M, Scholer H, Dobrinski I, Schlatt S. Sperm from neonatal mammalian testes grafted in mice. Nature. 2002;418(6899):778–81.

129. Schlatt S, Honaramooz A, Boiani M, Scholer HR, Dobrinski I. Progeny from sperm obtained after ectopic grafting of neonatal mouse testes. Biol Reprod. 2003;68(6):2331–5.

130. Honaramooz A, Li MW, Penedo MCT, Meyers S, Dobrinski I. Accelerated maturation of primate testis by xenografting into mice. Biol Reprod. 2004;70(5):1500–3.

131. Jamieson SW, Madani MM. The choice of valve protheses*. J Am Coll Cardiol. 2004;44(2):389–90.

132. Andreas M, Wallner S, Ruetzler K, Wiedemann D, Ehrlich M, Heinze G, Binder T, Moritz A, Hiesmayr MJ, Kocher A, Laufer G. Comparable long-term results for porcine and pericardial prostheses after isolated aortic valve replacement. Eur J Cardiothorac Surg. 2014;18:2014.

133. Cozzi E, White DJ. The generation of transgenic pigs as potential organ donors for humans. Nat Med. 1995;1(9):964–6.

134. Kimsa MC, Strzalka-Mrozik B, Kimsa MW, Gola J, Nicholson P, Lopata K, Mazurek U. Porcine endogenous retroviruses in xenotransplantation—molecular aspects. Viruses. 2014;6(5):2062–83.

135. Weiss RA. The discovery of endogenous retroviruses. Retrovirology. 2006;3:67.

136. Geens M, De Block G, Goossens E, Frederickx V, Van Steirteghem A, Tournaye H. Spermatogonial survival after grafting human testicular tissue to immunodeficient mice. Hum Reprod. 2006;21(2):390–6.

137. Goossens E, Geens M, De Block G, Tournaye H. Spermatogonial survival in long-term human prepubertal xenografts. Fertil Steril. 2008;90(5):2019–22.

138. Van Saen D, Goossens E, Bourgain C, Ferster A, Tournaye H. Meiotic activity in orthotopic xenografts derived from human postpubertal testicular tissue. Hum Reprod. 2011;26(2): 282–93.

139. Schlatt S, Honaramooz A, Ehmcke J, Goebell PJ, Rubben H, Dhir R, Dobrinski I, Patrizio P. Limited survival of adult human testicular tissue as ectopic xenograft. Hum Reprod. 2006;21(2):384–9.

140. Sato Y, Nozawa S, Yoshiike M, Arai M, Sasaki C, Iwamoto T. Xenografting of testicular tissue from an infant human donor results in accelerated testicular maturation. Hum Reprod. 2010;25(5):1113–22.

141. Wyns C, Van Langendonckt A, Wese FX, Donnez J, Curaba M. Long-term spermatogonial survival in cryopreserved and xenografted immature human testicular tissue. Hum Reprod. 2008;23(11):2402–14.

142. Luetjens CM, Stukenborg J-B, Nieschlag E, Simoni M, Wistuba J. Complete spermatogenesis in orthotopic but not in ectopic transplants of autologously grafted marmoset testicular tissue. Endocrinology. 2008;149(4):1736–47.

143. Sato T, Katagiri K, Gohbara A, Inoue K, Ogonuki N, Ogura A, Kubota Y, Ogawa T. In vitro production of functional sperm in cultured neonatal mouse testes. Nature. 2011; 471(7339):504–7.

144. Sato T, Katagiri K, Kubota Y, Ogawa T. In vitro sperm production from mouse spermatogonial stem cell lines using an organ culture method. Nat Protoc. 2013;8(11):2098–104.

145. Hayashi K, Ohta H, Kurimoto K, Aramaki S, Saitou M. Reconstitution of the mouse germ cell specification pathway in culture by pluripotent stem cells. Cell. 2011;146(4):519–32.

146. Sasaki K, Yokobayashi S, Nakamura T, Okamoto I, Yabuta Y, Kurimoto K, Ohta H, Moritoki Y, Iwatani C, Tsuchiya H, Nakamura S, Sekiguchi K, Sakuma T, Yamamoto T, Mori T, Woltjen K, Nakagawa M, Yamamoto T, Takahashi K, Yamanaka S, Saitou M. Robust in vitro induction of human germ cell fate from pluripotent stem cells. Cell Stem Cell. 2015;17(2):178–94.

147. Irie N, Weinberger L, Tang WW, Kobayashi T, Viukov S, Manor YS, Dietmann S, Hanna JH, Surani MA. SOX17 is a critical specifier of human primordial germ cell fate. Cell. 2015;160(1–2):253–68.

148. Teramura T, Takehara T, Kawata N, Fujinami N, Mitani T, Takenoshita M, Matsumoto K, Saeki K, Iritani A, Sagawa N, Hosoi Y. Primate embryonic stem cells proceed to early gametogenesis in vitro. Cloning Stem Cells. 2007;9(2):144–56.

149. Yamauchi K, Hasegawa K, Chuma S, Nakatsuji N, Suemori H. In vitro germ cell differentiation from cynomolgus monkey embryonic stem cells. PLoS ONE. 2009;4(4):e5338.

150. Park TS, Galic Z, Conway AE, Lindgren A, van Handel BJ, Magnusson M, Richter L, Teitell MA, Mikkola HK, Lowry WE, Plath K, Clark AT. Derivation of primordial germ cells from human embryonic and induced pluripotent stem cells is significantly improved by coculture with human fetal gonadal cells. Stem Cells. 2009;27(4):783–95.

151. Easley CA, Phillips BT, McGuire MM, Barringer JM, Valli H, Hermann BP, Simerly CR, Rajkovic A, Miki T, Orwig KE, Schatten GP. Direct differentiation of human pluripotent stem cells into haploid spermatogenic cells. Cell Rep. 2012;2(3):440–6.

152. Kee K, Gonsalves JM, Clark AT, Pera RA. Bone morphogenetic proteins induce germ cell differentiation from human embryonic stem cells. Stem Cells Dev. 2006;15(6):831–7.

153. Kee K, Angeles VT, Flores M, Nguyen HN, Reijo Pera RA. Human DAZL, DAZ and BOULE genes modulate primordial germ-cell and haploid gamete formation. Nature. 2009; 462(7270):222–5.

154. Durruthy Durruthy J, Ramathal C, Sukhwani M, Fang F, Cui J, Orwig KE, Reijo Pera RA. Fate of induced pluripotent stem cells following transplantation to murine seminiferous tubules. Hum Mol Genet. 2014;23(12):3071–84.

155. Ramathal C, Durruthy-Durruthy J, Sukhwani M, Arakaki JE, Turek PJ, Orwig KE, Reijo Pera RA. Fate of iPSCs derived from azoospermic and fertile men following xenotransplantation to murine seminiferous tubules. Cell Rep. 2014;7(4):1284–97.

156. Ramathal C, Angulo B, Sukhwani M, Cui J, Durruthy-Durruthy J, Fang F, Schanes P, Turek PJ, Orwig KE, Reijo Pera R. DDX3Y gene rescue of a Y chromosome AZFa deletion restores germ cell formation and transcriptional programs. Sci Rep. 2015;5:15041.
157. Panula S, Medrano JV, Kee K, Bergstrom R, Nguyen HN, Byers B, Wilson KD, Wu JC, Simon C, Hovatta O, Reijo Pera RA. Human germ cell differentiation from fetal- and adult-derived induced pluripotent stem cells. Hum Mol Genet. 2011;20(4):752–62.
158. Dominguez AA, Chiang HR, Sukhwani M, Orwig KE, Reijo Pera RA. Human germ cell formation in xenotransplants of induced pluripotent stem cells carrying X chromosome aneuploidies. Sci Rep. 2014;4:6432.
159. Easley CA, Simerly CR, Schatten G. Stem cell therapeutic possibilities: future therapeutic options for male-factor and female-factor infertility? Reprod Biomed Online. 2013;27(1):75–80.

Chapter 9
Assessing Testicular Reserve in the Male Oncology Patient

James A. Kashanian and Robert E. Brannigan

Abbreviations

AMH	Anti-Müllerian hormone
ASCO	American Society of Clinical Oncology
DSDs	Disorders of sexual development
FSH	Follicle-stimulating hormone
GnRH	Gonadotropin-releasing hormone
HPG	Hypothalamic-pituitary-gonadal
LH	Luteinizing hormone
WHO	World Health Organization

Overview

Over the past decade, numerous professional organizations have published fertility preservation recommendations that call for the seamless coordination of oncology care with concurrent fertility preservation care. For interested males, the cryopreservation of sperm prior to the initiation of cancer therapy has become an important aspect of comprehensive cancer care. Because fertility preservation is a major concern for many male patients diagnosed with malignancy, it is of utmost importance

J.A. Kashanian, MD (✉)
Weill Cornell Medicine – Urology, Weill Cornell Medical Center,
525 East 68th Street, Starr 900, New York, NY 10065, USA
e-mail: jak9111@med.cornell.edu

R.E. Brannigan, MD
Department of Urology, Northwestern University, Feinberg School of Medicine,
Galter Pavilion, Suite 20-150, 675 North Saint Clair Street, Chicago, IL 60611, USA

© Springer International Publishing Switzerland 2017
T.K. Woodruff, Y.C. Gosiengfiao (eds.), *Pediatric and Adolescent Oncofertility*,
DOI 10.1007/978-3-319-32973-4_9

for healthcare providers to discuss fertility preservation with affected patients as soon as possible after a cancer diagnosis is made.

In its updated guidelines published in 2013, the American Society of Clinical Oncology (ASCO) recommended that all patients should be counseled on the possibility of infertility arising as a consequence of oncology treatments. Additionally, these guidelines call for clinicians to offer early referral to fertility preservation specialists to further discuss these issues and help deliver fertility preservation care if the patient is interested [1].

Despite these guidelines, it is estimated that less than half of male pubertal cancer patients are referred for fertility preservation consultation or sperm cryopreservation. Furthermore, less than half of pediatric oncology specialists are familiar with the ASCO recommendations on fertility preservation. This marked disparity exists despite the fact that published studies demonstrate that one of the biggest regrets male cancer survivors have is not discussing the deleterious reproductive effects of cancer therapy and options for fertility preservation [2].

While some men may permanently lose the ability to produce viable sperm as a result of their cancer therapies, others will, over time, have the return of sperm to the ejaculate. The proper determination of posttreatment fertility is an important aspect of ongoing care and can be a fluid situation changing over weeks, months, and even years. Clinicians must be familiar with the reproductive toxicities associated with various cancer treatment regimens, as these side effects can impact the endocrine system driving male reproduction, the testes in which sperm production occurs, and the excurrent ductal system which is responsible for sperm transport into the female reproductive tract. Finally, clinicians must be capable of accurately counseling patients as they consider their reproduction options.

Normal testicular function is based on an intact hypothalamic-pituitary-gonadal (HPG) axis. The HPG axis drives male sexual development and fertility. This process is initiated by gonadotropin-releasing hormone (GnRH) that is secreted by the hypothalamus in a pulsatile manner. The distinct frequency and amplitude of these pulses directly stimulates luteinizing hormone (LH) and follicle-stimulating hormone (FSH) secretion by the anterior pituitary gland. FSH and LH support testicular Sertoli cell and Leydig cell function, respectively.

Testicular function is comprised of reproductive and androgenic function, and males may have a congenital or acquired defect in reproductive function (spermatogenesis), androgenic function (testosterone), or both. In the assessment of male reproductive and androgenic testicular function, it is important to delineate between primary and secondary causes. Etiologies of primary testicular dysfunction are vast and can include cryptorchidism, disorders of sexual development (DSDs), trauma, infection, iatrogenic causes, and medication use. Cancer therapies, including surgery, chemotherapy, and radiation therapy, can also cause primary testicular failure and adversely affect fertility. Causes of secondary testicular failure can include genetic abnormalities affecting the HPG axis, brain tumors, trauma, and iatrogenic causes. Again, cancer therapies such as surgery, chemotherapy, and radiation therapy can also impact the HPG axis, leading to secondary testicular failure and adversely affecting fertility. The effects of cancer therapy, whether causing primary or secondary testicular failure side effects, occur in a dose-dependent and treatment-dependent manner [3–6]. For example, spermatogenesis is often impacted by chemotherapy in a dose-dependent fashion [3]. A history of chemotherapy is also often associated with an increase in posttreatment gonadotropin (LH and FSH) levels, a sign that the pituitary gland is actively compensating for impaired testicular production of testosterone and sperm, respectively [7]. Likewise, radiation therapy can affect testicular function by potentially damaging both germ cells and Leydig cells. Transient effects on spermatogenesis are common at very low doses (≤2 Gy) of radiation therapy. Cumulative doses >2 Gy can result in transient or even permanent azoospermia [8]. At doses in excess of 20 Gy, Leydig cell testosterone production is commonly affected, with some men developing lasting primary hypogonadism [8].

Biomarkers are, by definition, measurable indicators of a physiological state within an organism. Sensitivity, specificity, low cost, and attainability are hallmark features of an ideal biomarker, including biomarkers to monitor male androgenic and reproductive function [9]. As will be detailed below, numerous biomarkers have been investigated in order to quantify animal and human reproductive function [9]. When assessing testicular reserve in a male cancer survivor, clinicians should keep in mind that the minimum initial evaluation of the patient should include a full medical history, physical examination, and measurement of serum testosterone and FSH levels [10].

Evaluation

A full medical history, including a detailed accounting of all oncology treatments, is the first step in a comprehensive reproductive evaluation of male cancer survivors. Modes of therapy, dosage, and duration of treatment often impact the severity and duration of testicular dysfunction. A complete genitourinary exam is also an essential component of the evaluation of a male cancer survivor. Particular attention should be paid to the patient's overall appearance, with an assessment for clinical signs of low androgen levels. This can include changes such as a decrease in muscle mass and body hair. A breast exam should be conducted to assess for gynecomastia, which is a common sign of hyperestrogenemia. Additionally, a careful scrotal exam should be performed. This includes documentation of the size, consistency, and location of the testicles bilaterally. Assessment for the presence and condition of the epididymis and vas deferens is also important. The clinician should assess these structures meticulously in order to assess for changes that might suggest evidence of inflammation and/or obstruction that can sometimes result in response to the tumor or iatrogenically as an outcome of cancer therapies. While not a foolproof determinant of reproductive potential, testicular size can be a meaningful predictor of testicular function (hormone and sperm production) [11].

Hormones

Serum testosterone and FSH levels are useful in determining reproductive potential and facilitating the differentiation between subtypes of subfertility and infertility [10]. Endocrine abnormalities are highly prevalent in the setting of certain types of cancer. For example, among testicular cancer survivors, half will have at least one abnormality long term in testosterone, LH, or FSH following treatment [7].

FSH acts on testicular Sertoli cells to support spermatogonial proliferation and maturation through meiosis. FSH levels have been shown to be inversely correlated to testicular spermatogenic function and are commonly used as a barometer for spermatogenesis. Schoor et al. published data demonstrating that 89 % of men with nonobstructive azoospermia will have a serum FSH level greater than 7.6 mIU/ml and a testicular long axis of <4.6 cm. These authors also showed that over 90 % of men with normal sperm production will have an FSH in the normal range [12]. Several other groups have critically assessed the role of FSH as a biomarker for spermatogenesis and have reported similar findings. These authors have collectively recommended FSH reference ranges for adult men with the upper limit of normal for FSH being between 7.5 and 7.8 mIU/ml [13, 14]. Since there is minimal diurnal variation in FSH levels, a single level is sufficient to assess spermatogenesis [15].

Occasionally, an oncology patient will be found to have an abnormally low serum FSH level. This can result from tumor involvement with the hypothalamus and/or pituitary gland or cancer treatments (especially radiation therapy or surgical procedures) involving these same structures. For patients affected by abnormally low FSH levels, recombinant FSH (r-FSH) therapy typically results in normalization of FSH levels and restoration of fertility potential.

LH stimulates testicular Leydig cell testosterone production. Serum levels of LH help to delineate if the origin of androgenic testicular failure is secondary to a central cause (low LH) or to a primary testicular cause (normal or increased LH). Sometimes, an oncology patient will be found to have abnormally low serum LH levels. As is the case for low FSH, this can result from tumor involvement with the hypothalamus and/or pituitary gland or cancer treatments involving these same structures. For patients affected by abnormally low LH levels, hCG therapy typically results in normalization of testosterone levels and restoration of fertility potential.

Testosterone is the male sex hormone that stimulates male muscle mass production, hair growth, libido, erections, bone health, and RBC production. Testosterone is also paramount in supporting spermatogenesis [16–18]. LH stimulates testicular Leydig cells to produce testosterone, which has autocrine, paracrine, and endocrine effects. Low levels of testosterone, although not necessarily predictive of spermatogenic failure, can potentiate poor sperm production and low sperm concentrations in the semen. Testosterone levels peak early in the morning, and AM levels are preferred for evaluation purposes. In the setting of post-cancer treatment, the best predictors of low testosterone are increasing patient age and low residual testicular volume <12 cc [19].

Inhibin B is a dimer molecule comprised of alpha and beta subunits and is secreted by Sertoli cells in the testicle. Inhibin B exerts negative feedback on FSH secretion by the anterior pituitary gland, and there is thus an inverse relationship between serum inhibin B and serum FSH levels. Inhibin B levels are positively correlated with testicle volume and sperm concentration. In infertile patients, inhibin B levels are decreased and FSH levels are increased. In general, the more pronounced the degree of spermatogenic impairment and the earlier the state of spermatogenic disruption, the lower the inhibin B level.

In patients with a history of receiving chemotherapy or radiation therapy, inhibin B levels are often diminished [20]. Some investigators postulate that inhibin B and inhibin B/FSH ratios are more sensitive markers of male infertility than FSH levels alone [21]. Others have shown that levels of inhibin B can predict basal and reserve Sertoli cell activity [22]. Despite these findings, inhibin B has a limited role in serving as a marker of spermatogenesis, with conflicting results being reported in the literature. For example, inhibin B levels are not reliable predictors of the presence of some foci of spermatogenesis in men with azoospermia [23]. Because of the inconsistent results, most clinicians do not routinely use serum inhibin B as a marker for predicting spermatogenesis.

Anti-Müllerian hormone (AMH) is another hormone that has garnered attention as a possible reproductive biomarker in males. In females, AMH serves as a biomarker for ovarian reserve. In males, some authors have suggested that this protein may be helpful to determine gonadal function, including FSH activity upon the testicle and androgen action within the testicle [24]. Several studies have specifically investigated the role of AMH as a marker for spermatogenesis [25] and, more specifically, chemotherapy-induced testicular toxicity [26]. To date, AMH has not been found to be a reliable predictor of spermatogenesis in men with infertility, including men with a history of cancer treatments. AMH is thus not routinely used to determine testicular reserve, in contrast to its effective role in determining ovarian reserve.

Estrogen is formed in males by the peripheral aromatization of testosterone in the adipose, brain, skin, and bone tissue. Estrogen's role in spermatogenic maturation is still being delineated. In excess levels, it inhibits GnRH and LH release. At this time, estrogen is not routinely used in the evaluation of testicular reserve following cancer therapy, but it is a lab value often checked in the clinical evaluation of an infertile male. For cancer survivors with obesity, estradiol serum levels should be assessed to ensure that levels are not elevated, which can result in suppression of testosterone production.

Semen Testing

Cryopreservation of sperm prior to the commencement of gonadotoxic cancer treatment is the preferred approach for fertility preservation in males. Sperm banking should be considered for all patients diagnosed with any malignancy, especially males diagnosed with testicular cancer, leukemia, and lymphoma. The importance of sperm cryopreservation is evident in studies revealing that most cancer patients remain interested in future fertility and continue storage of banked sperm even after completion of cancer treatment [27, 28]. Men who cryopreserve sperm are more likely to be young and single compared to those who opt against sperm banking. Additionally, men who bank sperm are more likely to father a child after treatment, whether it be by natural means or IVF [29, 30]. While interest in fertility preservation is high, approximately 10–15% of oncology patients who desire to bank sperm are unable to do so for a variety of reasons, including psychosocial issues, anejaculation, necrospermia, or azoospermia [28, 31]. For these males, sperm can often be surgically extracted from the testicles for cryopreservation. Also, while high percentages of patients opt to bank sperm, there are those men who choose not to do so. Proper reproductive counseling is imperative for these men who decide against sperm cryopreservation before commencing oncologic therapy, as they may put themselves at risk of permanent infertility.

At baseline, before initiation of cancer therapy, patients with certain malignancies may have significantly lower sperm concentration and worse semen quality compared to fertile controls [28, 31, 32]. Six to 11.8% of all oncology patients will be azoospermic at the time of presentation [31, 33–35]. This is in stark contrast to the incidence of azoospermia in the general population, which is 1% [36]. Overall tumor burden and tumor stage are factors that can impact these parameters in some men [37, 38]. Chemotherapeutic regimens can also have an array of effects on spermatogenesis. This can range from no or minimal impact on semen parameters to temporary oligospermia or azoospermia with significant recovery to normospermia [4], to irreversible oligospermia, or to azoospermia [3]. The latter outcome is particularly associated with alkylating agent chemotherapy. Similarly, radiation therapy can also affect quantitative semen characteristics in the short and long term, but semen parameters will often return to baseline by 24 months after treatment [32]. The ultimate effects on spermatogenesis, however, depend largely on the dose and location of radiation therapy being delivered. Bujan et al. demonstrated that 6% of men remained azoospermic at 12 months and 2% at 24 months following radiation therapy for testicular cancer [32].

Unlike in females, where ovarian reserve is established in utero and declines over time, spermatogenesis commences at puberty and continues throughout life. Because of this, the semen analysis is currently the gold standard for assessing fertility status in the male. This test is readily available at most tertiary care centers and can be performed at any age after puberty. Semen analysis testing is an easy, cost-effective, and noninvasive mode of determining fertility potential in the male. Important parameters that comprise a formal semen analysis include the semen volume, sperm concentration, sperm motility, and sperm morphology.

In 2010 the World Health Organization (WHO) published the fifth edition of the *Laboratory Manual for the Examination and Processing of Human Semen*. Normal reference ranges were based on semen parameters of men whose partners became pregnant within 12 months of trying to conceive. Cutoffs above the fifth percentile

Table 9.1 Bulk semen parameters

	WHO fourth edition	WHO fifth edition
Volume	≥ 2.0 ml	≥ 1.5 ml
Sperm concentration	≥ 20 million sperm per ml	≥ 15 million sperm per ml
Sperm motility	$\geq 50\%$ total motility	$\geq 40\%$ total motility
Sperm morphology	$\geq 14\%$ normal forms	$>4\%$ normal forms
White blood cells	$\leq 1.0 \times 10^6$ per ml	$<1.0 \times 10^6$ per ml

were considered normal [39]. Table 9.1 represents normal reference ranges of bulk semen parameters for the WHO IV and WHO V editions.

Although these values are all taken into account when discussing male fertility, there is no algorithm available to reliably predict future fertility in men based on varying levels of sperm concentration, motility, and morphology. Calculations of the total sperm count, total motile sperm count, and morphology cutoffs have all been fraught with inaccuracy in predicting absolute fertility potential.

Future Direction

In this evolving age of personalized medicine, increasing attention has been focused on the genetics of male fertility. As in other disease states, biomarkers are frequently used for diagnosis and stratification, treatment selection, monitoring of disease progression, and establishing patients' responses to therapy [40]. Although semen analysis testing is still recognized as a surrogate marker of male fertility, the exponential growth of biomarkers derived from proteomics, epigenomics, and genomics has contributed to a new direction of male fertility research. This shift in investigative focus could prove to be the next frontier in directed personalized medicine. However, although many studies have evaluated the genetic basis of male fertility, basic science and translational research have not resulted in a wealth of clinically useful diagnostic tests. Ideally, insights would be gained into genetic susceptibility to various cancer therapies, as well as propensity of an individual to regain reproductive function after completion of cancer treatment.

More than 3,000 genes (about 4% of human genome) are expressed in the testicles alone, and hundreds of these genes influence reproductive function in humans [41]. Additionally, there are over 4,000 proteins expressed in the seminal plasma. Because of this, significant attention has been focused on the proteomes of the testicles, sperm, seminal fluid, and epididymis [42]. It is thought that these proteins might represent a rich source of potential biomarkers for male fertility [43], and characterization of the reproductive proteome might ultimately lead to significant improvement in the evaluation of the male reproductive tract [44, 45].

This enhanced understanding of fertility markers at the level of the individual might facilitate the development of more comprehensive prognostic models for patients. The benefit of this approach would be potentially enhanced diagnostic capabilities, reduced cost, and personalized fertility treatments that anticipate reproductive success at baseline (before cancer treatment) and post-cancer therapy. This field is still quite young, and it is estimated that more than 1,000 biomarkers would be needed to accurately evaluate male fertility potential [46]. Although much more clinical insight is needed, the implications of a more personalized approach to infertility risk stratification would be an enormously useful tool for clinicians and patients alike.

In conclusion, a serum testosterone level, a serum FSH level, and a semen analysis are currently the most robust biomarkers for assessing testicular reserve in the male cancer survivor. As the era of "personalized medicine" progresses, panels of biomarkers that stratify baseline fertility potential and posttreatment infertility risk will facilitate clinical decision-making for both healthcare providers and their patients.

References

1. Loren AW, Mangu PB, Beck LN, Brennan L, Magdalinski AJ, Partridge AH, et al. Fertility preservation for patients with cancer: American Society of Clinical Oncology clinical practice guideline update. J Clin Oncol Off J Am Soc Clin Oncol. 2013;31(19):2500–10.
2. Stein DM, Victorson DE, Choy JT, Waimey KE, Pearman TP, Smith K, et al. Fertility preservation preferences and perspectives among adult male survivors of pediatric cancer and their parents. J Adolesc Young Adult Oncol. 2014;3(2):75–82.
3. Green DM, Liu W, Kutteh WH, Ke RW, Shelton KC, Sklar CA, et al. Cumulative alkylating agent exposure and semen parameters in adult survivors of childhood cancer: a report from the St Jude Lifetime Cohort Study. Lancet Oncol. 2014;15(11):1215–23.
4. Howell SJ, Shalet SM. Testicular function following chemotherapy. Hum Reprod Update. 2001;7(4):363–9.
5. De Mas P, Daudin M, Vincent MC, Bourrouillou G, Calvas P, Mieusset R, et al. Increased aneuploidy in spermatozoa from testicular tumour patients after chemotherapy with cisplatin, etoposide and bleomycin. Hum Reprod (Oxford, Engl). 2001;16(6):1204–8.
6. Stahl O, Eberhard J, Cavallin-Stahl E, Jepson K, Friberg B, Tingsmark C, et al. Sperm DNA integrity in cancer patients: the effect of disease and treatment. Int J Androl. 2009;32(6):695–703.
7. Sprauten M, Brydoy M, Haugnes HS, Cvancarova M, Bjoro T, Bjerner J, et al. Longitudinal serum testosterone, luteinizing hormone, and follicle-stimulating hormone levels in a population-based sample of long-term testicular cancer survivors. J Clin Oncol Off J Am Soc Clin Oncol. 2014;32(6):571–8.
8. Shalet SM. Effect of irradiation treatment on gonadal function in men treated for germ cell cancer. Eur Urol. 1993;23(1):148–51. discussion 52.
9. Dere E, Anderson LM, Hwang K, Boekelheide K. Biomarkers of chemotherapy-induced testicular damage. Fertil Steril. 2013;100(5):1192–202.
10. The optimal evaluation of the infertile male: best practice statement. American Urological Association. Reviewed and validity confirmed 2011.
11. Bahk JY, Jung JH, Jin LM, Min SK. Cut-off value of testes volume in young adults and correlation among testes volume, body mass index, hormonal level, and seminal profiles. Urology. 2010;75(6):1318–23.
12. Schoor RA, Elhanbly S, Niederberger CS, Ross LS. The role of testicular biopsy in the modern management of male infertility. J Urol. 2002;167(1):197–200.

13. Barbotin AL, Ballot C, Sigala J, Ramdane N, Duhamel A, Marcelli F, et al. The serum inhibin B concentration and reference ranges in normozoospermia. Eur J Endocrinol/Eur Fed Endocr Soc. 2015;172(6):669–76.
14. Gordetsky J, van Wijngaarden E, O'Brien J. Redefining abnormal follicle-stimulating hormone in the male infertility population. BJU Int. 2012;110(4):568–72.
15. Spratt DI, O'Dea LS, Schoenfeld D, Butler J, Rao PN, Crowley Jr WF. Neuroendocrine-gonadal axis in men: frequent sampling of LH, FSH, and testosterone. Am J Phys. 1988;254(5 Pt 1):E658–66.
16. Huang HF, Boccabella AV. Dissociation of qualitative and quantitative effects of the suppression of testicular testosterone upon spermatogenesis. Acta Endocrinol. 1988;118(2):209–17.
17. Jarow JP, Zirkin BR. The androgen microenvironment of the human testis and hormonal control of spermatogenesis. Ann N Y Acad Sci. 2005;1061:208–20.
18. Tsai MY, Yeh SD, Wang RS, Yeh S, Zhang C, Lin HY, et al. Differential effects of spermatogenesis and fertility in mice lacking androgen receptor in individual testis cells. Proc Natl Acad Sci U S A. 2006;103(50):18975–80.
19. Puhse G, Secker A, Kemper S, Hertle L, Kliesch S. Testosterone deficiency in testicular germ-cell cancer patients is not influenced by oncological treatment. Int J Androl. 2011;34(5 Pt 2):e351–7.
20. Marchetti C, Hamdane M, Mitchell V, Mayo K, Devisme L, Rigot JM, et al. Immunolocalization of inhibin and activin alpha and betaB subunits and expression of corresponding messenger RNAs in the human adult testis. Biol Reprod. 2003;68(1):230–5.
21. Grunewald S, Glander HJ, Paasch U, Kratzsch J. Age-dependent inhibin B concentration in relation to FSH and semen sample qualities: a study in 2448 men. Reproduction (Cambridge, England). 2013;145(3):237–44.
22. Adamopoulos D, Kapolla N, Nicopoulou S, Pappa A, Koukkou E, Gregoriou A. Assessment of Sertoli cell functional reserve and its relationship to sperm parameters. Int J Androl. 2003;26(4):215–25.
23. Tunc L, Kirac M, Gurocak S, Yucel A, Kupeli B, Alkibay T, et al. Can serum Inhibin B and FSH levels, testicular histology and volume predict the outcome of testicular sperm extraction in patients with non-obstructive azoospermia? Int Urol Nephrol. 2006;38(3–4):629–35.
24. Grinspon RP, Rey RA. New perspectives in the diagnosis of pediatric male hypogonadism: the importance of AMH as a Sertoli cell marker. Arq Bras Endocrinol Metabologia. 2011;55(8):512–9.
25. Tuttelmann F, Dykstra N, Themmen AP, Visser JA, Nieschlag E, Simoni M. Anti-Mullerian hormone in men with normal and reduced sperm concentration and men with maldescended testes. Fertil Steril. 2009;91(5):1812–9.
26. Levi M, Hasky N, Stemmer SM, Shalgi R, Ben-Aharon I. Anti-Mullerian hormone is a marker for chemotherapy-induced testicular toxicity. Endocrinology. 2015;156:3818–27. en20151310.
27. Johnson MD, Cooper AR, Jungheim ES, Lanzendorf SE, Odem RR, Ratts VS. Sperm banking for fertility preservation: a 20-year experience. Eur J Obstet Gynecol Reprod Biol. 2013;170(1):177–82.
28. Bizet P, Saias-Magnan J, Jouve E, Grillo JM, Karsenty G, Metzler-Guillemain C, et al. Sperm cryopreservation before cancer treatment: a 15-year monocentric experience. Reprod Biomed Online. 2012;24(3):321–30.
29. Girasole CR, Cookson MS, Smith Jr JA, Ivey BS, Roth BJ, Chang SS. Sperm banking: use and outcomes in patients treated for testicular cancer. BJU Int. 2007;99(1):33–6.
30. Pacey A, Merrick H, Arden-Close E, Morris K, Rowe R, Stark D, et al. Implications of sperm banking for health-related quality of life up to 1 year after cancer diagnosis. Br J Cancer. 2013;108(5):1004–11.
31. van Casteren NJ, Boellaard WP, Romijn JC, Dohle GR. Gonadal dysfunction in male cancer patients before cytotoxic treatment. Int J Androl. 2010;33(1):73–9.
32. Bujan L, Walschaerts M, Moinard N, Hennebicq S, Saias J, Brugnon F, et al. Impact of chemotherapy and radiotherapy for testicular germ cell tumors on spermatogenesis and sperm DNA: a multicenter prospective study from the CECOS network. Fertil Steril. 2013;100(3):673–80.

33. Crha I, Ventruba P, Zakova J, Huser M, Kubesova B, Hudecek R, et al. Survival and infertility treatment in male cancer patients after sperm banking. Fertil Steril. 2009;91(6):2344–8.
34. Molnar Z, Benyo M, Bazsane Kassai Z, Levai I, Varga A, Jakab A. Influence of malignant tumors occurring in the reproductive age on spermiogenesis: studies on patients with testicular tumor and lymphoma. Orv Hetil. 2014;155(33):1306–11.
35. Zakova J, Lousova E, Ventruba P, Crha I, Pochopova H, Vinklarkova J, et al. Sperm cryopreservation before testicular cancer treatment and its subsequent utilization for the treatment of infertility. TheScientificWorldJournal. 2014;2014:575978.
36. Gangel EK, American Urological Association Inc, American Society for Reproductive Medicine. AUA and ASRM produce recommendations for male infertility. American Urological Association, Inc and American Society for Reproductive Medicine. Am Fam Physician. 2002;65(12):2589–90.
37. Smit M, van Casteren NJ, Wildhagen MF, Romijn JC, Dohle GR. Sperm DNA integrity in cancer patients before and after cytotoxic treatment. Hum Reprod (Oxford, Engl). 2010;25(8):1877–83.
38. Gandini L, Lombardo F, Salacone P, Paoli D, Anselmo AP, Culasso F, et al. Testicular cancer and Hodgkin's disease: evaluation of semen quality. Hum Reprod (Oxford, Engl). 2003;18(4):796–801.
39. World Health Organization. WHO laboratory manual for the examination and processing of human semen. 5th ed. Geneva: World Health Organization; 2010. xiv, 271 p. p.
40. Plebani M. Proteomics: the next revolution in laboratory medicine? Clin Chim Acta Int J Clin Chem. 2005;357(2):113–22.
41. Zorrilla M, Yatsenko AN. The genetics of infertility: current status of the field. Curr Genet Med Rep. 2013;1(4):1–22.
42. Upadhyay RD, Balasinor NH, Kumar AV, Sachdeva G, Parte P, Dumasia K. Proteomics in reproductive biology: beacon for unraveling the molecular complexities. Biochim Biophys Acta. 2013;1834(1):8–15.
43. Gilany K, Minai-Tehrani A, Savadi-Shiraz E, Rezadoost H, Lakpour N. Exploring the human seminal plasma proteome: an unexplored gold mine of biomarker for male infertility and male reproduction disorder. J Reprod Infertility. 2015;16(2):61–71.
44. Kolialexi A, Mavrou A, Spyrou G, Tsangaris GT. Mass spectrometry-based proteomics in reproductive medicine. Mass Spectrom Rev. 2008;27(6):624–34.
45. Fernandez-Encinas A, Garcia-Peiro A, Ribas-Maynou J, Abad C, Amengual MJ, Navarro J, et al. Characterization of nuclease activity in human seminal plasma and its relationship with semen parameters, sperm DNA fragmentation and male infertility. J Urol. 2016;195(1):213–9.
46. Zhu WB, Long XY, Fan LQ. Male fecundity prognosis and infertility diagnosis in the era of personalised medicine. Asian J Androl. 2010;12(4):463–7.

Chapter 10
Male Sexuality

Brooke Cherven, Linda Ballard, Chad Ritenour, and Lillian Meacham

Sexuality includes both physical and emotional components, has influences from societal norms and values, and plays a role in quality of life. Disorders of male sexual function have been attributed to many etiologic categories. In the mid- to late 1900s, male sexual dysfunction was thought to be primarily of psychogenic origin. Subsequently, perhaps in part due to a focus on medical and surgical interventions for sexual dysfunction, physiologic causes of sexual dysfunction progressively came into consideration. Now sexual health is realized to be multidimensional and an important contributor to overall health and quality of life. One of the most common forms of male sexual dysfunction, erectile dysfunction, has prevalence ranges from 10 to 55 % in various study populations [1, 2]. The National Health and Social Life Survey (NHSLS) subclassifies sexual dysfunction into problems associated with (1) desire for sex, (2) arousal difficulties, (3) inability to achieve climax or ejaculation, (4) anxiety about sexual performance, (5) climaxing or ejaculating too rapidly, (6) physical pain during intercourse, and (7) not finding sex pleasurable [1]. From this comprehensive definition, it is clear that sexual dysfunction includes physiologic, psychological, and social factors. Publications on sexual dysfunction in survivors of pediatric and adolescent cancer are limited and most focus on the psychosocial dimensions of sexual dysfunction in this population. In a recent publication, one-third of male and half of female survivors of childhood cancer reported problems with sexual function [3].

B. Cherven, MPH, RN, CPON (✉) • L. Ballard, APRN, CPNP
Aflac Cancer and Blood Disorders Center, Children's Healthcare of Atlanta,
Atlanta, GA, USA
e-mail: Brooke.Cherven@choa.org

C. Ritenour, MD
Division of Men's Health/Infertility and General Urology, Department of Urology
Emory University, Atlanta, GA, USA

L. Meacham, MD
Aflac Cancer Center/Children's Healthcare of Atlanta, Pediatrics Emory University,
Atlanta, GA, USA

© Springer International Publishing Switzerland 2017   153
T.K. Woodruff, Y.C. Gosiengfiao (eds.), *Pediatric and Adolescent Oncofertility*,
DOI 10.1007/978-3-319-32973-4_10

Of interest in this study, males were more likely to report sexual symptoms as distressing. In another study of childhood cancer survivors compared to the general population, male survivors but not female survivors reported problems with interest and satisfaction with sex [4]. It is important that male survivors of childhood cancer be educated about, and screened for, potential sexual dysfunction and provided options for treatment, so as to mitigate its impact on quality of life.

Normal Sexual Development and Function

A review the anatomy of the male reproductive system as well as endocrinology and physiology is important in the consideration of sexual function in male survivors of pediatric and adolescent cancer. Sexual differentiation occurs in the fetus at 6–12 weeks gestation. In the presence of hormonally functioning testes, the phallus and scrotum form and the Wolffian ducts emerge while the Mullerian ducts regress. In mid-gestation the hypothalamic-pituitary-testicular axis matures. Gonadotropin-releasing hormone (GnRH) produced in the medial basal hypothalamus is released into the hypophyseal portal circulation and regulates the secretion of luteinizing hormone (LH) and follicle-stimulating hormone (FSH). LH regulates testosterone production from the Leydig cells in the testes, while FSH is important for spermatogenesis. The hypothalamic-pituitary axis is quiescent after a brief burst of activity in early infancy until puberty which begins at age 11.5–12 years in males. As the physical transition from child to adult occurs with the acquisition of secondary sexual characteristics, sexual behaviors also emerge. Although the average age of ejacularche is 13 years, the onset of masturbation and sexual activities with others is modified by social mores, family beliefs, and the individual's health and beliefs.

To understand the pathophysiologic causes of sexual dysfunction, it is important to know the male genitourinary anatomy and normal physiologic functions related to sexual activity [5]. The penis is composed of a single corpus spongiosum surrounding the urethra and paired corpora cavernosa which fill with blood during an erection. The innervation to the penis is through somatic, parasympathetic, and sympathetic nerves. The somatic nerves have both sensory and motor functions. The parasympathetic nerves which arise from the sacral cord at S2 and S4 and traverse the retroperitoneal space as the nervi erigentes signal vasodilation of the corpora, and this initiates an erection. The counterbalancing sympathetic nervous system regulates contraction of the vasa deferentia, seminal vesicles, prostate, and bladder neck during sexual activity which results in emission. In addition, the sympathetic nervous system mediates detumescence.

The male sexual response has been divided into various stages and substages which can be summarized into the following: desire or libido, erection, emission/ejaculation, and detumescence [6–9]. Psychological factors, social factors, chronic health conditions, medications, and substance use can alter normal sexual function (Table 10.1). Much is published on disorders of sexual function in the normal adult male population with the bulk of the studies focused on erectile dysfunction. It is

Table 10.1 Male sexual dysfunction

Dysfunction by the activities of the sexual cycles	Causes of sexual dysfunction
Libido/desire:	Psychogenic
Hypoactive sexual desire	Androgen deficiency
15 % adult men	Major psychological disorders
	Chronic medical conditions
	Drugs (antihypertensives, psychotropics, dopamine blockers)
	Substance abuse (alcohol, narcotics)
Erection/erectile dysfunction:	Psychogenic
12 % in >18 years old	Androgen deficiency
25–50 % in 60–70 years old	Major psychological disorders
52 % in mass male aging study	Chronic medical conditions (diabetes, vascular, cardiac, hepatic, renal, pulmonary cancer)
	Penile disease (Peyronie's disease, congenital malformations)
	Drugs (antihypertensives, anticholinergics, psychotropics)
	Substance abuse (cigarette smoking, alcohol, narcotics)
Ejaculation:	Psychogenic
Premature ejaculation	Poor health status
Prevalence 20 30 %	Sympathetic denervation (diabetes, surgery, or radiation)
Problems of emission or retrograde ejaculation	Drugs (sympatholytic, antihypertensive, MAO inhibitors, CNS depressants, antipsychotics)
	Androgen deficiency
Orgasm:	Psychogenic
Orgasmic dysfunction	Drugs (SSRI, TCA, MAO inhibitors)
Relatively rare – prevalence 3–10 %	Substance abuse
	CNS nervous system disease (multiple sclerosis, Parkinson's disease, Huntington's chorea, lumbar sympathectomy)
Detumescence:	Structural abnormalities (Peyronie's disease, phimosis)
Failure of detumescence (priapism)	Primary priapism (idiopathic)
	Secondary priapism due to disease (sickle cell, amyloidosis, inflammatory, solid tumors, trauma) or due to drugs (phenothiazine, trazodone, cocaine)

estimated that 322 million patients will experience ED by the year 2025 [10]. An overview of male sexual dysfunction in the general population, as well as the limited studies published on survivors of pediatric and adolescent cancer, will be included in this chapter.

Erectile Dysfunction (ED)

Erectile dysfunction has been defined by the NIH as the "persistent inability to attain and maintain an erection sufficient to permit satisfactory sexual performance" [11]. Erectile function is the result of a complex interplay between vascular, neurologic, hormonal, and psychological factors and may significantly impact quality of life. Epidemiological data have shown a high prevalence and incidence of ED worldwide. The first large, community-based study of ED was the Massachusetts Male Aging Study (MMAS) [2]. The study reported an overall prevalence of 52% ED in noninstitutionalized men aged 40–70 years in the Boston area; Furlow reported a rate of 12% in males above age 18 [12], while other surveys reported ranges of 25–30% in men aged 60–70 [13, 14].

Etiology

The pathophysiology of ED may be vascular, neurogenic, anatomical, hormonal, drug induced, and/or psychogenic. ED may also be a result of a mix of etiologies (see Table 10.1). Systemic diseases such as chronic liver, kidney disease, diabetes, or cancer have been associated with ED [5]. Cardiovascular diseases are strongly associated with ED, which may be the complaint that leads to discovery of an underlying diagnosis of hypertension or coronary artery disease. Anatomical disorders include Peyronie's disease, congenital malformations, and genitourinary trauma. Hormonal disorders include hypogonadism and hyperprolactinemia. Medications associated with ED include primarily antihypertensive agents and psychogenic drugs. In addition, the normal aging process has been shown to result in a decrease in sexual responsiveness and is reflected in the increased incidence of complaints of ED in older age groups [2].

Diagnosis

The first step in screening for ED is a detailed sexual and medical history of the patient. Partners, when available, should be included.

Sexual History

The sexual history should include information about previous and current sexual relationships, onset, severity and duration of the erectile problem, and previous consultations and treatments. A detailed description should be made of the rigidity and duration of both sexually stimulated and morning erections and of problems with arousal, ejaculation, and orgasm [15]. Assessment of other areas of sexual dysfunction such as ejaculation, libido, and orgasm should be included in the history. Several patient questionnaires have been developed for assessment of ED, including the Sexual Health Inventory for Men (SHIM) and the International Index of Erectile Function (IIEF) [15]. Either of these questionnaires may be used as an adjunct to diagnosis of ED.

Medical History

Patients with ED should be screened for symptoms of possible hypogonadism, including decreased energy, libido, and fatigue, as well as for symptomatic lower urinary tract infections. Any history of heart disease, hypertension, diabetes mellitus, neurologic disorders, and renal disease should be reviewed. Lifestyle factors that include smoking, obesity, high-fat diet, use of recreational drugs and alcohol, and lack of exercise may be contributing factors. Mental health history and current psychological status are important considerations as depression is a common comorbidity in ED. Medications, including antihypertensive, cardiac, psychotropic, and hypoglycemic agents, are often associated with ED. It may be difficult, however, to separate the medication from the underlying disease as the causative agent of the ED. History of cancer of the pelvic organs, testes, prostate, central nervous system, and spinal tumors and associated treatments including surgery and radiation may contribute to ED.

Physical Examination

The physical examination should be focused on the genitourinary, endocrine, vascular, and neurological systems. The exam may reveal unsuspected diagnoses, such as Peyronie's disease (an acquired, localized fibrotic disorder of the tunica albuginea resulting in penile deformity, mass, and/or pain), or hypogonadism. Signs of hypogonadism include decreased volume and/or turgor of the testes, alterations in secondary sexual characteristics, and gynecomastia. Blood pressure and femoral and peripheral pulses can reflect vascular health. A thorough neurological exam, including visual fields, should be assessed for symptoms of pituitary tumors.

Laboratory Testing

Laboratory testing should be tailored to the patient's complaints and risk factors. Testing may include fasting glucose or HbA1c, urinalysis, blood chemistry panel, and lipid profile. ED may be an early manifestation of coronary artery disease [16]. Concern for associated cardiovascular disease may warrant further investigation and/or referral to a cardiologist. Hormonal tests include a morning sample for a total testosterone. However, the threshold of testosterone to maintain erectile function is low, and ED is usually a symptom of more severe cases of hypogonadism. Additional hormonal tests, such as prolactin and luteinizing hormone, are performed when low testosterone levels are detected. If any abnormality is observed, referral to an endocrinologist may be indicated.

Specialized Diagnostic Tests

While most patients with ED can be diagnosed with a thorough history and physical exam, some patients may need referral to a urologist for specific diagnostic tests. These may include nocturnal penile tumescence and rigidity test, intracavernosal injection test, duplex ultrasound of the penis, arteriography, and dynamic infusion cavernosometry or cavernosography.

Treatment Options

The primary goal in the management strategy of a patient with ED is to determine and treat its underlying etiology when possible. The American Urological Association (AUA) has issued evidence-based guidelines for the diagnosis and treatment of erectile dysfunction [17]. Originally written in 1996, the guidelines have been reviewed and revised in 2005 and 2011 and provide detailed descriptions of recommended strategies for ED management.

ED may be associated with modifiable or reversible risk factors, including lifestyle and/or medications. These factors may be modified either before or in conjunction with specific therapies. Screening for cardiovascular disease must be done prior to treatment, due to the potential risks associated with sexual activity in patients with heart disease [18]. Guidelines developed by the Princeton Consensus Panel [17] describe three levels (high, intermediate, low) of cardiovascular risk factors. Patients in the high and intermediate categories should be evaluated by a cardiologist prior to initiating therapies for ED.

The currently available therapies that should be considered for the treatment of erectile dysfunction include the following: pharmacologic (oral phosphodiesterase type 5 [PDE-5] inhibitors), intraurethral alprostadil, intracavernous vasoactive drug injection, vacuum constriction devices, and penile prosthesis implantation. These appropriate treatment options should be applied in a stepwise fashion with increasing invasiveness and risk balanced against the likelihood of efficacy [17], and referral for management by urology may be appropriate. PDE-5 inhibitors are contraindicated in men taking nitrates and should be used cautiously in men taking alpha-adrenergic blocker medications. The choice of a specific PDE-5 inhibitor (short or long acting) depends on the frequency of intercourse and the patient's personal experience.

Surgical correction may be needed for patients with ED due to penile abnormalities, e.g., hypospadias, congenital curvature, or Peyronie's disease, with preserved rigidity. Endocrine therapy for hypogonadism or hyperprolactinemia is an appropriate intervention for patients with a definite endocrinopathy. Combination therapy of a PDE-5 inhibitor and testosterone may be useful for hypogonadal men who do not respond to PDE-5 therapy alone. Testosterone therapy should be supervised by an endocrinologist and requires close monitoring for side effects (liver, prostate). Testosterone should be used cautiously in patients with unstable cardiac disease or concern for prostate disease [19].

Psychosexual therapy may be useful in combination with both medical and surgical treatment for men with ED. For some patients, brief education, support, and reassurance may be sufficient to restore sexual function, and for others, referral for more specialized and intensive counseling may be necessary.

Ejaculatory Dysfunction

Premature Ejaculation

Premature ejaculation (PE) is a common male sexual dysfunction. Prevalence rates are quite variable ranging from 20 to 30 % in multiple studies of adult males [15, 20], while European studies indicate an approximate prevalence of 5 % [16]. PE can be difficult to define, and few men present for treatment. It is defined in the DSM-VI as persistent or recurrent ejaculation with minimal sexual stimulation that occurs before or shortly after penetration and, importantly, before the person wishes it.

Etiology

The etiology and pathophysiology of PE are unknown. A significant proportion of men with ED also experience PE, and it can be difficult to distinguish between them. Other potential risk factors for PE include a genetic predisposition, poor overall health status and obesity, prostate inflammation, thyroid hormone disorders, emotional problems and stress, and traumatic sexual experiences [16].

Diagnosis

The diagnosis of PE is based on the patient's medical and sexual history. Important criteria include whether PE is situational, such as with a specific partner or certain circumstances, and lifelong or acquired and impact on sexual activity and quality of life for both the patient and partner. Physical exam may assist in identifying associated underlying conditions, such as endocrinopathies and urological disorders.

There are several patient questionnaires for use in diagnosing PE. The most commonly used is the Premature Ejaculation Diagnostic Tool (PEDT) [21].

Treatment

Treatment approaches may include behavioral modification therapies and/or psychotherapy, decrease in sensory input, or controlled use of medications that have delayed ejaculation as part of their side effect profile. Although not approved by the FDA for this indication, oral antidepressants (SSRIs) and topical anesthetic agents have been shown to delay ejaculation in men with PE and have minimal side effects when used for the treatment of PE. Treatment with oral antidepressants should be started at the lowest possible dose that is compatible with a reasonable chance of success. In patients with concomitant PE and ED, the ED should be treated first [20]. Regular follow-up is important to evaluate efficacy and side effects. Support and education of the patient and, when possible, the partner are an integral part of PE therapy [20].

Inhibited Ejaculation

The prevalence of inhibited ejaculation is estimated at 1.5 in 1000 of the general male population [15]. Rates of inhibited ejaculation increase with age, with an overall incidence of 3% in men aged 50–54 years [22]. This disorder may be lifelong or acquired and situational or partner specific and is described as delayed or absent ejaculation.

Etiology

The majority of patients who report inhibited ejaculation have no clear etiology. There is an association with reports of personal or relationship distress and general health issues [15]. Any medical disease, drug, or surgical procedure that interferes with either central (including spinal or supraspinal) control of ejaculation or the autonomic innervation to the seminal tract, including the sympathetic innervation to the seminal vesicles, the prostatic urethra, and the bladder neck, or sensory innervation to the anatomical structures involved in the ejaculation process, can result in delayed ejaculation, anejaculation, and anorgasmia [23]. Specific causes of delayed or absent ejaculation include medications, sympathetic denervation, hormone deficiency, lower urinary tract infections, and spinal cord injury.

Treatment

Treatments include psychosexual counseling, medication therapy or discontinuation of interfering medication, hormone replacement, and vibratory stimulation.

Retrograde Ejaculation (RE)

Etiology

Retrograde ejaculation results from damage to the sympathetic innervation of the ejaculatory system and bladder neck. RE may be caused by anatomic abnormalities such as urethral strictures, bladder neck resection, or fibrosis. Neurologic causes include multiple sclerosis, spinal cord injury, retroperitoneal lymphadenectomy, prostate or colorectal surgery, or diabetic neuropathy. Pharmacologic agents can also result in RE, primarily antihypertensive drugs, alpha-adrenergic blocking drugs, antipsychotics, and antidepressants [15].

Diagnosis

Patients with absent or low-volume ejaculate should be tested using semen analysis and urinalysis. Diagnosis is confirmed by the presence of sperm in a post-ejaculation urine sample. Diagnosis may result following evaluation for infertility due to azoospermia.

Treatment

In cases of pharmacologic etiology, discontinuation of the medication may resolve the problem. Pharmacotherapy is most often used for neurologic causes, particularly if partial nerve damage exists. Current drugs include alpha-adrenergic agents such as ephedrine, or tricyclic antidepressants with anticholinergic effects. Successful response is most likely found in patients with partial nerve damage.

Painful Ejaculation

Ejaculatory pain, although rare, may result from epididymal congestion after vasectomy, duct infection or obstruction, testicular torsion, mass lesion, lower urinary tract infection, or prostatitis. Psychogenic causes should also be considered.

Psychosexual Problems

Sexual dysfunction often has psychosocial components as an underlying cause and/ or a consequence. Relationship status, strain with partner, life changes, and stress can all impact sexual function. Any patients with sexual dysfunction problems should be evaluated for psychological issues. Even if a problem is found to have a known physical cause, there may still be underlying psychological causes or implications.

Erectile dysfunction and ejaculatory problems can often be associated with psychological problems, particularly depression and anxiety. In the Massachusetts Male Aging Study, researchers found that ED was associated with depressive symptoms (OR 1.82, 95 % CI, 1.21–2.73) [2].

Hypoactive sexual desire (HSD), or decreased libido, is a subjective report of the absence or decrease in frequency of sexual desire. It is often associated with other sexual dysfunctions, such as ED, and is influenced by social and cultural norms [15]. Depression and relationship conflict can influence sexual desire, and patients reporting HSD may benefit from referral to a psychologist.

Sexuality in Survivors of Childhood Cancer

Risk for Sexual Dysfunction in Survivors of Childhood Cancer

Survivors of childhood cancer should receive lifelong, specialized follow-up for late effects of cancer treatment. Survivorship care is individualized based on diagnosis and treatment exposures and is best directed by a Survivorship Healthcare Plan (SHP) which includes a detailed medical summary of cancer treatment, individualized late effect risk profile, and surveillance plan for early detection of late effects. An SHP is created using the Children's Oncology Group Long-Term Follow-Up Guidelines for Survivors of Childhood, Adolescent, and Young Adult Cancer [24]. These guidelines are evidence-based screening recommendations created by multidisciplinary teams of expert clinicians in the field of childhood cancer survivorship. In addition to screening recommendations for a variety of health problems, the guidelines detail specific treatments which are associated with potential sexual dysfunction, such as radiation and surgery (Table 10.3) [25].

The impact of cancer treatment on sexuality has not been studied extensively in survivors of childhood cancer. Relander [26] found that among male survivors, 60% reported normal sexual function, with higher rates of sexual dysfunction reported in patients treated for tumors of the hypothalamic-pituitary region and patients who received testicular radiation or high doses of alkylating agents. The self-report of sexual function, however, in general is not specific to types of problems. The limited evidence of association of childhood cancer treatment with erectile dysfunction, ejaculatory problems, and psychosexual problems as well as psychosocial implications of sexual dysfunction in survivors will be discussed below.

Erectile Dysfunction

Etiology in Survivors

Specific treatment-related risk factors in survivors include cranial, pelvic, or spinal surgery, radiation, and hormonal deficiency, as well as those risk factors found in the general population such as increasing age and emotional distress [27]. Untreated hypoandrogenism may impact erectile function. In a report from the Childhood Cancer Survivor Study, radiation therapy to the testes was associated with ED as was pelvic radiation, thought to be caused by effects on the corpora cavernosa or penile bulb [28]. The study found that exposures as low as 10 Gy were associated with ED, suggesting that males treated at a young age may be vulnerable to permanent changes of the penile structure [28]. Treatment-related comorbidities such as obesity, diabetes mellitus, hyperlipidemia, renal disease, cardiac dysfunction, and/or depression and anxiety may cause or worsen ED, and many survivors are at higher risk than their peers for these conditions [29, 30]. See Table 10.2 for a list of health conditions associated with sexual dysfunction with bolded items those that can be seen in survivors depending on their treatment exposure history. Specific

Table 10.2 Health condition associated with sexual dysfunction

Vascular disease	*Cardiovascular disease (hypertension, atherosclerosis, hyperlipidemia)*
	Diabetes mellitus
Neurogenic	*Central causes*
	Degenerative disorders (multiple sclerosis, Parkinson's disease, etc.)
	Stroke
	Central nervous system tumors
	Peripheral causes
	Spinal cord trauma or diseases
	Polyneuropathy
	Types 1 and 2 diabetes mellitus
	Chronic renal failure
Anatomic or structural	Hypospadias/epispadias
	Micropenis
	Congenital curvature of the penis
	Peyronie's disease
Hormonal	*Hypogonadism*
	Hyperprolactinemia
Medication side effect	Antihypertensives (diuretics are the most common medication causing ED)
	Antidepressants (selective serotonin reuptake inhibitors, tricyclics)
	Antipsychotics (including neuroleptics)
	Antiandrogens
	GnRH analogues and antagonists
	Recreational drugs (alcohol, heroin, cocaine, marijuana, methadone)
Psychogenic	*Generalized*
	Lack of arousability and disorders of sexual intimacy
	Situational
	Partner-related, performance-related issues due to distress
Trauma	Penile fracture
	Peyronie's disease

Italics indicates conditions for which many survivors are at risk because of their treatment history
See the Children's Oncology Group Long-term Follow-up Guidelines for treatment exposures associated with risk for various health conditions. www.survivorshipguidelines.org

Table 10.3 Cancer treatment exposures associated with increased risk for sexual dysfunction[a]

Chemotherapy	Radiation sites	Surgery
None	Pelvis	Spinal cord surgery
	Spine	Pelvic surgery
	Testicular	Cystectomy
		Retroperitoneal tumor or node dissection

[a]According to the Children's Oncology Group Long-term Follow-up Guidelines

childhood cancer treatments which may increase risk for sexual dysfunction are found in Table 10.3.

Incidence in Survivors

The specific incidence of ED in childhood cancer survivors has not been well studied. Some studies report an incidence to be around 20% in survivors [3, 28, 31]. In a study of 1622 adult survivors of childhood cancer, Ritenour et al, using the International Index of Erectile Function, found that 12% met the criteria for erectile dysfunction, compared with only 4% of their healthy siblings (Relative Risk 2.66, 95% CI (1.41, 5.01)). Survivors were also twice as likely than their siblings to report treatment for ED [28]. Similar to the general population, sexual dysfunction was more common in older survivors, regardless of previous treatment [31].

Ejaculatory Problems

Etiology in Survivors

Surgical procedures and/or pelvic radiation involving the bladder or other pelvic organs may also impact nerve and blood vessel function. Retroperitoneal lymph node dissection techniques have been known to cause retrograde ejaculation, and while procedures have been improved, they continue to carry a risk. Patients with impaired spinal cord function may have difficulty with ejaculation [15].

Patients with comorbid conditions related to their cancer diagnosis and treatments may experience ejaculatory dysfunction due to medication therapy such as antihypertensives and antidepressants.

Incidence in Survivors

Sundberg compared young adult male survivors with healthy peers and found survivors more frequently reported sexual dysfunction compared with peers; this includes premature ejaculation in 9% of survivors compared to 7% of peers and orgasmic difficulty during intercourse among 10% of survivors compared with 3% of peers [4].

Jonker-Pool et al. conducted a meta-analysis of research focused on survivors of testicular cancer, a common diagnosis in the young adult population, which revealed that ejaculatory dysfunction was reported in 44% of survivors and was related to surgery in the retroperitoneal area [32].

Psychosexual Issues in Survivors

Much of what is known about sexual dysfunction in survivors of childhood cancer has been assessed through the lens of sexuality, satisfaction with sexuality, impact on quality of life, and life satisfaction. A recent study examined body image and sexual satisfaction in a group of 87 survivors and age-/gender-matched controls [33]. While results from this study indicate comparable satisfaction and psychosexual development, other studies have found that survivors report problems in categories of the NHSLS such as decreased desire and arousal as well as a negative impact from health problems on sexual satisfaction.

Zebrack surveyed 599 survivors of childhood cancer aged 18–39 and found that 20% of males reported lack of sexual interest and being unable to relax and enjoy sex and 16% reported at least some difficulty in becoming sexually aroused [3]. Van Dijk et al. surveyed 60 survivors (31 male) between the ages of 16 and 40 who were diagnosed under the age of 21 to assess the relationship of psychosexual function and quality of life and found that many survivors experienced problems [34]. Sexual problems included just over 40% of respondents who seldom or were never able to feel themselves sexually attractive and 44% felt almost no sexual attraction and seldom satisfied with their sexual lives. Forty-four percent were seldom/never able to see themselves as sexually attractive toward others [34].

Those who reported sexual dysfunction also had poorer health-related quality of life, and the association between the two was stronger among males than females [3]. When comparing survivors by gender, females were more likely to report sexual function problems, but having a sexual function problem had a larger impact on quality of life in males. This finding is echoed by van Dijk's study where 18% of male survivors surveyed felt a limitation in their sexual life due to their illness, mainly associated with uncertainty about their own body, difficulty with emotions, scars, and possible fertility problems [34]. Interestingly a study of survivors of cancer to the lower bone extremity found that those who had an amputation or Van Nes rotationplasty reported better sexual functioning than those who had a limb salvage procedure [35].

Cancer's Impact on Normal Sexual Development

The cancer diagnosis can often impact the trajectory of typical childhood development, especially for those patients whose treatment may interrupt normal adolescence. Research has found that survivors have fewer sexual partners and often reach sexual milestones later than healthy peers. Survivors are often older at the time of the first relationship and at time of the first sexual intercourse [36]. Van Dijk found this to be true especially for survivors who had received their cancer treatment during adolescence [34]. These findings are echoed through qualitative study of adolescent survivors who describe the challenges of forming romantic relationships while undergoing treatment and the need to prioritize getting through treatment over dating [37].

Relationships and Intimacy

A cancer diagnosis and treatment can have effects on future relationships. Over one-third of adolescent and young adult cancer survivors report cancer having a negative impact on dating, and 40–60 % report a negative impact on their sexual function/intimate relations, with a larger perceived impact seen in older childhood cancer survivors (30–39 years of age) compared with adolescents aged 15–20 years [38]. In a qualitative study of adolescent survivors, Stinson et al. found that the adolescents expected cancer to have little impact on future sexual relationships, but parents in the same study worried that their child's history of cancer could impact future relations [37]. Survivors often struggle with the disclosure of their cancer history with a new romantic partner, and this can be particularly stressful if they are concerned about their future fertility and its potential impact on forming a relationship [39].

How to Approach Cancer Survivors

It is crucial that providers who are caring for survivors of childhood cancer obtain a thorough history to assess for any sexual functioning problems. Bolte et al. suggest using the Permission, Limited Information, Specific Suggestions, Intensive Therapy (PLISSIT) model when communicating with adolescent and young adult survivors about sexuality after cancer treatment [40, 41] (Table 10.4). Talking about sexuality and sexual functioning can be uncomfortable for providers but they may find general open-ended questions helpful in initiating the conversation. Using language such as "tell me what your friends are talking about with sex…what are you wondering about…" can help providers quickly gauge where patients are developmentally and identify their concerns (see Table 10.4 for more suggestions).

When referring to a urologist, providers should ensure the urologist is familiar with the context of the patient's health in terms of previous treatment by providing a thorough health history and risk for late effects, such as that provided in a Survivorship Healthcare Plan. Survivors may also benefit from a referral to psychology.

Challenges and Future Directions

Assessing the true incidence of sexual dysfunction is difficult. Many survivors transition to adult care which makes it difficult to ascertain the prevalence of late effects and the impact of late effects on the quality of life. Since these are not

Table 10.4 Using the PLISSIT model for communicating with male cancer survivors

PLISSIT model	Example question
Permission: offering permission for sexual challenges to exist and permission to initiate discussion and legitimize concerns	*Some survivors experience sexual problems after cancer treatment. Is that something you would like to talk more about today?*
Limited information: address myths, reeducate patients about sexual health, provide resources	*You received radiation to your pelvis which can sometimes cause erectile dysfunction. Have you experienced this at all?*
Specific suggestions: individualize recommendations, avoid medical jargon	*Many people benefit from treatment with medication or other interventions. Are you interested in hearing more about treatment options today?*
Intensive therapy: provide opportunities for patients to express feelings of fear and frustration around changes in sexuality after cancer treatment	*Having erectile dysfunction can often be stressful and impact relationships. Would you like to see a counselor who specializes in this?*

problems often seen in the pediatric realm, many survivors are not aware that they might be at increased risk of developing sexual health problems. Ensuring that survivors, especially as they transition to adult care, are aware of their risk and confident in talking with a healthcare provider about sexual function will be important to empower them to receive the care they need. Educating adult providers about the risks for sexual dysfunction associated with cancer treatment in childhood and its long-lasting impact on health is always important.

References

1. Laumann EO, Paik A, Rosen RC. Sexual dysfunction in the United States: prevalence and predictors. JAMA. 1999;281(6):537–44.
2. Feldman HA, et al. Impotence and its medical and psychosocial correlates: results of the Massachusetts Male Aging Study. J Urol. 1994;151(1):54–61.
3. Zebrack BJ, et al. Sexual functioning in young adult survivors of childhood cancer. Psychooncology. 2010;19(8):814–22.
4. Sundberg KK, et al. Sexual function and experience among long-term survivors of childhood cancer. Eur J Cancer. 2011;47(3):397–403.
5. Kandeel FR, Koussa VK, Swerdloff RS. Male sexual function and its disorders: physiology, pathophysiology, clinical investigation, and treatment. Endocr Rev. 2001;22(3):342–88.
6. Kolodyn RC, Masters WH, Johnson VE. Textbook of sexual medicine. Boston: Little Brown and Co; 1979. p. 1–28.
7. Govier FE, et al. Timing of penile color flow duplex ultrasonography using a triple drug mixture. J Urol. 1995;153(5):1472–5.
8. Lue TF, Tanagho E. Contemporary management of impotence and infertility. Baltimore: Williams & Wilkins; 1988.
9. Walsh PC, Wilson J. Harrison's principles of internal medicine. 11th ed. New York: McGraw-Hill Book Co.; 1987.
10. Ayta IA, McKinlay JB, Krane RJ. The likely worldwide increase in erectile dysfunction between 1995 and 2025 and some possible policy consequences. BJU Int. 1999;84(1):50–6.
11. Online, N.C.S., Impotence. 1992. 10(4):1–31.

12. Furlow WL. Prevalence of impotence in the United States. Med Aspects Hum Sex. 1985;19: 13–6.
13. Schiavi RC, et al. Healthy aging and male sexual function. Am J Psychiatry. 1990;147(6): 766–71.
14. Diokno AC, Brown MB, Herzog AR. Sexual function in the elderly. Arch Intern Med. 1990;150(1):197–200.
15. Porst H, Buvat J. Standard practice in sexual medicine. Maiden: Blackwell Publishing; 2006.
16. Wespes E, et al. EAU guidelines on erectile dysfunction: an update. Eur Urol. 2006;49(5): 806–15.
17. Montague DK, et al. Clinical guidelines panel on erectile dysfunction: summary report on the treatment of organic erectile dysfunction. The American Urological Association. J Urol. 1996;156(6):2007–11.
18. Nehra A, et al. The Princeton III Consensus recommendations for the management of erectile dysfunction and cardiovascular disease. Mayo Clin Proc. 2012;87(8):766–78.
19. Bhasin S, et al. Testosterone therapy in adult men with androgen deficiency syndromes: an endocrine society clinical practice guideline. J Clin Endocrinol Metab. 2006;91(6):1995–2010.
20. Montague DK, et al. AUA guideline on the pharmacologic management of premature ejaculation. J Urol. 2004;172(1):290–4.
21. Symonds T, et al. Development and validation of a premature ejaculation diagnostic tool. Eur Urol. 2007;52(2):565–73.
22. Blanker MH, et al. Erectile and ejaculatory dysfunction in a community-based sample of men 50 to 78 years old: prevalence, concern, and relation to sexual activity. Urology. 2001;57(4):763–8.
23. Coolen LM, et al. Central regulation of ejaculation. Physiol Behav. 2004;83(2):203–15.
24. Children's Oncology Group. Long-term follow-up guidelines for survivors of childhood, adolescent and young adult cancers, Version 4.0. Monrovia, CA: Children's Oncology Group. 2013. Retrieved from http://www.survivorshipguidelines.org.
25. Landier W, et al. Development of risk-based guidelines for pediatric cancer survivors: the Children's Oncology Group Long-Term Follow-Up Guidelines from the Children's Oncology Group Late Effects Committee and Nursing Discipline. J Clin Oncol. 2004;22(24):4979–90.
26. Relander T, et al. Gonadal and sexual function in men treated for childhood cancer. Med Pediatr Oncol. 2000;35(1):52–63.
27. Kenney LB, et al. Male reproductive health after childhood, adolescent, and young adult cancers: a report from the Children's Oncology Group. J Clin Oncol. 2012;30(27):3408–16.
28. Ritenour CW, et al. Sexual health in male childhood cancer survivors: a report from the childhood cancer survivor study (CCSS). 13th international conference on long-term complications of treatment of children and adolescents for cancer poster presentation. Memphis, TN. 2014.
29. Oeffinger KC, et al. Chronic health conditions in adult survivors of childhood cancer. N Engl J Med. 2006;355(15):1572–82.
30. Hudson MM, et al. Clinical ascertainment of health outcomes among adults treated for childhood cancer. JAMA. 2013;309(22):2371–81.
31. Bober SL, et al. Sexual function in childhood cancer survivors: a report from Project REACH. J Sex Med. 2013;10(8):2084–93.
32. Jonker-Pool G, et al. Sexual functioning after treatment for testicular cancer – review and meta-analysis of 36 empirical studies between 1975–2000. Arch Sex Behav. 2001;30(1):55–74.
33. Lehmann V, et al. Body issues, sexual satisfaction, and relationship status satisfaction in long-term childhood cancer survivors and healthy controls. Psychooncology. 2015;25(2):210–6.
34. van Dijk EM, et al. Psychosexual functioning of childhood cancer survivors. Psychooncology. 2008;17(5):506–11.
35. Barrera M, et al. Sexual function in adolescent and young adult survivors of lower extremity bone tumors. Pediatr Blood Cancer. 2010;55(7):1370–6.
36. Stam H, Grootenhuis MA, Last BF. The course of life of survivors of childhood cancer. Psychooncology. 2005;14(3):227–38.

37. Stinson J, et al. A qualitative study of the impact of cancer on romantic relationships, sexual relationships, and fertility: perspectives of Canadian adolescents and parents during and after treatment. J Adolesc Young Adult Oncol. 2015;4(2):84–90.
38. Bellizzi KM, et al. Positive and negative psychosocial impact of being diagnosed with cancer as an adolescent or young adult. Cancer. 2012;118(20):5155–62.
39. Thompson AL, Long KA, Marsland AL. Impact of childhood cancer on emerging adult survivors' romantic relationships: a qualitative account. J Sex Med. 2013;10 Suppl 1:65–73.
40. Bolte S, Zebrack B. Sexual issues in special populations: adolescents and young adults. Semin Oncol Nurs. 2008;24(2):115–9.
41. Annon J. The PLISSIT model: a proposed conceptual scheme for the behavioral treatment of sexual problems. J Sex Educ Ther. 1976;2:1–15.

Chapter 11
Fertility Preservation in Patients with Disorders of Sex Development

Courtney A. Finlayson

Strides made in fertility preservation for cancer patients have inspired the expansion of the field of oncofertility to other medical conditions associated with infertility. One of the emerging areas is that of disorders of sex development (DSDs).

DSDs are conditions in which there is incongruence in an individual's chromosomal, gonadal, or phenotypic sex [1]. There are three main steps in sex development: establishment of chromosomal sex, determination of gonadal sex, and differentiation to phenotypic sex. Errors in meiosis or translocation of genetic material may result in sex chromosome DSDs. Abnormalities in transcription factors determining gonadal development into the testes or ovaries may lead to disorders of gonadal development. Finally, disorders of androgen synthesis, androgen excess, or androgen action account for most of the remaining DSDs [2].

DSDs are commonly thought of as conditions presenting with ambiguous genitalia in an infant, but there are many other presentations as well. Children may present with premature virilization, adolescents with primary amenorrhea, or adults with infertility. Table 11.1 categorizes DSDs based on a consensus statement on intersex disorders and their management published in 2006 [2]. This landmark paper changed the approach to this group of patients. In the 50 preceding years, the "optimal gender policy" was followed, in which sex reassignment surgery was favored at a young age. It was thought that individuals were psychosexually neutral and that early surgery, without the knowledge of the patient, facilitated stable gender identity and appropriate gender role behavior [3]. Over time, doubt grew about this approach [4]. Patients treated according to the earlier approach grew up and began voicing discontent about the secrecy, the surgical outcomes, and the common terminology such as intersex and hermaphrodite. Molecular genetics was also advancing and changing the understanding of many of the conditions. These factors

C.A. Finlayson, MD
Division of Endocrinology, Department of Pediatrics, Ann and Robert H. Lurie Children's Hospital of Chicago, 225 E. Chicago Ave. Box 54, Chicago, IL 60611, USA
e-mail: cfinlayson@luriechildrens.org

© Springer International Publishing Switzerland 2017   171
T.K. Woodruff, Y.C. Gosiengfiao (eds.), *Pediatric and Adolescent Oncofertility*,
DOI 10.1007/978-3-319-32973-4_11

Table 11.1 Categorization of disorders of sex development

Sex chromosome DSD	46,XY DSD	46,XX DSD
Disorders of gonadal development		
45,X, 45,X/46,XX, 45,X/46,XY Turner syndrome	Complete gonadal dysgenesis	Ovotesticular DSD
47,XYY	Partial gonadal dysgenesis	Testicular DSD
Klinefelter syndrome		
45,X/46,XY	Gonadal regression	Gonadal dysgenesis
Mixed gonadal dysgenesis, ovotesticular DSD		
46,XX/46,XY	Ovotesticular DSD	
Chimeric, ovotesticular DSD		
	Disorders of androgen synthesis or action	Disorders of androgen excess
	Androgen biosynthesis defect (e.g., 5-alpha reductase deficiency)	Fetal androgen excess (e.g., 21-hydroxylase deficiency congenital adrenal hyperplasia)
	Defect in androgen action (e.g., complete androgen insensitivity or partial androgen insensitivity syndrome)	Fetoplacental androgen excess (e.g., aromatase deficiency)
	LH receptor defects	Maternal (e.g., luteoma)
	Others	
	Cloacal exstrophy	Cloacal exstrophy
	Disorders of anti-Mullerian hormone	Vaginal atresia
	Severe hypospadias	Mayer-Rokitansky-Kuster-Hauser syndrome

led to the 2006 Consensus Statement that acknowledged the controversial issues in management and made recommendations about nomenclature, evaluation, and management and care for these patients as part of a multidisciplinary team including surgeons, endocrinologists, behavioral health experts, ethicists, and geneticists. There is increasing availability of such programs for patients with DSDs around the world.

Nomenclature remains a controversial issue in this field, however. The 2006 Consensus Statement modified the overarching terms of intersex and hermaphrodite to DSD in an effort to make the term less pejorative. Other terms, such as variation in sex development and difference in sex development, were also considered, but ultimately, DSD was chosen. Some affected individuals continue to prefer the term intersex, while others prefer DSD and yet others dislike both terms. Presumably, the words "disorder" and "sex" have negative connotations to some individuals, and there is anecdotal evidence to this end. There are few studies addressing this topic.

In a study of 19 affected individuals' parents and 25 providers, overall the term DSD was considered preferable to intersex [5]. The parents considered it a term which made it easier to understand their child's condition and to explain it to their child, but only 36.8 % reported DSD as an acceptable term to describe an individual's condition when it is not possible to assign sex at birth as a result of atypical genitalia. Conclusions to make from this study, however, are limited by sample size. In 2015, Lin-Su et al. reported results from a survey of 589 patients with congenital adrenal hyperplasia who are members of the CARES support group [6]. In this group, 71 % disliked or strongly disliked the DSD term. This study, however, is of a very specific diagnosis and support group; therefore, these results may not reflect those of the population as a whole. There have been no large-scale studies of individuals and the medical community as a whole to determine whether a universally acceptable term may be found. The term DSD is used in this chapter as it is the currently accepted medical terminology, but with the understanding that this is not the preferred term for many affected individuals.

Medical, surgical, and psychosocial care is improving, but fertility preservation has rarely been addressed despite the number of conditions associated with a fertility/sterility risk. The fertility concerns, however, are different from those faced in cancer patients. Fertility issues facing individuals with specific DSD diagnoses are shown in Table 11.2. First, some DSDs are associated with abnormal gonadal development resulting in streak gonads or dysgenetic testes and ovaries [7]. This may result in gonadal failure from birth or progressive gonadal failure in childhood or adolescence. As such, the presence and quality of germs cells may vary, but we have no ability to assess numbers of germ cells at birth. Furthermore, the rate of failure of gonads differs within and between conditions. While there is uncertainty in the oncofertility patient as well, there is a known time for surgical resection of gonads or initiation of gonadotoxic chemotherapy which makes the care of DSD patients distinct.

Second, the presence of abnormal gonads, specifically in 46,XY DSDs, increases risk for development of gonadal tumors [8]. Screening of intra-abdominal gonads by radiology techniques is not sufficient to rule out tumor [9]. To prevent the development of cancer, gonadectomy has been recommended in most 46,XY DSD conditions at the time of diagnosis, often in infancy or early childhood. However, this practice is changing and, increasingly, gonadal tumor risk is assessed for each specific condition. A recent review by Abaci et al. estimated tumor risk for each DSD type. High-risk conditions included gonadal dysgenesis with intra-abdominal gonad, 15–35 % risk, and PAIS with non-scrotal gonad, 50 %. Intermediate risk included Turner syndrome with Y chromosome, 12 %; PAIS with scrotal gonad, unknown risk; and gonadal dysgenesis with scrotal gonad, unknown risk. Low-risk conditions were CAIS and ovotesticular DSD [10]. Thus, there is evidence that in some conditions, gonadectomy should be performed at diagnosis, whereas in others, it may be safe to delay [11]. One reason for delaying gonadectomy may be to preserve the possibility for biological fertility. The consideration of gonadectomy is a challenging one for most patients and families and is often considered in infancy through adolescence.

Table 11.2 Fertility issues by DSD diagnosis

Category	Disorder	Karyotype	Fertility issues	Malignancy concern	Common discordance between gender identity and gonadal type
Sex chromosome DSD					
	Turner syndrome	45,X 45,X/46,XX 45,X/46,XY	Premature ovarian failure, streak gonads	Yes, if Y chromosome material	No
	Klinefelter syndrome	47,XXY	Testicular failure	No	No
	Mixed gonadal dysgenesis	45,X/46,XY	Gonadal failure	Yes	Yes
46,XY DSD					
	Complete or partial gonadal dysgenesis (e.g., SRY, SOX9)	46,XY	Potential streak gonads or gonadal failure	Yes	Yes
	Ovotesticular DSD	46,XY	Potential streak gonads or gonadal failure	Yes	Yes
	LH receptor mutations	46,XY	Testes slightly reduced in size but mature Leydig cells absent/scarce (Leydig cell hypoplasia)	No	No
	5-alpha reductase deficiency	46,XY	Oligospermia, azoospermia	No	Yes
	Complete androgen insensitivity syndrome	46,XY	Not much evidence, suspect azoospermia or oligospermia	Yes	Yes
	Partial androgen insensitivity syndrome	46,XY	Not much evidence, suspect azoospermia or oligospermia	Yes	Yes

Table 11.2 (continued)

Category	Disorder	Karyotype	Fertility issues	Malignancy concern	Common discordance between gender identity and gonadal type
	Persistent Mullerian duct syndrome	46,XY	Maybe (if prolonged cryptorchidism or anatomic obstruction) but likely normal sperm production	Possibly (cryptorchidism or of Mullerian remnants)	No
46,XX DSD					
	Gonadal dysgenesis	46,XX	Potential streak gonads or gonadal failure	Yes	Yes
	Ovotesticular DSD	46,XX	Potential streak gonads or gonadal failure	Possibly	Yes
	Testicular DSD (SRY+, dup SOX9)	46,XX	Potential infertility	Possibly	No
	Congenital adrenal hyperplasia	46,XX	Often due to anovulation, but treated medically with success	No	No
	Aromatase deficiency	46,XX	Hypergonadotropic hypogonadism	No	Yes

Third, due to the nature of disorders of sex development, the gonads and germ cells may not match the patient's gender identity. In complete androgen insensitivity syndrome, for example, patients have a 46,XY karyotype and gonads are testicles, but due to mutations in the gene encoding the androgen receptor, the body is unable to respond to androgen. Thus, internally the individual has testes, Wolffian structures, and no Mullerian structures, but externally the genitalia appear completely female with a blind-ending vagina. The vast majority of the individuals have a female gender identity. There is a risk of gonadoblastoma; thus, many undergo gonadectomy, which may be done at any age, but increasingly is performed after puberty. If fertility preservation options were to be considered, this would involve preservation of sperm for an individual who otherwise identifies, appears, and is a woman.

In two conditions, Turner syndrome and Klinefelter syndrome, fertility preservation has begun to gain some momentum. Spontaneous fertility in Turner syndrome is rare, estimated at about 2–5 % [12]. There is an accelerated loss of oocytes from the ovaries after the 18th week of fetal life or over a few postnatal months or years such that most have lost all of their germ cells before completing puberty [12]. Parenting options for women with Turner syndrome historically focused on adoption, but increasingly there is emphasis on expanding biological options. These have included heterologous in vitro fertilization with ovum donation or homologous IVF with embryo transfer resulting in live births in women with Turner syndrome. Other modalities are considered, but have not yet resulted in live births. This includes homologous IVF with oocyte cryopreservation, which is scientifically possible at this time, and ovarian tissue cryopreservation from prepubertal individuals, which remains experimental [13]. Controversy has arisen about women with Turner syndrome carrying pregnancies because their risk of morbidity is much higher than for women without Turner syndrome [14]. Of primary concern is the increased risk of circulatory complications such as aortic dissection. The American Society for Reproductive Medicine has stated that Turner syndrome is a relative contraindication to pregnancy and that in a patient with Turner syndrome and a documented cardiac anomaly, Turner syndrome is an absolute contraindication to pregnancy [15]. Thus, patients with Turner syndrome are advised to use a gestational carrier for the term of their pregnancy.

Classical Klinefelter syndrome is characterized by germ cell regression which begins in utero, accelerating during spontaneous puberty leading to testicular fibrosis and hyalinization of the seminiferous tubules and hyperplasia of the interstitium in late adolescence and adults [16]. Often, pubertal development is incomplete and testosterone production fails during this period. Additionally, it usually leads to infertility. Many men are azoospermic, but successful assisted reproduction in adult men with Klinefelter syndrome has been achieved by testicular sperm extraction followed by ICSI. It has been suggested that cryopreservation of spermatozoa might be best achieved early in adolescence. This has proven difficult as age and rate of pubertal maturation vary, as does ability of an adolescent boy to produce ejaculate with masturbation [16]. Studies of testicular tissue in 13–16-year-old boys with Klinefelter syndrome showed massive fibrosis and hyalinization and only showed tubular spermatogonia in the youngest patient suggesting that testicular tissue cryopreservation is most likely to be successful at younger ages [17].

Infertility and sterility is clearly a risk and a complicated issue for individuals with DSDs and their parents, who may make decisions before a child is mature enough to participate in that process. It is presumed that these are important considerations, but there is no clear understanding of the DSD community's views of fertility as the issue has not been comprehensively studied [18, 19]. A better appreciation of the views of the affected individuals is necessary to guide the field. Working on the assumption that some individuals with DSDs will desire fertility preservation, there are many more questions that arise. Which patients with DSD conditions are likely to benefit, and when this should be offered for optimal chances of preservation? Again, there is little to no evidence about the presence and quality of germ cells in patients with DSDs, and this requires evaluation. Should a surgical procedure and its associated risks should be undertaken in an otherwise healthy child for cryopreservation of tissue, when this procedure remains experimental? Whereas some DSD patients may be undergoing gonadectomy during which fertility preservation techniques can be done simultaneously, others may not. In traditional 45,X or 45,X/45,XX mosaic Turner syndrome, for example, there is progressive loss of germ cells, but no indication for gonadectomy. Should parents have the option to choose that surgery be undertaken in early childhood because more germ cells are present for preservation? In Turner syndrome, with a higher risk of pregnancy-associated morbidity, should efforts for fertility preservation be pursued? As gender identity may not match an individual's gonads and potential production of sperm versus ova, how does this affect considerations of fertility preservation? If a parent acts as the proxy for the child in fertility preservation decision-making, how is responsibility for preservation and ownership of the reproductive material delineated? Many DSDs are caused by genetic mutations; thus, there is a risk of offspring inheriting the same condition. How should this affect decisions about fertility preservation, and how should preimplantation genetics be employed in these cases? There are many complicated questions facing the field of fertility preservation for DSD patients. Future research efforts must address these questions to better serve this patient population.

References

1. Ohnesorg T, Vilain E, Sinclair AH. The genetics of disorders of sex development in humans. Sex Dev Genet Mol Biol Evol Endocrinol Embryol Pathol Sex Determination Diff. 2014;8(5):262–72.
2. Houk CP, Hughes IA, Ahmed SF, Lee PA, Writing Committee for the International Intersex Consensus Conference Participants. Summary of consensus statement on intersex disorders and their management. International Intersex Consensus Conference. Pediatrics. 2006;118(2):753–7.
3. Wiesemann C, Ude-Koeller S, Sinnecker GH, Thyen U. Ethical principles and recommendations for the medical management of differences of sex development (DSD)/intersex in children and adolescents. Eur J Pediatr. 2010;169(6):671–9.
4. Diamond M, Sigmundson HK. Sex reassignment at birth. Long-term review and clinical implications. Arch Pediatr Adolesc Med. 1997;151(3):298–304.
5. Davies JH, Knight EJ, Savage A, Brown J, Malone PS. Evaluation of terminology used to describe disorders of sex development. J Pediatr Urol. 2011;7(4):412–5.
6. Lin-Su K, Lekarev O, Poppas DP, Vogiatzi MG. Congenital adrenal hyperplasia patient perception of 'disorders of sex development' nomenclature. Int J Pediatr Endocrinol. 2015;2015(1):9.
7. Cools M, van Aerde K, Kersemaekers AM, Boter M, Drop SL, Wolffenbuttel KP, et al. Morphological and immunohistochemical differences between gonadal maturation delay and early germ cell neoplasia in patients with undervirilization syndromes. J Clin Endocrinol Metab. 2005;90(9):5295–303.
8. Cools M, Looijenga LH, Wolffenbuttel KP, T'Sjoen G. Managing the risk of germ cell tumourigenesis in disorders of sex development patients. Endocr Dev. 2014;27:185–96.
9. Nakhal RS, Hall-Craggs M, Freeman A, Kirkham A, Conway GS, Arora R, et al. Evaluation of retained testes in adolescent girls and women with complete androgen insensitivity syndrome. Radiology. 2013;268(1):153–60.
10. Abaci A, Catli G, Berberoglu M. Gonadal malignancy risk and prophylactic gonadectomy in disorders of sexual development. J Pediatr Endocrinol Metab. 2015;28:1019–27.

11. van der Zwan YG, Biermann K, Wolffenbuttel KP, Cools M, Looijenga LH. Gonadal malde-velopment as risk factor for germ cell cancer: towards a clinical decision model. Eur Urol. 2015;67(4):692–701.
12. Hovatta O. Pregnancies in women with Turner's syndrome. Ann Med. 1999;31(2):106–10.
13. Hewitt JK, Jayasinghe Y, Amor DJ, Gillam LH, Warne GL, Grover S, et al. Fertility in Turner syndrome. Clin Endocrinol (Oxf). 2013;79(5):606–14.
14. Hagman A, Kallen K, Bryman I, Landin-Wilhelmsen K, Barrenas ML, Wennerholm UB. Morbidity and mortality after childbirth in women with Turner karyotype. Hum Reprod. 2013;28(7):1961–73.
15. Practice Committee of American Society For Reproductive Medicine. Increased maternal car-diovascular mortality associated with pregnancy in women with Turner syndrome. Fertil Steril. 2012;97(2):282–4.
16. Aksglaede L, Juul A. Testicular function and fertility in men with Klinefelter syndrome: a review. Eur J Endocrinol. 2013;168(4):R67–76.
17. Van Saen D, Gies I, De Schepper J, Tournaye H, Goossens E. Can pubertal boys with Klinefelter syndrome benefit from spermatogonial stem cell banking? Hum Reprod. 2012;27(2):323–30.
18. Rives N, Milazzo JP, Perdrix A, Castanet M, Joly-Helas G, Sibert L, et al. The feasibility of fertility preservation in adolescents with Klinefelter syndrome. Hum Reprod. 2013;28(6):1468–79.
19. Sanders C, Carter B, Lwin R. Young women with a disorder of sex development: learning to share information with health professionals, friends and intimate partners about bodily differences and infertility. J Adv Nurs. 2015;71(8):1904–13.

Chapter 12
Fertility Preservation in Patients with Gender Dysphoria

Jason Jarin, Emilie Johnson, and Veronica Gomez-Lobo

Abbreviations

BPA	Bisphenol A
DES	Diethylstilbestrol
DHEA	Didehydroepiandrosterone
GD	Gender dysphoria
GnRH	Gonadotropin-releasing hormone
PCBs	Polychlorinated biphenyls
PCOS	Polycystic ovarian syndrome
PESA	Percutaneous sperm aspiration
TESA	Testicular sperm aspiration
TESE	Testicular sperm extraction
WPATH	World Professional Association for Transgender Health

J. Jarin, MD (✉) • V. Gomez-Lobo, MD
Department of Women and Infant Services, Department of Surgery, MedStar Washington
Hospital Center, Children's National Medical Center,
110 Irving St NW, Washington, DC 20010, USA
e-mail: Jason.D.Jarin@medstar.net

E. Johnson, MD, MPH
Division of Urology Chicago, Department of Urology and Center for Healthcare Studies, Ann
& Robert H. Lurie Children's Hospital of Chicago, Northwestern University, Feinberg School
of Medicine, 225 E. Chicago Ave, Chicago, IL 60616, USA

© Springer International Publishing Switzerland 2017
T.K. Woodruff, Y.C. Gosiengfiao (eds.), *Pediatric and Adolescent Oncofertility*,
DOI 10.1007/978-3-319-32973-4_12

Introduction

Recent events have demonstrated increasing media attention to the issue of transgender individuals. The *Diagnostic and Statistical Manual of Mental Disorders* (DSM-5) changed the nomenclature for transgender individuals from gender identity disorder to gender dysphoria in 2013. Gender dysphoria refers to the psychological distress encountered in persons whose gender at birth is contrary to the one they identify with. The psychiatric focus is on the distress experienced due to the incongruence between assigned and affirmed gender, and current evidence supports that gender affirming therapy greatly improves outcomes [1]. The American Psychiatric Association further states that such individuals should be able to obtain care without fear of discrimination and that treatment options for this condition include counseling, cross-sex hormones, gender reassignment surgery, and social and legal transition to the desired sex [1]. In 2009, the Endocrine Society along with the Pediatric Endocrine Society, World Professional Association for Transgender Health (WPATH), European Society of Endocrinology, and the European Society for Pediatric Endocrinology published the "Endocrine treatment of transsexual persons: an Endocrine Society clinical practice guideline" [2]. These groups and the guidelines support the use of "cross-sex" hormones to further the gender affirming process and recommend counseling regarding fertility and options for fertility preservation, as cross-sex hormone therapy may impair future fertility.

Nomenclature

Although this chapter is titled "Fertility Preservation in Patients with Gender Dysphoria," the information and concepts presented herein apply to the spectrum of individuals who exhibit gender variance and desire medical interventions to facilitate transition to a gender other than the one assigned at birth. As mentioned above, these medical interventions include pubertal suppression, cross-gender hormone therapy, and gonadectomy, all of which have the potential to affect future fertility. For consistency in this chapter, the authors have chosen to use the terms "trans," "trans-woman," and "trans-man." However, a much larger range of terminology is applicable and relevant to the mental and physical health of individuals with gender variance, many of whom may pursue medical interventions which have the potential to affect fertility in the future.

The authors recognize that terminology related to the transgender experience is in evolution, and aim to provide some basic information about relevant nomenclature. It is important to note that some of the terms used may be offensive to some individuals, while preferable to others. Additionally, there have been recent shifts in language use that may not be fully reflected in the terms defined in this chapter.

However, assembling the non-exhaustive list below was thought to be important to provide clarity and context for the remainder of the chapter:

Sex vs. gender

> *Sex* – Anatomy of a person's reproductive system and secondary sex characteristics.
>
> *Gender* – Social roles based on sex, typically culturally based.

Gender-related terms

> *Biological sex/natal sex* – Sex assigned at birth, based on both anatomy and chromosomes.
>
> *Gender identity/affirmed gender* – An individual's internal sense of their[1] own gender, may it be male, female, or another gender. May not be aligned with biological/natal sex.
>
> *Gender expression* – Physical manifestation of an individual's gender identity (e.g., clothing, mannerisms, pronouns, chosen name).
>
> *Gender role* – Societal norms regarding how men and women should think, behave, speak, and dress.
>
> *Gender variance, gender nonconforming* – Closely related terms describing behavior not conforming to socially defined male or female norms (e.g., dress, activities) based on sex.

Gender identity

> *Cisgender* – Individuals for whom internal gender identity agrees with their anatomy and the gender they were assigned at birth.
>
> *Transgender, trans* – A person whose gender identity does not match their anatomy and gender assigned at birth. Often also abbreviated as *trans** to emphasize the range of individuals who do not identify as a traditional cisgender man or woman.
>
> *Transsexual* – A person who has the strong desire to assume the physical characteristics and gender role of the opposite sex. This term has a more binary connotation than transgender and has been viewed somewhat negatively in recent years, and thus is being used less often than terms such as transgender, and trans.
>
> *Trans-woman, male-to-female (MTF) transgender* – Individuals with a male natal gender, but female gender identity. For this chapter, the authors have chosen the term trans-woman, as it affirms the individual's gender identity.
>
> *Trans-man, female-to-male (FTM) transgender* – Individuals with a female natal gender, but male gender identity. For this chapter, the authors have chosen the term trans-man, as it affirms the individual's gender identity.

---

[1] Intentionally grammatically incorrect to avoid using binary gender-based terminology.

Genderqueer – Individuals who identify with both male and female genders, or
who identify with neither gender.
Gender fluid – A dynamic mix between male and female gender identities.

Other helpful terminology

Gender dysphoria– The DSM-V diagnosis used by medical and mental health
professionals to describe psychological distress caused by discontent with
one's natal sex. *Gender identity disorder (GID)* was the terminology previously used by the DSM-IV and has largely been abandoned.
Transitioning – The process of physically and permanently changing external
gender presentation to align with one's internal gender identity. Genital surgery is not a requirement.
Sexual orientation – Pattern of romantic or sexual attraction; separate from gender identity and gender expression. For example, a trans-man is not necessarily
romantically attracted only to women. Traditional categories include heterosexual, homosexual, and bisexual. Newer classifications include asexual,
polysexual, and pansexual.

Current Treatment Guidelines

Psychological Evaluation

It is essential that individuals with GD be evaluated and managed by a mental health
provider with experience in order to assess whether they indeed qualify for the diagnosis as well as evaluate for confounding psychological factors. The mental health
provider may also provide psychotherapy and evaluate for psychological readiness
for medical interventions such as puberty blockers and/or cross-sex hormones.
Persons with GD are at high risk of adverse mental health including anxiety, depression, self-harm and suicide, poor school performance, and drug and alcohol abuse
[3]. Thus, ideally a mental health provider will continue to evaluate and support the
individual during social and biological transition.

Puberty Suppression

Some children with GD experience increasing distress during puberty as their body
begins to change. The Endocrine Society Guidelines supports the use of puberty
blockers starting when the child reaches Tanner 2 stage (breast budding in natal girls
and testicular volume of 4 cc in natal boys) [2]. The mental health provider needs to
assess whether the patient meets medical eligibility and provides a letter of support
for the pediatric endocrinologist or gynecologist to begin puberty blockers. Such
treatment not only addresses the mental distress of the child but also prevents

secondary sexual characteristics from developing which may later be difficult to alter, such as the Adam's apple or large breasts. In general, puberty suppression is usually achieved with gonadotropin-releasing hormone (GnRH) agonists such as a histrelin rod or Depo-Lupron.

Cross-Sex Hormones

Regardless of whether puberty suppression was undertaken, the Endocrine Society Guidelines support initiation of cross-sex hormones around the age of 16 years. Individuals considering cross-sex hormones need to be counseled extensively regarding the expected results of feminizing/masculinizing medications and their possible adverse health effects. Such a discussion should include the effects on fertility and options for fertility preservation, as cross-sex hormone therapy may impair future fertility. In addition, prior to initiation of cross-sex hormone therapy, the WPATH recommends that a qualified mental health professional should provide documentation (such as a referral letter) of the patient's personal and treatment history, eligibility, and need for cross-sex hormone.

Testosterone Treatment for Trans-boys and Trans-men

Testosterone is recommended to achieve the desired masculinization of a natal female with gender dysphoria. In cases where an adolescent has received puberty suppression, it is given in low doses and increased slowly (as done with induction of puberty). In both prepubertal and postpubertal individuals, testosterone is generally administered subcutaneously or intramuscularly every 1–2 weeks at the lowest dose needed to maintain the desired clinical result and levels within normal male physiologic levels (320–1000 ng/dl) [4]. This requires discussion prior to initiation not only of the risks of masculinizing hormone therapy but also of the timing of development of the desired effects, so the patient has reasonable expectations. Monitoring for adverse effects includes both clinical and laboratory evaluation specific to the risks of hormone therapy and the patient's individual risks/comorbidities [5]. The most concerning morbidity noted in trans-men is polycythemia which can be treated with reduction of the testosterone and/or phlebotomy with blood donation.

Estrogen Treatment for Trans-girls and Trans-women

Hormone therapy for adolescents desiring feminizing therapy is more complex, with most clinical studies reporting the concurrent use of antiandrogens with estrogen therapy if the patient has not undergone puberty suppression [6]. Puberty induction, in suppressed individuals, may be undertaken with oral estrogen as well as transdermal (patch) and parenteral formulations. While the inherent risk of VTE within the adolescent population is less than in adults, transdermal preparations may offer an advantage by lowering these risks [3]. Following puberty induction, serum estradiol should be maintained at premenopausal levels (<200 pg/ml), and testosterone should be in the physiologic female range (<55 ng/dl). In individuals who have experienced puberty, this treatment may require high doses of estradiol (2–6 mg) as well as androgen blockers such as spironolactone. As with testosterone therapy, regular clinical and laboratory assessment should be performed to monitor for adverse effects.

Cross-Sex Hormones Effect on Fertility

Estrogen and Fertility in Trans-women

Although some estrogen is necessary for spermatogenesis, an overabundance of estrogen can be detrimental to fertility. Specific data regarding the effect of exogenous estrogen on sperm production in trans-women are lacking. However, data from animal studies, human epidemiologic studies, and studies related to the effect of obesity on human male reproductive function are relevant to trans-women who may desire biological children in the future.

Animal Data

There is a large body of literature demonstrating reduced fertility parameters and alterations in genital anatomy in male rodents exposed to estrogenic compounds in utero. Of more relevance to the trans-women who may begin estrogen supplementation during adolescence or adulthood, several studies of adult rodents have explored the impact of exogenous estrogens on multiple different measures of fertility potential. For example, increasing doses of exogenous estrogens have been associated with alteration in sperm counts and motility [7], testicular histology [8], and epididymal sperm content [9] in adult male rats. High doses of exogenous estrogens administered to adult male rats have also been associated with lower fertility rates, as measured by litter size [7–9]; one study even demonstrated a complete loss of potency at the highest dose of an estrogen receptor-α agonist [8]. Reversibility of the effects of estrogen on testicular histology has been demonstrated, suggesting that the effects of estrogen on fertility potential may not be permanent [9].

Evidence in Humans

Environmental Estrogens

In addition to the animal data, concern has existed for many years that environmental estrogens may be contributing impairments in male reproductive health and functioning, including an increase in male factor infertility [10]. To a great extent, concern regarding the effects of environmental estrogens on male fertility is a result of studies evaluating the link between in utero diethylstilbestrol (DES) exposure and adult male infertility. Although there have been several studies suggesting a link between fetal DES exposure and reduced adult semen parameters, the data are far from definitive [11]. Similarly, concern exists that exposure to endocrine disruptors with estrogenic properties such as phthalates, polychlorinated biphenyls (PCBs), and bisphenol A (BPA) may be associated with male infertility [12], although clear causality has not been established.

A few studies have attempted to link environmental endocrine disrupters to male factor infertility. For example, one Argentinian study demonstrated an association between exposure to pesticides and solvents (as measured by self-report) and lower semen parameters [13]. In that study, pesticide exposure was also associated with higher serum estrogen concentrations and lower luteinizing hormone concentrations compared with men not exposed to pesticides [13]. This suggests that any effect of chemical exposure on fertility may be at least partially hormonally mediated.

In a study of men presenting to an infertility clinic in India, infertile men were found to have detectable PCBs in their seminal plasma, whereas normal controls were not [14]. Seminal plasma phthalates were also found to be higher in infertile men compared with controls [14]. Not surprisingly, total motile sperm count was lower in the infertile men as well, although a causal relationship between estrogenic chemicals and fertility was only suggested, not proven, by this investigation.

Elevated Estrogen in Obese Men

Obesity has been associated with male infertility, and the mechanisms are likely multifactorial. In addition to hormonal abnormalities, obesity is also associated with erectile dysfunction and increased intrascrotal temperatures, all of which can cause difficulties with fertility [15]. From an endocrinologic standpoint, increasing BMI is associated with both infertility and hormonal derangements including low testosterone, elevated estradiol, and low inhibin B levels [16]. Additionally, semen parameters have been found to be altered in some studies of infertile obese men, although results have been inconsistent [15–17].

The exact relationship between hormonal profiles and semen parameters and paternity among obese men remains to be fully elucidated. A decreased serum testosterone to estradiol ratio has also been associated with infertility in a subset of men presenting with this complaint regardless of BMI, again suggesting that elevated estradiol can have a detrimental effect on fertility [18]. However, the relative contribution of elevated estrogen to fertility has not been determined.

Summary

• Although low levels of estrogen are necessary for male fertility, higher levels of exogenous estrogen administration appear to have a detrimental effect on the fertility potential of male gametes, as supported by both rodent data and human clinical and epidemiologic studies.

- The negative effects of estrogen on the testis appear to be at least partially reversible.
- Threshold levels for the amount and duration of exogenous estrogen exposure necessary to have a negative effect on fertility have yet to be established.

Testosterone and Fertility in Trans-men

Analogous to the role estrogen plays in male fertility, some testosterone is necessary for normal reproductive functioning in women. Also similar to the effect of estrogen on testicular function, exogenous testosterone can cause negative effects on ovarian function leading to fertility problems. However, there is a paucity of data specifically examining the effects of testosterone on future fertility on trans-men. Reviewed below, relevant animal data do exist, and information regarding the effects of elevated testosterone in women with polycystic ovarian syndrome (PCOS) may also be extrapolated to trans-men who use exogenous testosterone.

Animal Data

Data from animal studies has established that supraphysiologic androgen levels have a negative effect on the ovary. For example, exogenous testosterone administration has been associated with reduced ovarian weight in both adult female rats [19] and homing pigeons [20]. Suggested mechanisms include delayed follicular maturation [20] and follicular atresia potentially due to an antiestrogenic effect of testosterone [19]. Administration of a potent androgen, didehydroepiandrosterone (DHEA) to adult female rats has also been associated with follicular atresia [21]. Additionally, DHEA administration may cause local ovarian testosterone production and inflammation, leading to reductions in fertility potential [21].

Evidence in Humans

PCOS Data

PCOS is characterized by endocrine and reproductive dysfunction. Women with PCOS have manifestations of hyperandrogenism including challenges with fertility. In addition to elevated androgens, other endocrine abnormalities are also present, including elevated levels of insulin, inhibin B, and luteinizing hormone [22]. Through a multifactorial pathway, folliculogenesis is impaired, potentially due to a delay or arrest in follicular maturation [22, 23]. Although androgens certainly play a role in PCOS-related ovarian dysfunction, infertility related to PCOS is not solely due to androgen effects. One key factor associated with infertility in women with

PCOS may be the estradiol-to-testosterone ratio, with lower ratios being associated with anovulation [24].

Reports of Pregnancy in Trans-men

Despite the evidence from human and animal data, pregnancy (as documented by self-report) has been reported in trans-men who have previously used testosterone [25, 26]. This suggests that the effects of testosterone (at the doses typically used by trans-men) on ovarian function are incomplete and/or at least partially reversible.

Summary

- Low levels of testosterone are necessary for female fertility, although higher levels are associated with changes in ovarian histology and function that can lead to infertility.
- The effects of exogenous testosterone on the ovaries do not cause sterility, as pregnancies have been reported in trans-men who have previously used testosterone.
- Threshold levels for the amount and duration of exogenous testosterone exposure necessary to have a negative effect on fertility have yet to be established.

Ethics of Fertility Preservation Options for Trans-individuals

Because of the potential effects of treatment on fertility, loss of reproductive potential has long been viewed as an inexorable consequence to transition [27]. It was not until 2001 that the Endocrine Society explicitly stated that reproductive issues need to be discussed prior to the initiation of treatment. Furthermore, the American Academy of Child and Adolescent Psychiatry has maintained that there has been no credible evidence that shows that a parent's sexual orientation or gender identity will adversely affect the development of offspring, further supporting the need to discuss the reproductive needs of transgender individuals and their potential as parents [28].

Current established methods of fertility preservation include sperm, oocyte, and embryo cryopreservation, all of which have been considered standard of care for patients receiving gonadotoxic therapy [29]. It is reasonable to extend this standard to trans-men and trans-women receiving cross-gender hormones. Informed consent to access assisted reproductive technology poses further ethical questions in the adolescent population, as they are still considered minors. However, research on cognition and capacity suggests that adolescents show significant ability to provide informed consent, suggesting that content and wording of informed consent forms for adolescents should resemble those used with adults [30]. The American

Academy of Pediatrics state that children and adolescents need to be involved in decisions involving their health care in a developmentally appropriate manner [31]. This includes obtaining parental consent in matters involving adolescents as well as obtaining assent in minors who are able to understand the choices presented prior to treatment.

Experimental procedures such as ovarian or testicular cryopreservation may be reasonable to perform in adult trans-individuals in research settings with institutional review board (IRB) oversight [29]. Their use in the transgender adolescent population, however, is precluded by current WPATH recommendations not to perform irreversible surgery in trans-adolescents as well as the current paucity of data regarding the actual risk of gonadal toxicity of these treatments.

Fertility Preservation Options Prior to Initiation of Cross-Sex Hormones

Trans-women

Trans-women who have undergone male puberty prior to initiating estrogen therapy may opt for fertility preservation through sperm cryopreservation. Sperm cryopreservation was first reported in 1953 by Bunge and Sherman and has since become the most widely used method of fertility preservation for men faced with fertility challenges [32]. This can be easily accomplished at sperm-banking facilities, with sperm classically obtained through masturbation [33]. In cases in which sperm is not possible to be obtained through ejaculation, surgical techniques also exist that may retrieve sperm for cryopreservation including testicular sperm aspiration (TESA), percutaneous sperm aspiration (PESA), and testicular sperm extraction (TESE). Please refer to Chap. 7 for a detailed discussion of these options.

Trans-men

Trans-men who have undergone female puberty can choose to preserve fertility through embryo cryopreservation or oocyte cryopreservation. The success of embryo cryopreservation in achieving viable pregnancies has long been documented. Furthermore, oocyte cryopreservation has improved dramatically over the past decade so much so that it is currently recommended by the American Society for Reproductive Medicine for patients undergoing chemotherapy or other potentially gonadotoxic therapies [34]. Both methods are discussed in detail in Chap. 6. It is important to note that while pregnancies resulting from assisted reproductive technology have been reported in trans-men undergoing testosterone therapy, there is still no available data about pregnancies in trans-men achieved using cryopre-served oocytes obtained prior to initiating testosterone [25]. There has, however, been a case report of a transgender male undergoing ovarian stimulation and subsequent oocyte retrieval and cryopreservation before initiating androgen therapy [35].

Ovarian tissue cryopreservation is currently an experimental option, but one that possibly carries the most potential and has been offered to women undergoing chemotherapy [36]. Ovarian tissue cryopreservation does not require hormonal stimulation; however, as previously discussed, this is not recommended for transgender adolescents given the irreversibility of oophorectomy.

Special Considerations

Fertility Preservation After Puberty Suppression

Fertility preservation after puberty suppression presents unique issues as the gonads (both testes and ovary) have not matured at Tanner stage 2, which is when the Endocrine Society recommends starting puberty suppression. There have been reports of successful sperm retrieval either by electroejaculation or testicular sperm extraction in adolescents scheduled to undergo gonadotoxic therapy for malignancy; however, successful extraction was documented only in adolescents with at least Tanner stage 3 development [37]. Ovulation induction in adolescents also presents a similar challenge, with only one case report of successful ovarian stimulation and oocyte retrieval on a premenarcheal natal female with Tanner stage 3 breast development and Tanner stage 1 pubic hair [38].

To circumvent this, the Endocrine Society Guidelines recommends fertility preserving measures to be performed after cessation of gonadotropin suppression but prior to cross-gender hormone treatment [2]. Pubertal suppression with GnRH analogues is reversible and should not prevent resumption of pubertal development upon cessation of treatment; however, patients need to be counseled that there is no data in this population concerning the time required for sufficient spermatogenesis or for resumption of ovulation following pubertal suppression [39]. Furthermore, cessation of suppression without subsequent cross-gender hormone therapy may result in irreversible and undesirable sex characteristics, depending on the length treatment is to be withheld [2].

Fertility Preservation Options at Time of Gonadectomy

Currently in the United States, there are several investigational protocols for ovarian or testicular tissue freezing in young men and women whose fertility is threatened by needed cancer therapy. These involve removal of a portion or the entire gonad with cryopreservation of the tissue for possible thawing and future use. These procedures are discussed in Chaps. 6 and 7. The American Society of Clinical Oncology currently recommends that these procedures be performed under institutional review board oversight as they are experimental [39]. As discussed above the Endocrine Society Guidelines state that it is reasonable to perform gonadectomy after age 18 as part of gender-affirming surgery in transgender adolescents and adults, and at this time tissue freezing under IRB protocol could be considered [2]. Most patients undergo surgery after they have initiated hormonal therapy, and thus their gonadal function may already be affected. This highlights the need for all transgender individuals to be informed and counseled regarding options for fertility prior to medical or surgical treatment.

Future Research Priorities

The field of oncofertility has heightened awareness about fertility concerns in oncology patients; however, the application of fertility preservation in transgender medicine is just emerging. While we know that prolonged use of cross-sex hormones can have negative effects on both ovarian and testicular function, there is no data examining the amount and duration of exposure that guarantees infertility in both transmen and trans-women. Establishing the extent of gonadotoxicity of cross-gender hormone therapy would allow clinicians to better inform their patients about their options for fertility preservation and future. Furthermore, puberty suppression raises the possibility of ovulation induction and sperm extraction in adolescents who may be in mid- or late adolescence but very early in their pubertal development [37, 38]. Further research is needed to ascertain the safety of these interventions in children who are in Tanner stages 2–3.

Conclusion

Advances in the field of oncofertility have opened doors to fertility preservation in other populations, including transgender kids and adolescents. However, this population presents its own unique set of challenges because of the early timing of puberty suppression and the unknown extent of cross-gender hormone gonadotoxicity. Furthermore, while there is available data on the views of both parents and children regarding fertility preservation in the setting of cancer, there is little to no literature describing the attitudes of transgender kids and adolescents regarding their potential for future childbearing [40]. Nevertheless, all transgender individuals need to be informed and counseled regarding their options for fertility prior to initiation of puberty suppression or cross-gender hormones.

References

1. American Psychiatric Association. Diagnostic and statistical manual of mental disorders. 5th ed. Arlington: American Psychiatric Association; 2013.
2. Hembree WC, Cohen-Kettenis P, Delemarre-van de Waal HA, Endocrine Society, et al. Endocrine treatment of transsexual persons: an Endocrine Society clinical practice guideline. J Clin Endocrinol Metab. 2009;94(9):3132–54.
3. World Professional Association for Transgender Health (WPATH). Standards of Care for the Health of Transsexual, Transgender, and Gender-Nonconforming People. 7th Version. World Professional Association for Transgender Health. 2012.
4. de Delemarre-Van de Waal HA, Cohen-Kettenis PT. Clinical management of gender identity disorder in adolescents. Eur J Endocrinol. 2006;155 Suppl 1:S131–7.
5. Feldman J, Safer J. Hormone therapy in adults: suggested revisions to the sixth version of the standards of care. Int J Transgenderism. 2009;11(3):146–82.
6. Gooren L. Hormone treatment of the adult transsexual patient. Horm Res. 2005;64 Suppl 2:31–6.
7. Dumasia K, et al. Effect of estrogen receptor-subtype-specific ligands on fertility in adult male rats. J Endocrinol. 2015;225(3):169–80.
8. Gill-Sharma MK, et al. Antifertility effects of estradiol in adult male rats. J Endocrinol Invest. 2001;24(8):598–607.
9. Robaire B, Duron J, Hales BF. Effect of estradiol-filled polydimethylsiloxane subdermal implants in adult male rats on the reproductive system, fertility, and progeny outcome. Biol Reprod. 1987;37(2):327–34.
10. Sharpe RM, Skakkebaek NE. Are oestrogens involved in falling sperm counts and disorders of the male reproductive tract? Lancet. 1993;341(8857):1392–5.
11. Fisch H, Hyun G, Golden R. The possible effects of environmental estrogen disrupters on reproductive health. Curr Urol Rep. 2000;1(4):253–61.
12. Skakkebaek NE, et al. Is human fecundity declining? Int J Androl. 2006;29(1):2–11.
13. Oliva A, Spira A, Multigner L. Contribution of environmental factors to the risk of male infertility. Hum Reprod. 2001;16(8):1768–76.
14. Rozati R, et al. Role of environmental estrogens in the deterioration of male factor fertility. Fertil Steril. 2002;78(6):1187–94.
15. Du Plessis SS, et al. The effect of obesity on sperm disorders and male infertility. Nat Rev Urol. 2010;7(3):153–61.
16. Pauli EM, et al. Diminished paternity and gonadal function with increasing obesity in men. Fertil Steril. 2008;90(2):346–51.
17. Palmer NO, et al. Impact of obesity on male fertility, sperm function and molecular composition. Spermatogenesis. 2012;2(4):253–63.
18. Pavlovich CP, et al. Evidence of a treatable endocrinopathy in infertile men. J Urol. 2001;165(3):837–41.
19. Hillier SG, Ross GT. Effects of exogenous testosterone on ovarian weight, follicular morphology and intraovarian progesterone concentration in estrogen-primed hypophysectomized immature female rats. Biol Reprod. 1979;20(2):261–8.
20. Goerlich VC, Dijkstra C, Groothuis TG. Effects of in vivo testosterone manipulation on ovarian morphology, follicular development, and follicle yolk testosterone in the homing pigeon. J Exp Zool A Ecol Genet Physiol. 2010;313(6):328–38.
21. Velez LM, et al. Effect of hyperandrogenism on ovarian function. Reproduction. 2015;149(6):577–85.
22. van der Spuy ZM, Dyer SJ. The pathogenesis of infertility and early pregnancy loss in polycystic ovary syndrome. Best Pract Res Clin Obstet Gynaecol. 2004;18(5):755–71.

23. Dumesic DA, Padmanabhan V, Abbott DH. Polycystic ovary syndrome and oocyte developmental competence. Obstet Gynecol Surv. 2008;63(1):39–48.
24. Amato MC, et al. Low estradiol-to-testosterone ratio is associated with oligo-anovulatory cycles and atherogenic lipidic pattern in women with polycystic ovary syndrome. Gynecol Endocrinol. 2011;27(8):579–86.
25. Light AD, et al. Transgender men who experienced pregnancy after female-to-male gender transitioning. Obstet Gynecol. 2014;124(6):1120–7.
26. Ellis SA, Wojnar DM, Pettinato M. Conception, pregnancy, and birth experiences of male and gender variant gestational parents: it's how we could have a family. J Midwifery Womens Health. 2015;60(1):62–9.
27. Lawrence AA, Shaffer JD, Snow WR. Healthcare needs of transgendered patients. J Am Med Assoc. 1996;276:874.
28. American Academy of Child & Adolescent Psychiatry. Facts for Families: Children with Lesbian, Gay, Bisexual and Transgender Parents. Washington, DC; 2013.
29. The Ethics Committee of the American Society for Reproductive Medicine. Fertility Preservation and Reproduction in patients facing gonadotoxic therapies. Birmingham, AL; 2013.
30. Santelli JS, et al. Guidelines for adolescent health research. J Adolesc Health. 2003;33(5):396–409.
31. Fallat ME, Hutter J, American Academy of Pediatrics Committee on Bioethics, American Academy of Pediatrics Section on Hematology/Oncology, American Academy of Pediatrics Section on Surgery. Preservation of fertility in pediatric and adolescent patients with cancer. Pediatrics. 2008;121(5):e1461–9.
32. Bunge RG, Sherman JK. Fertilizing capacity of frozen human spermatozoa. Nature. 1953;172:767–8.
33. Wang JH, Muller CH, Lin K. Optimizing fertility preservation for pre- and postpubertal males with cancer. Semin Reprod Med. 2013;31:274–85.
34. Practice Committees of American Society for Reproductive Medicine, Society for Assisted Reproductive Technology. Mature oocyte cryopreservation: a guideline. Fertil Steril. 2013;99:37–43.
35. Wallace SA, Blough KL, Kondapalli LA. Fertility preservation in the transgender patient: expanding oncofertility care beyond cancer. Gynecol Endocrinol. 2014;30:1–4.
36. De Sutter P. Gender reassignment and assisted reproduction: present and future reproductive options for transsexual people. Hum Reprod. 2001;16(4):612–4.
37. Berookhim BM, Mulhall JP. Outcomes of operative sperm retrieval strategies for fertility preservation among males scheduled to undergo cancer treatment. Fertil Steril. 2014;101(3):805–11.
38. Reichman DE, Davis OK, Zaninovic N, Rosenwaks Z, Goldschlag DE. Fertility preservation using controlled ovarian hyperstimulation and oocyte cryopreservation in a premenarcheal female with myelodysplastic syndrome. Fertil Steril. 2012;98(5):1225–8.
39. Loren AW, Mangu PB, Beck LN, Brennan L, Magdalinski AJ, Partridge AH, Quinn G, Wallace WH, Oktay K, American Society of Clinical Oncology. Fertility preservation for patients with cancer: American Society of Clinical Oncology clinical practice guideline update. J Clin Oncol. 2013;31(19):2500–10.
40. Schover LR. Patient attitudes toward fertility preservation. Pediatr Blood Cancer. 2009;53(2):281–4.

Chapter 13
The Importance of Disclosure for Sexual Minorities in Oncofertility Cases

Christina Tamargo, Gwen Quinn, Matthew B. Schabath, and Susan T. Vadaparampil

Laura 33 years old, is seeing oncologist Dr. Smith to discuss results of her recent biopsy. Dr. Smith has reviewed Laura's social and medical history, which includes a previous benign biopsy for testicular cancer and says, "Your name is Laura? That's an unusual name for guy?" The patient responds, "I identify as female and chose the name Laura." Dr. Smith, uncertain of how to respond, proceeds to explain the cancer diagnosis. "You have colorectal cancer and your treatment will include both alkylating agents and radiation. This type of treatment can render you sterile but that is probably not a concern with folks like you. "Laura responds, "Why would you say that? I've always wanted to have children." Dr. Smith, still uncertain how to address his patient says "I'm going to call my nurse in here to talk to you, her son is gay and she knows more about this stuff than I do." Laura, reeling from the cancer diagnosis is crying and says with anger "I'm not gay, I'm transgender, and I am still a human being."

Abbreviations

AAP   American Academy of Pediatrics
ACOG   American College of Obstetricians and Gynecologists
ART   Assisted Reproductive technology
ASCO   American Society of Clinical Oncology
AYA   Adolescent and young adult
CDC   Centers for disease control and prevention
ESHRE   European Society for Human Reproduction and Embryology

C. Tamargo • G. Quinn (✉) • M.B. Schabath, Ph.D. • S.T. Vadaparampil, Ph.D.
Obstetrics and Gynecology, Northwestern University, Feinberg School of Medicine, Chicago, IL, USA

H. Lee Moffitt Cancer Center & Research Institute, University of South Florida, Tampa, FL, USA
e-mail: Christina.Tamargo@moffitt.org; Gwen.Quinn@moffitt.org

© Springer International Publishing Switzerland 2017
T.K. Woodruff, Y.C. Gosiengfiao (eds.), *Pediatric and Adolescent Oncofertility*,
DOI 10.1007/978-3-319-32973-4_13

FP   Fertility preservation
IOM   Institute of Medicine
LGBTQ   Lesbian, gay, bisexual, transsexual/transgender, queer/questioning
NCCN   National Comprehensive Cancer Network
QoL   Quality of life

Overview

The lesbian, gay, bisexual, transsexual/transgender, and queer/questioning (LGBTQ) population is an understudied and underserved population often referred to as sexual minorities [1]. The labels "lesbian, gay, and bisexual" refer to sexual orientation [2, 3]. The terms "transsexual" and "transgender" refer to gender identities where an individual does not identify with the sex assigned to him or her at birth (i.e., biological sex) [2, 3]. The labels "queer" and "questioning" may be used to refer to either sexual orientation or gender identity [4, 5]. There are several other terms associated with this community (e.g., "gender fluid, genderqueer, two-spirit") as well as nomenclature used within these groups that is typically not acceptable to be used by nonmembers (e.g., dyke) [6, 7]. It is estimated that 3–12 % of the United States population identifies as gay, lesbian, or bisexual and 1–3 % are transgender [8].

Each of the subpopulations under the term sexual minorities is likely to be unique, with varied health risk factors, communication preferences, and medical and social histories [4, 9]. It is common for all LGBTQ communities to perceive discrimination and lack of acceptance by society in general and in the healthcare setting in particular [4]. Several recent studies have identified that LGBTQ patients avoid preventive healthcare due to fear of perceived discrimination or because they cannot find an LGBTQ-friendly provider [1, 10–16]. LGBTQ individuals experience a variety of health disparities including higher rates of suicide attempts, higher prevalence of mental health issues, and increased risk for certain cancers [17–22].

LGBTQ Populations and Cancer

Because LGBTQ status is not collected in national surveys and registries [23], at present there are limited published data on cancer rates in LGBTQ populations [19, 24, 25]. As such, the cancer burden among the community is not known despite researchers utilizing novel approaches to estimate prevalence, density, incidence, and mortality of cancer among sexual minorities [26–29]. A recent review by Quinn et al. [19] synthesized the current literature on seven cancer sites that may disproportionately affect LGBTQ populations, specifically cancers of the anus, breast, uterine cervix, colon, endometrium, lung, and prostate. The authors noted that cancer health disparities in the LGBTQ community are likely attributed to multiple factors including social and economic factors, lower rates of access to healthcare and screening, and higher rates of risk factors and deleterious behaviors [19].

Disclosure of Gender Identify and Sexual Orientation in Healthcare

The increased risks for cancer associated with LGBTQ individuals are further exacerbated by nondisclosure of gender identity and sexual orientation by patients and failure to inquire by providers, which can lead to failure to screen, diagnose, or treat important medical problems [30–36]. The American Academy of Pediatrics, the American Medical Association, and the Society for Adolescent Health and Medicine all recommend providers discuss sexuality with all adolescents and offer nonjudgmental communication about sexual orientation [33, 37–39]. Patient disclosure of sexual orientation is associated with increased patient satisfaction and improved quality of care [33]. The majority of studies on LGBTQ disclosure have focused on older adults. Quinn et al. [40] surveyed 632 LGBTQ individuals, with a mean age of 58, about experiences with healthcare providers and reported 67 % always or often disclosed their status to their provider. Further, less than 10 % had ever experienced discrimination in a healthcare setting [40]. In a study of 291 LGBT patients with cancer, with a mean age of 62, 79 % reported disclosing their identity to their cancer provider; 34 % reported making this disclosure to correct a heteronormative assumption [32].

Very little is known about LGBTQ youth, especially those with cancer and their healthcare experiences [19, 24, 25, 33, 41–43]. The limited data that are available suggest younger sexual minorities may be less likely to disclose their sexual orientation or gender identity preferences to a healthcare provider [9]. A study of LGBTQ 18- to 23-year-olds without cancer found only 13 % had disclosed to a provider [33]. This finding is particularly important given the documented reproductive health needs and concerns regarding infertility and fertility experienced by adolescent and young adult (AYA) oncology patients [44–52]. The vast majority of studies focused on AYA concerns in these areas have not included assessments of sexual orientation and/or gender identity. The remainder of this chapter provides an overview of the potential unique concerns related to fertility.

Discussion of Fertility Considerations for LGBTQ AYA Cancer Patients

AYAs with cancer may experience permanent or temporary infertility [53–57]. The risk of infertility depends on a variety of factors such as cancer type, stage, chemotherapy regimen and dose, use of endocrine therapy, radiation site and dose, surgical site, and/or use of bone marrow or stem cell transplantation [58–67]. There are several excellent reviews that discuss these factors in greater detail [68–73]. Generally, younger patients are less likely to experience infertility [66, 67]. The American Society of Clinical Oncology (ASCO), the National Comprehensive Cancer Network (NCCN), and the American Academy of Pediatrics (AAP) have all issued guidelines urging oncology healthcare providers to discuss infertility risk and fertility options with AYA patients and to refer them to fertility specialists [58, 74, 75]. ASCO and NCCN guidelines also suggest further reproductive health discussions such as the use of contraception and referrals to genetic counselors in the case of familial cancer syndromes [58, 75].

However, studies suggest these discussions are either not occurring, as evidenced by lack of documentation in the medial record, or not recalled by AYA patients, as shown in retrospective studies of cancer survivors' satisfaction with and recall of discussion of fertility with oncology healthcare providers [76–80]. Several recent studies recognized that discussions with a healthcare provider about fertility risk, regardless of whether preservation methods were used, were associated with higher quality of life (QoL) and less regret than patients who did not report such discussions [51, 76, 81–84].

LGBTQ AYAs with a cancer diagnosis face the same serious threats to QoL due to temporary or permanent fertility issues as heterosexual and gender-aligned AYA [68, 71, 85–89]. Impaired fertility can have a ripple effect on other QoL issues such as romantic partnering, body image, and sexuality [71, 86]. Although this has not been empirically validated in populations with cancer, surveys and case studies of men and women with infertility issues suggest a relationship between poor self-image and the inability to procreate/produce biological children [90–92]. Although many AYAs have strong ideas about having children in their future, equal numbers may not have seriously thought about it, and may not consider it unless a healthcare provider brings it up [45, 46, 79, 93–100].

Available studies suggest that sexual minority AYAs with cancer are likely to be interested in discussion of fertility preservation at similar rates as heterosexual and gender-aligned patients. T'Sjoen [87] reported that prior to initiating cross-sex hormones, some transgender persons elect to preserve fertility so that a future biological child may be possible. Wierckx [88] interviewed 50 transsexual men to identify reproductive wishes; 54 % desired children and 37 % had considered banking sperm prior to beginning cross-sex hormones. A single case study of a 33-year-old gay man with prostate cancer identified that fertility was a key issue in making his treatment choices [89].

While discussing risks of infertility and fertility preservation (FP) options is important for this population, it is also important to consider the unique psychosocial and developmental issues of LGBTQ AYAs diagnosed with cancer. Unique experiences and considerations of LGBTQ individuals may cause them to have different desires regarding future childbearing and thus FP. For example, one transgender male-to-female child desired to have children in the future, but not with the sperm that could have been stored from her male body [101]. Given such situations, it may be useful for healthcare providers to focus on more diverse family building options, rather than solely on biological parenting – for example, surrogacy and adoption may be of interest to LGBTQ individuals like this child.

Multiple studies of AYA cancer patients and survivors have identified several reasons why discussions about fertility and reproductive health do not take place with newly diagnosed patients. These reasons include the severity of the cancer diagnosis, a provider's discomfort or lack of knowledge on the topic, and a perception that a patient is not interested in fertility if he or she does not initiate a conversation about it [46, 79, 93, 94, 98–100]. To date there have been very limited studies on LGBTQ AYAs with cancer and their fertility concerns, their childbearing intentions, or oncology healthcare providers' attitudes toward recommending fertility preservation to these patients. One of the first studies assessing oncologists' knowledge of the need to discuss fertility risks with patients identified many would not recommend sperm banking to a gay male patient [98]. It is not clear from this study if the perception is that gay male patients are perceived to be uninterested in having children, or if a value judgment is being made that this population should not have children.

Availability of and Challenges to Accessing FP and Biological Parenting Options for LGBTQ AYA Patients

For LGBTQ patients who wish to pursue FP options, it is important to consider the unique challenges that they may face. The American College of Obstetricians and Gynecologists (ACOG) acknowledges that lesbian and bisexual women experience barriers in the healthcare system due to concerns about confidentiality, need to disclose, and fear of discrimination [102]. ACOG urges providers to consider that any patient, even one who is pregnant, may be a lesbian or bisexual woman [102]. ACOG also sees refusal to provide reproductive health services to same-sex couples or transgender individuals as a form of discrimination [102–104]. The European Society for Health Reproduction Ethics (ESHRE) also stresses that denying any group access to assisted reproduction "cannot be reconciled with a human rights perspective" [105]. Yet, a recent study showed sexual minority women seek fertility services at half the rate of heterosexual women [106]. However, Grover et al. [107] report the number of same-sex male couples seeking reproductive health services has had a 21-fold increase since 2003. Yager et al. [108] report that lesbian and bisexual women trying to conceive perceive reduced lack of support and heterosexism in fertility healthcare systems.

A survey of 41 transgender men who had become pregnant showed 36 (88%) achieved this pregnancy through their own oocytes despite having used testosterone prior to the pregnancy. Only half of the men reported receiving prenatal care, and all subjects reported low levels of provider knowledge of transgender health. However, what the study also reveals is that many transgender men who have transitioned socially, and in some case medically, still desire a biological child [109].

However, studies of healthcare providers suggest some bias in dealing with LGBTQ patients. A study of Canadian providers showed 11% did not offer sperm banking to gay men [99]. A study of nine transgender individuals living in Canada who attempted to use ART reported all had a negative experience with providers [110]. A US study of obstetrics and gynecology providers revealed 14% would not suggest ART to women in same-sex relationships or unmarried women [111]. In a 2012 analysis of the websites of US fertility clinics, 11% of clinics did not accept lesbian and single women, and only 10 % of all clinic websites had an explicit non-discrimination disclosure [112]. Several legal studies have examined the juxtaposition between a provider's right not to provide medical care that he or she deems contrary to moral values or conscientious refusal, and discrimination in the context of reproductive medicine [113–117]. The AMA guidelines, however, state, "Physicians cannot refuse to care for patients based on race, gender, sexual orientation, gender identity or any other criteria that would constitute invidious discrimination" [118], nor can they discriminate against patients with infectious diseases [119].

Ongoing advances in assisted reproductive technology (ART) such as uterine transplants for successful pregnancy will continue to raise new ethical issues about the ability for transgender females to carry a pregnancy. For example, Murphy [120] explored this ethical conundrum in a recent commentary and concluded there are no strong arguments to preclude either the state from developing a line of research to explore the medical feasibility of this or for a transgender woman to pursue a uterine transplant with the goal of carrying a pregnancy.

Policy and Practice

Institutional policies and practices as well as healthcare providers' verbal and nonverbal communication provide a foundation for AYA LGBTQ patients to disclose their status [30, 121, 122]. Implementing systems-level approaches to routinely collecting relevant information for LGBTQ populations can provide an important starting point to facilitate optimal care [30, 122]. However, health intake forms with binary categories of gender and sexual orientation may dissuade patients from providing this important piece of their social and medical history. Inclusive health forms allow patients to use their own language to describe their gender, romantic relationship, and sexual history [30]. For example, the *Fenway Guide to Lesbian, Gay, Bisexual, and Transgender Health* suggests providers should consider the possibility that "every new patient may have any gender identity or sexual orientation or engage in any sexual behavior: avoid making assumptions based on stereotypes or generalizing from your own experience" [123]. As shown in Table 13.1, taking a sexual history can involve multiple questions that may be different than most providers leaned in medical school [4, 124, 125]. Table 13.1 provides suggestions for taking a sexual history. Table 13.2 offers considerations for healthcare providers when asking these questions such as examining your own values and being aware of nonverbal body language.

The Joint Commission, the Centers for Disease Control and Prevention (CDC), and the Institute of Medicine (IOM) all recommend sexual orientation, and gender identity should be collected in patient medical records [5, 126–129]. CDC and IOM further recommend the aggregation of these data to ensure these populations are represented in clinical research and to reduce health disparities in the population [5, 129]. Figure 13.1 below provides sample wording for the collection of sexual orientation and gender identity on a medical form.

Table 13.1 Suggested sexual health history questions for face-to-face interview (Makadon et al. [123])

Are you having sex?
Are you sexually active with men, women, or both?
What type of sex do you have?   Prompts: oral, vaginal, anal
For each type of sex, are you using barriers or condoms? If yes, how often do you use them?   Prompts: every time, not with primary partner
Do you have any questions about the use of barriers?
What keeps you from using barriers?

Table 13.2 Dos and don'ts in taking a sexual history (Makadon et al. [123])

Do begin with a statement explaining that you ask these questions of all your patients and that the questions are vital to the patient's overall health	*Don't* make assumptions about past, current, or future sexual behavior
Do avoid language that presumes heterosexuality	*Don't* assume that a person who identifies as lesbian or gay has never had an opposite-sex partner
Do check yourself for judgmental facial expressions, body language, and tone of speech	*Don't* assume that an LGBTQ person does not have (or lacks the desire to have) children or has never been pregnant
Do be prepared to answer questions about STI and HIV transmission risk for various sexual activities relevant to LGBTQ people	–
Do note that transgender individuals, men who have sex with men, and those who engage in high-risk sexual activities are at increased risk for contracting HIV and certain STIs	–
Do screen and treat according to the CDC guidelines (www.cdc.gov/std/treatment)	–
Do realize that although STIs are less common among lesbians, clinicians should still screen all women for STI risk, regardless of sexual orientation. The more sexual partners a woman has (female or male), the greater her risk. Bacterial vaginosis may be more common in women who have sex with women than in the general population	–
Do consider the overall health of patients who present with sexual functioning concerns, including their psychological status, physical wellness, and relationship health	–

Conclusion

Healthcare providers in the oncology care setting are increasingly called to understand the unique needs of, and provide care to, a diverse patient population [19, 130]. While great strides have been made over the last decade with respect to cultural

Please provide the following information so that providers and staff may address you correctly and bill for services correctly.

a. Name on Insurance or Legal Government Records:
_____

b. Preferred Name/Nickname (if different):   _____

c. What is your current gender identity (check all that apply):
Male   Female   Transgender Male/Trans Man/FTM
Transgender Female/Trans Woman/ MTF   Genderqueer
Additional Category, please specify: _____
Decline to Answer

d. What sex were you assigned at birth on your original birth certificate (check one)
Male   Female   Decline to Answer

e. What sex is listed on your health insurance of government records
Male   Female

f. What gender pronoun do you prefer (he, she, they, zie etc):_____

g. Do you think of yourself as:
Lesbian
                        Gay   Homosexual
Straight or heterosexual   Bisexual   Something else_____
Don't know

Fig. 13.1 Sample language for a medical form (Makadon et al. [123])

competence, there is a growing awareness that diversity spans beyond minority groups solely based on race and ethnicity and includes sexual minority groups that have long been marginalized in the US healthcare system. Our review specifically discusses the challenges of AYA LGBTQ patients in the context of cancer-related infertility and fertility preservation. However, many of the issues and considerations that we have discussed as well as the suggestions we provide can be used to more broadly impact and improve healthcare for sexual minority groups.

References

1. Fredriksen-Goldsen KI, Kim HJ, Barkan SE, Muraco A, Hoy-Ellis CP. Health disparities among lesbian, gay, and bisexual older adults: results from a population-based study. Am J Public Health. 2013;103(10):1802–9. Pubmed Central PMCID: Pmc3770805, Epub 2013/06/15. eng.
2. Spectrum Center. LGBT terms and definitions [internet]. Ann Arbor: Spectrum Center; 2015. [cited 2015 Jul 20], Available from: http://internationalspectrum.umich.edu/life/definitions.

3. Johnson CV, Mimiaga MJ, Bradford J. Health care issues among lesbian, gay, bisexual, transgender and intersex (LGBTI) populations in the United States: introduction. J Homosex. 2008;54(3):213–24. Epub 2008/10/02. eng.
4. Institute of Medicine. The health of lesbian, gay, bisexual, and transgender people: building a foundation for better understanding. Washington, DC: National Academies Press; 2011.
5. Institute of Medicine. Collecting sexual orientation and gender identity data in electronic health records. Washington, DC: National Academies Press; 2013.
6. UC Berkeley Gender Equity Resource Center. Definition of Terms [Internet]. Berkeley: UC Berkeley Gender Equity Resource Center; c2014 [updated 2013 Jul; cited 2015 Jul 21]. Available from: http://geneq.berkeley.edu/lgbt_resources_definiton_of_terms.
7. Gender and Sexuality Center. LGBT Vocab 101 [Internet]. Northfield: Gender and Sexuality Center; [date unknown] [updated 2014 May 27; cited 2015 Jul 21]. Available from: https://apps.carleton.edu/campus/gsc/students/ally/lgbtvocab/.
8. Gates GJ. How many people are lesbian, gay, bisexual, and transgender? Los Angeles: The Williams Institute, University of California, Los Angeles School of Law; 2011.
9. Durso LE, Meyer IH. Patterns and predictors of disclosure of sexual orientation to healthcare providers among lesbians, gay men, and bisexuals. Sex Res Social Policy. 2013;10(1): 35–42.
10. Hart SL, Bowen DJ. Sexual orientation and intentions to obtain breast cancer screening. J Womens Health (Larchmt). 2009;18(2):177–85. Pubmed Central PMCID: Pmc2945722, Epub 2009/02/03. eng.
11. Tracy JK, Lydecker AD, Ireland L. Barriers to cervical cancer screening among lesbians. J Womens Health (Larchmt). 2010;19(2):229–37. Pubmed Central PMCID: Pmc2834453, Epub 2010/01/26. eng.
12. Tracy JK, Schluterman NH, Greenberg DR. Understanding cervical cancer screening among lesbians: a national survey. BMC Public Health. 2013;13:442. Pubmed Central PMCID: Pmc3693978, Epub 2013/05/07. eng.
13. Newman PA, Roberts KJ, Masongsong E, Wiley DJ. Anal cancer screening: barriers and facilitators among ethnically diverse gay, bisexual, transgender, and other men who have sex with men. J Gay Lesbian Soc Serv. 2008;20(4):328–53. Pubmed Central PMCID: Pmc3002049, Epub 2008/10/01. Eng.
14. Potter J, Peitzmeier SM, Bernstein I, Reisner SL, Alizaga NM, Agenor M, et al. Cervical cancer screening for patients on the female-to-male spectrum: a narrative review and guide for clinicians. J Gen Intern Med. 2015;30(12):1857–64. Epub 2015/07/15. Eng.
15. Lutz AR. Screening for asymptomatic extragenital gonorrhea and chlamydia in men who have Sex with men: significance, recommendations, and options for overcoming barriers to testing. LGBT Health. 2015;2(1):27–34.
16. Dodge B, Van Der Pol B, Rosenberger JG, Reece M, Roth AM, Herbenick D, et al. Field collection of rectal samples for sexually transmitted infection diagnostics among men who have sex with men. Int J STD AIDS. 2010;21(4):260–4. Epub 2010/04/10. eng.
17. McKay B. Lesbian, gay, bisexual, and transgender health issues, disparities, and information resources. Med Ref Serv Q. 2011;30(4):393–401. Epub 2011/11/02. eng.
18. National Alliance on Mental Illness. Mental health issues among gay, lesbian, bisexual, and transgender (GLBT) people [Internet]. Arlington: National Alliance on Mental Illness Multicultural Action Center; 2007 [cited 2015 Jul 21]. Available from: http://www.nami.org/Content/ContentGroups/Multicultural_Support1/Fact_Sheets1/GLBT_Mental_Health_07.pdf.
19. Quinn GP, Sanchez JA, Sutton SK, Vadaparampil ST, Nguyen GT, Green BL, et al. Cancer and lesbian, gay, bisexual, transgender/transsexual, and queer/questioning (LGBTQ) populations. CA Cancer J Clin. 2015;65:384.
20. Almeida J, Johnson RM, Corliss HL, Molnar BE, Azrael D. Emotional distress among LGBT youth: the influence of perceived discrimination based on sexual orientation. J Youth Adolesc. 2009;38(7):1001–14. Pubmed Central PMCID: Pmc3707280, Epub 2009/07/29. eng.

21. Burgess D, Tran A, Lee R, van Ryn M. Effects of perceived discrimination on mental health and mental health services utilization among gay, lesbian, bisexual and transgender persons. J LGBT Health Res. 2007;3(4):1–14. Epub 2008/12/02. eng.
22. National Institutes of Health. Plans for Advancing LGBT Health Research [Internet]. Bethesda: U.S. Department of Health and Human Services; 2013 [updated 2013 Jan 4; cited 2015 Jul 21]. Available from: http://nih.gov/about/director/01032013_lgbt_plan.htm.
23. Margolies L. Bisexual Women and Breast Cancer [Internet]. Santa Monica: National LGBT Cancer Network; c2015 [updated 2013 Oct 7; cited 2015 Jul 21]. Available from: http://cancer-network.org/cancer_information/bisexuals_and_cancer/bisexual_women_and_breast_cancer.php.
24. Brown JP, Tracy JK. Lesbians and cancer: an overlooked health disparity. Cancer Causes Control. 2008;19(10):1009–20.
25. NIH LGBT Research Coordinating Committee. Consideration of the institute of medicine (IOM) report on the health of lesbian, gay, bisexual, and transgender (LGBT) individuals. Washington, DC: National Institutes of Health; 2013.
26. Boehmer U, Miao X, Maxwell NI, Ozonoff A. Sexual minority population density and incidence of lung, colorectal and female breast cancer in California. BMJ Open. 2014;4(3):e004461. Pubmed Central PMCID: Pmc3975738, Epub 2014/03/29. eng.
27. Boehmer U, Miao X, Ozonoff A. Cancer survivorship and sexual orientation. Cancer. 2011;117(16):3796–804. Epub 2011/05/11. eng.
28. Boehmer U, Ozonoff A, Miao X. An ecological analysis of colorectal cancer incidence and mortality: differences by sexual orientation. BMC Cancer. 2011;11:400. Pubmed Central PMCID: Pmc3188512, Epub 2011/09/23. eng.
29. Boehmer U, Ozonoff A, Miao X. An ecological approach to examine lung cancer disparities due to sexual orientation. Public Health. 2012;126(7):605–12. Pubmed Central PMCID: Pmc3389196, Epub 2012/05/15. eng.
30. Quinn GP, Schabath MB, Sanchez JA, Sutton SK, Green BL. The importance of disclosure: lesbian, gay, bisexual, transgender/transsexual, queer/questioning, and intersex individuals and the cancer continuum. Cancer. 2015;121(8):1160–3.
31. Dahan R, Feldman R, Hermoni D. Is patients' sexual orientation a blind spot of family physicians? J Homosex. 2008;55(3):524–32. Epub 2008/12/02. eng.
32. Kamen CS, Smith-Stoner M, Heckler CE, Flannery M, Margolies L, editors. Social support, self-rated health, and lesbian, gay, bisexual, and transgender identity disclosure to cancer care providers. Oncol Nurs Forum. 2015;42(1):44–51: NIH Public Access.
33. Meckler GD, Elliott MN, Kanouse DE, Beals KP, Schuster MA. Nondisclosure of sexual orientation to a physician among a sample of gay, lesbian, and bisexual youth. Arch Pediatr Adolesc Med. 2006;160(12):1248–54.
34. Bjorkman M, Malterud K. Being lesbian–does the doctor need to know? A qualitative study about the significance of disclosure in general practice. Scand J Prim Health Care. 2007;25(1):58–62.
35. Boehmer U, Case P. Physicians don't ask, sometimes patients tell. Cancer. 2004;101(8):1882–9.
36. Johnson MJ, Nemeth LS. Addressing health disparities of lesbian and bisexual women: a grounded theory study. Womens Health Issues. 2014;24(6):635–40.
37. American Medical Association. AMA Policy Regarding Sexual Orientation [Internet]. Chicago: American Medical Association; c1995-2015 [cited 2015 Jul 22]. Available from: http://www.ama-assn.org/ama/pub/about-ama/our-people/member-groups-sections/glbt-advisory-committee/ama-policy-regarding-sexual-orientation.page.
38. Frankowski BL. Sexual orientation and adolescents. Pediatrics. 2004;113(6):1827–32. Epub 2004/06/03. eng.
39. Society for Adolescent Health and Medicine. Recommendations for promoting the health and well-being of lesbian, gay, bisexual, and transgender adolescents: a position paper of the Society for Adolescent Health and Medicine. J Adolesc Health. 2013;52(4):506–10. Epub 2013/03/26. eng.

40. Quinn GP, Sutton SK, Winfield B, Breen S, Canales J, Shetty G, et al. Lesbian, gay, bisexual, transgender, queer/questioning (LGBTQ) perceptions and health care experiences. J Gay Lesbian Soc Serv. 2015;27(2):246–61.
41. Fisher CB, Mustanski B. Reducing health disparities and enhancing the responsible conduct of research involving LGBT youth. Hastings Cent Rep. 2014;44 Suppl 4:S28–31. Epub 2014/09/19. eng.
42. Mayer KH, Bradford JB, Makadon HJ, Stall R, Goldhammer H, Landers S. Sexual and gender minority health: what we know and what needs to be done. Am J Public Health. 2008;98(6):989–95.
43. Mustanski B. Future directions in research on sexual minority adolescent mental, behavioral, and sexual health. J Clin Child Adolesc Psychol. 2015;44(1):204–19. Pubmed Central PMCID: Pmc4314941, Epub 2015/01/13. eng.
44. Carter J, Penson R, Barakat R, Wenzel L. Contemporary quality of life issues affecting gynecologic cancer survivors. Hematol Oncol Clin North Am. 2012;26(1):169–94.
45. Partridge AH, Gelber S, Peppercorn J, Sampson E, Knudsen K, Laufer M, et al. Web-based survey of fertility issues in young women with breast cancer. J Clin Oncol. 2004;22(20):4174–83.
46. Schover LR. Patient attitudes toward fertility preservation. Pediatr Blood Cancer. 2009;53(2):281–4.
47. Howard-Anderson J, Ganz PA, Bower JE, Stanton AL. Quality of life, fertility concerns, and behavioral health outcomes in younger breast cancer survivors: a systematic review. J Natl Cancer Inst. 2012;104(5):386–405.
48. Bleyer A, Barr R, Hayes-Lattin B, Thomas D, Ellis C, Anderson B, et al. The distinctive biology of cancer in adolescents and young adults. Nat Rev Cancer. 2008;8(4):288–98.
49. Levine J, Canada A, Stern CJ. Fertility preservation in adolescents and young adults with cancer. J Clin Oncol. 2010;28(32):4831–41.
50. Canada AL, Schover LR. The psychosocial impact of interrupted childbearing in long-term female cancer survivors. Psychooncology. 2012;21(2):134–43. Pubmed Central PMCID: 3123665.
51. Letourneau JM, Ebbel EE, Katz PP, Katz A, Ai WZ, Chien AJ, et al. Pretreatment fertility counseling and fertility preservation improve quality of life in reproductive age women with cancer. Cancer. 2012;118(6):1710–7. Pubmed Central PMCID: 3235264.
52. Gorman JR, Usita PM, Madlensky L, Pierce JP. Young breast cancer survivors: their perspectives on treatment decisions and fertility concerns. Cancer Nurs. 2011;34(1):32–40. Pubmed Central PMCID: 2980796.
53. Bahadur G. Fertility issues for cancer patients. Mol Cell Endocrinol. 2000;169(1–2):117–22. Epub 2001/01/13. eng.
54. Padron OF, Sharma RK, Thomas Jr AJ, Agarwal A. Effects of cancer on spermatozoa quality after cryopreservation: a 12-year experience. Fertil Steril. 1997;67(2):326–31. Epub 1997/02/01. eng.
55. Drasga RE, Einhorn LH, Williams SD, Patel DN, Stevens EE. Fertility after chemotherapy for testicular cancer. J Clin Oncol. 1983;1(3):179–83. Epub 1983/03/01. eng.
56. Carter J, Rowland K, Chi D, Brown C, Abu-Rustum N, Castiel M, et al. Gynecologic cancer treatment and the impact of cancer-related infertility. Gynecol Oncol. 2005;97(1):90–5. Epub 2005/03/26. eng.
57. Crawshaw M, Sloper P. A qualitative study of the experiences of teenagers and young adults when faced with possible or actual fertility impairment following cancer treatment. York: Department of Social Policy and Social Work, University of York; 2006.
58. Loren AW, Mangu PB, Beck LN, Brennan L, Magdalinski AJ, Partridge AH, et al. Fertility preservation for patients with cancer: American Society of Clinical Oncology clinical practice guideline update. J Clin Oncol. 2013;31(19):2500–10. Epub 2013/05/30. eng.
59. Gracia CR, Sammel MD, Freeman E, Prewitt M, Carlson C, Ray A, et al. Impact of cancer therapies on ovarian reserve. Fertil Steril. 2012;97(1):134–40.e1. Pubmed Central PMCID: Pmc4005036. Epub 2011/12/06. eng.

60. Critchley HO, Wallace WH. Impact of cancer treatment on uterine function. J Natl Cancer Inst Monogr. 2005;34:64–8. Epub 2005/03/24. eng.
61. Littley MD, Shalet SM, Beardwell CG, Ahmed SR, Applegate G, Sutton ML. Hypopituitarism following external radiotherapy for pituitary tumours in adults. Q J Med. 1989;70(262):145–60. Epub 1989/02/01. eng.
62. Su HI, Sammel MD, Velders L, Horn M, Stankiewicz C, Matro J, et al. Association of cyclophosphamide drug-metabolizing enzyme polymorphisms and chemotherapy-related ovarian failure in breast cancer survivors. Fertil Steril. 2010;94(2):645–54. Pubmed Central PMCID: Pmc2891284, Epub 2009/04/21. eng.
63. van Dorp W, van den Heuvel-Eibrink MM, Stolk L, Pieters R, Uitterlinden AG, Visser JA, et al. Genetic variation may modify ovarian reserve in female childhood cancer survivors. Hum Reprod. 2013;28(4):1069–76. Epub 2013/01/31. eng.
64. American Cancer Society. Fertility and women with cancer [internet]. Atlanta: American Cancer Society; 2013. [cited 2015 Jul 22]. Available from: http://www.cancer.org/acs/groups/cid/documents/webcontent/acspc-041244-pdf.pdf.
65. LIVESTRONG. LIVESTRONG Fertility [Internet]. Austin: LIVESTRONG; c2014 [cited 2015 Jul 22]. Available from: http://assets.livestrong.org/we-can-help/LIVESTRONG-Fertility-Brochure.pdf.
66. Cancer.net. Fertility Concerns and Preservation for Men [Internet]. [place unknown]: American Society of Clinical Oncology; c2005-2015 [cited 2015 Jul 22]. Available from: http://www.cancer.net/coping-and-emotions/sexual-and-reproductive-health/fertility-concerns-and-preservation-men.
67. Cancer.net. Fertility Concerns and Preservation for Women [Internet]. [place unknown]: American Society of Clinical Oncology; c2005-2015 [cited 2015 Jul 22]. Available from: http://www.cancer.net/coping-and-emotions/sexual-and-reproductive-health/fertility-concerns-and-preservation-women.
68. Levine JM, Kelvin JF, Quinn GP, Gracia CR. Infertility in reproductive-age female cancer survivors. Cancer. 2015;121(10):1532–9. Epub 2015/02/05. eng.
69. Hulvat MC, Jeruss JS. Maintaining fertility in young women with breast cancer. Curr Treat Options Oncol. 2009;10(5-6):308–17. Pubmed Central PMCID: Pmc2908234, Epub 2010/03/20. eng.
70. Duffy C, Allen S. Medical and psychosocial aspects of fertility after cancer. Cancer J. 2009;15(1):27–33. Pubmed Central PMCID: Pmc2719717, Epub 2009/02/07. eng.
71. Goldfarb S, Mulhall J, Nelson C, Kelvin J, Dickler M, Carter J. Sexual and reproductive health in cancer survivors. Semin Oncol. 2013;40(6):726–44. Epub 2013/12/18. eng.
72. Tournaye H, Dohle GR, Barratt CL. Fertility preservation in men with cancer. Lancet. 2014;384(9950):1295–301. Epub 2014/10/07. eng.
73. Ginsberg JP. Educational paper: the effect of cancer therapy on fertility, the assessment of fertility and fertility preservation options for pediatric patients. Eur J Pediatr. 2011;170(6):703–8. Epub 2010/12/04. eng.
74. Fallat ME, Hutter J. Preservation of fertility in pediatric and adolescent patients with cancer. Pediatrics. 2008;121(5):e1461–9. Epub 2008/05/03. eng.
75. Coccia P, Pappo A, Altman J, Bhatia S, Borges V, Borinstein S, et al. The NCCN adolescent and young adult (AYA) oncology clinical practice guideline, version 2.2015 [internet]. Cold Spring Harbor: Harborside Press, LLC; 2015. [cited 2015 Jul 22]. Available from: http://www.nccn.org/professionals/physician_gls/pdf/aya.pdf.
76. Quinn GP, Block RG, Clayman ML, Kelvin J, Arvey SR, Lee JH, et al. If you did not document it, it did not happen: rates of documentation of discussion of infertility risk in adolescent and young adult oncology patients' medical records. J Oncol Pract. 2015;11(2):137–44. Epub 2015/01/01. eng.
77. Vadaparampil ST, Quinn GP. Improving communication between oncologists and reproductive specialists to promote timely referral of patients with cancer. J Oncol Pract. 2013;9(6):300–2. Epub 2013/08/15. eng.

78. Banerjee R, Tsiapali E. Occurrence and recall rates of fertility discussions with young breast cancer patients. Support Care Cancer. 2015;24(1):163–71. Epub 2015/05/15. eng.
79. Quinn GP, Vadaparampil ST, Lee JH, Jacobsen PB, Bepler G, Lancaster J, et al. Physician referral for fertility preservation in oncology patients: a national study of practice behaviors. J Clin Oncol. 2009;27(35):5952–7. Epub 2009/10/15. eng.
80. Yeomanson DJ, Morgan S, Pacey AA. Discussing fertility preservation at the time of cancer diagnosis: dissatisfaction of young females. Pediatr Blood Cancer. 2013;60(12):1996–2000. Epub 2013/07/10. eng.
81. Partridge AH, Gelber S, Peppercorn J, Ginsburg E, Sampson E, Rosenberg R, et al. Fertility and menopausal outcomes in young breast cancer survivors. Clin Breast Cancer. 2008;8(1):65–9. Epub 2008/05/27. eng.
82. Bastings L, Baysal O, Beerendonk CC, IntHout J, Traas MA, Verhaak CM, et al. Deciding about fertility preservation after specialist counselling. Hum Reprod. 2014;29(8):1721–9. Epub 2014/06/12. eng.
83. Wilkes S, Coulson S, Crosland A, Rubin G, Stewart J. Experience of fertility preservation among younger people diagnosed with cancer. Hum Fertil (Camb). 2010;13(3):151–8. Epub 2010/09/21. eng.
84. Jeruss JS, Woodruff TK. Preservation of fertility in patients with cancer. N Engl J Med. 2009;360(9):902–11. Pubmed Central PMCID: Pmc2927217, Epub 2009/02/28. eng.
85. Rowan K. Fertility preservation during treatment is a growing issue for women. J Natl Cancer Inst. 2010;102(5):294–6. Epub 2010/02/23. eng.
86. Murphy D, Klosky JL, Reed DR, Termuhlen AM, Shannon SV, Quinn GP. The importance of assessing priorities of reproductive health concerns among adolescent and young adult patients with cancer. Cancer. 2015;121(15):2529–36. Epub 2015/06/05. eng.
87. T'Sjoen G, Van Caenegem E, Wierckx K. Transgenderism and reproduction. Curr Opin Endocrinol Diabetes Obes. 2013;20(6):575–9.
88. Wierckx K, Van Caenegem E, Pennings G, Elaut E, Dedecker D, Van de Peer F, et al. Reproductive wish in transsexual men. Hum Reprod. 2012;27(2):483–7.
89. Santillo VM. Prostate cancer diagnosis and treatment of a 33-year-old gay man. J Gay Lesbian Ment Health. 2005;9(1-2):155–71.
90. [author unknown]. New Survey Finds Infertility Delivers a Serious Blow to Self-Esteem [Internet]. Whitehouse Station: PR Newswire; 2010 [cited 2015 Jul 24]. Available from: http://www.prnewswire.com/news-releases/new-survey-finds-infertility-delivers-a-serious-blow-to-self-esteem-82242177.html.
91. Faramarzi M, Pasha H, Esmailzadeh S, Kheirkhah F, Hajian-Tilaki K, Salmalian H. A survey of correlation infertility self-efficacy with behavioral health scales in infertile women. Health (N Y). 2014;6(10):943.
92. Wischmann T, Schilling K, Toth B, Rosner S, Strowitzki T, Wohlfarth K, et al. Sexuality, self-esteem and partnership quality in infertile women and men. Geburtshilfe Frauenheilkd. 2014;74(8):759–63. Pubmed Central PMCID: Pmc4153818, Epub 2014/09/16. Eng.
93. Jukkala AM, Azuero A, McNees P, Bates GW, Meneses K. Self-assessed knowledge of treatment and fertility preservation in young women with breast cancer. Fertil Steril. 2010;94(6):2396–8. Epub 2010/05/08. eng.
94. Oosterhuis BE, Goodwin T, Kiernan M, Hudson MM, Dahl GV. Concerns about infertility risks among pediatric oncology patients and their parents. Pediatr Blood Cancer. 2008;50(1):85–9. Epub 2007/05/22. eng.
95. Burns KC, Boudreau C, Panepinto JA. Attitudes regarding fertility preservation in female adolescent cancer patients. J Pediatr Hematol Oncol. 2006;28(6):350–4. Epub 2006/06/24. eng.
96. Maltaris T, Seufert R, Fischl F, Schaffrath M, Pollow K, Koelbl H, et al. The effect of cancer treatment on female fertility and strategies for preserving fertility. Eur J Obstet Gynecol Reprod Biol. 2007;130(2):148–55. Epub 2006/09/19. eng.
97. Klock SC, Zhang JX, Kazer RR. Fertility preservation for female cancer patients: early clinical experience. Fertil Steril. 2010;94(1):149–55. Epub 2009/05/02. eng.

98. Schover LR, Brey K, Lichtin A, Lipshultz LI, Jeha S. Oncologists' attitudes and practices regarding banking sperm before cancer treatment. J Clin Oncol. 2002;20(7):1890–7. Epub 2002/03/29. eng.
99. Achille MA, Rosberger Z, Robitaille R, Lebel S, Gouin JP, Bultz BD, et al. Facilitators and obstacles to sperm banking in young men receiving gonadotoxic chemotherapy for cancer: the perspective of survivors and health care professionals. Hum Reprod. 2006;21(12):3206–16. Epub 2006/08/05. eng.
100. Quinn GP, Vadaparampil ST, Gwede CK, Miree C, King LM, Clayton HB, et al. Discussion of fertility preservation with newly diagnosed patients: oncologists' views. J Cancer Surviv. 2007;1(2):146–55. Epub 2008/07/24. eng.
101. Navasky M, O'Connor K. Growing up trans [television broadcast]. FRONTLINE. Boston: Public Broadcasting Service; 2015.
102. ACOG Committee on Health Care for Underserved Women. ACOG Committee Opinion No. 525: health care for lesbians and bisexual women. Obstet Gynecol. 2012;119(5):1077.
103. ACOG Committee on Health Care for Underserved Women. Committee opinion no. 512: health care for transgender individuals. Obstet Gynecol. 2011;118(6):1454–8. Epub 2011/11/23. eng.
104. American College of Obstetricians Gynecologists. ACOG Committee Opinion No. 385 November 2007: the limits of conscientious refusal in reproductive medicine. Obstet Gynecol. 2007;110(5):1203.
105. De Wert G, Dondorp W, Shenfield F, Barri P, Devroey P, Diedrich K, et al. ESHRE task force on ethics and Law 23: medically assisted reproduction in singles, lesbian and gay couples, and transsexual people. Hum Reprod. 2014;29(9):1859–65.
106. Blanchfield BV, Patterson CJ. Racial and sexual minority women's receipt of medical assistance to become pregnant. Health Psychol. 2015;34(6):571.
107. Grover SA, Shmorgun Z, Moskovtsev SI, Baratz A, Librach CL. Assisted reproduction in a cohort of same-sex male couples and single men. Reprod Biomed Online. 2013;27(2): 217–21.
108. Yager C, Brennan D, Steele LS, Epstein R, Ross LE. Challenges and mental health experiences of lesbian and bisexual women who are trying to conceive. Health Soc Work. 2010;35(3):191–200.
109. Light AD, Obedin-Maliver J, Sevelius JM, Kerns JL. Transgender men who experienced pregnancy after female-to-male gender transitioning. Obstet Gynecol. 2014;124(6):1120–7.
110. James-Abra S, Tarasoff L, Epstein R, Anderson S, Marvel S, Steele L, et al. Trans people's experiences with assisted reproduction services: a qualitative study. Hum Reprod. 2015;30(6):1365–74.
111. Lawrence RE, Rasinski KA, Yoon JD, Curlin FA. Obstetrician–gynecologists' beliefs about assisted reproductive technologies. Obstet Gynecol. 2010;116(1):127–35.
112. Johnson KM. Excluding lesbian and single women? An analysis of US fertility clinic websites. Womens Stud Int Forum. 2012;35(5):394–402.
113. Lumpkin CA. Does a pharmacist have the right to refuse to fill a prescription for birth control. U Miami Law Rev. 2005;60:105.
114. Smearman CA. Drawing the line: the legal, ethical and public policy implications of refusal clauses for pharmacists. Ariz Law Rev. 2006;48:469.
115. Storrow RF. Medical conscience and the policing of parenthood. William & Mary J Women Law. 2009;16:369.
116. Dickens B. Legal protection and limits of conscientious objection: when conscientious objection is unethical. Med Law. 2009;28(2):337.
117. Langlois N. Life-sustaining treatment law: a model for balancing a woman's reproductive rights with a pharmacist's conscientious objection. BCL Rev. 2005;47:815.
118. American Medical Association. Opinion 9.12 – Patient-physician relationship: respect for law and human rights [Internet]. Chicago: American Medical Association; c1995-2015 [updated 2008 Jun; cited 2015 Jul 23]. Available from: http://www.ama-assn.org/ama/pub/physician-resources/medical-ethics/code-medical-ethics/opinion912.page.

119. American Medical Association. Opinion 2.23 – HIV testing [internet]. Chicago: American Medical Association; 2010. [cited 2015 Jul 23]. Available from: http://www.ama-assn.org/ama/pub/physician-resources/medical-ethics/code-medical-ethics/opinion223.page.
120. Murphy TF. Assisted gestation and transgender women. Bioethics. 2015;29(6):389–97. Epub 2014/12/17. eng.
121. The Fenway Institute. Asking patients questions about sexual orientation and gender identity in clinical settings: a study in four health centers. Boston: The Fenway Institute and the Center for American Progress; 2013.
122. Makadon HJ. Ending LGBT invisibility in health care: the first step in ensuring equitable care. Cleve Clin J Med. 2011;78(4):220–4.
123. Makadon HJ, Mayer KH, Potter J, Goldhammer H. The Fenway guide to lesbian, gay, bisexual, and transgender health. 2nd ed. Philadelphia: ACP Press; 2015.
124. White W, Brenman S, Paradis E, Goldsmith ES, Lunn MR, Obedin-Maliver J, et al. Lesbian, gay, bisexual, and transgender patient care: medical students' preparedness and comfort. Teach Learn Med. 2015;27(3):254–63. Epub 2015/07/15. eng.
125. Sequeira GM, Chakraborti C, Panunti BA. Integrating lesbian, gay, bisexual, and transgender (LGBT) content into undergraduate medical school curricula: a qualitative study. Ochsner J. 2012;12(4):379–82. Pubmed Central PMCID: Pmc3527869, Epub 2012/12/26. eng.
126. Cahill S, Makadon H. Sexual orientation and gender identity data collection in clinical settings and in electronic health records: a key to ending LGBT health disparities. LGBT Health. 2014;1(1):34–41.
127. The Joint Commission. Advancing effective communication, cultural competence, and patient- and family-centered care for the lesbian, gay, bisexual, and transgender (LGBT) community: a field guide. Oak Brook 2011.
128. Institute of Medicine Board on the Health of Select Populations. The national academies collection: reports funded by National Institutes of Health. Collecting sexual orientation and gender identity data in electronic health records: workshop summary. Washington, DC: National Academies Press (US); 2013.
129. Ward BW, Dahlhamer JM, Galinsky AM, Joestl SS. Sexual orientation and health among U.S. adults: national health interview survey, 2013. Natl Health Stat Report. 2014 Jul 15(77):1–10. Epub 2014/07/16. eng.
130. Davey MP, Waite R, Nunez A, Nino A, Kissil K. A snapshot of patients' perceptions of oncology providers' cultural competence. J Cancer Educ. 2014;29(4):657–64. Epub 2014/02/08. eng.

Chapter 14
Fertility Issues in Transfusion-Dependent Thalassemia Patients: Pathophysiology, Assessment, and Management

Sylvia T. Singer

Introduction

Thalassemia, an inherited hemoglobin synthesis disorder, is one of the most common genetic conditions worldwide. It is characterized by a wide variation in clinical phenotypes; the most severe form, β-thalassemia major (TM), is manifested by severe anemia in early childhood, bone changes, and splenomegaly. TM requires regular blood transfusion therapy for survival, frequently referred to as transfusion-dependent thalassemia (TDT). Since transfused blood entails high iron concentration, it results in iron overload and multi-organ dysfunction if excess iron is not adequately removed. In contrast, thalassemia intermedia (TI) is associated with milder mutations resulting in a milder phenotype and patients, though anemic, are not transfusion dependent and have lower iron burden. Occasionally, patients with TI will have progressive anemia and clinical findings necessitating regular transfusion therapy.

Inadequate control of transfusion-induced iron overload is the primary impediment to the long-term health and management of TM patients; iron accumulation through the transfused blood (and some from increased intestinal absorption) is present in a significant number of patients, and is a primary cause of end-organ dysfunction. While cardiac and hepatic iron-induced damage can result in premature death, the endocrinopathies, including delayed puberty and subfertility, can pose serious debilitating complications with major impact on patients' quality of life (QOL). Despite significant progress in iron chelation regimens and methods for measurement of organ-specific hemosiderosis, impairment of reproductive capacity is well documented among patients with TDT and is still prevalent. Though spontaneous fertility can occur in adequately transfused and well-chelated patients, many

S.T. Singer, MD
UCSF Benioff Children's Hospital Oakland,
747 Fifty Second Street, Oakland, CA 94609, USA
e-mail: tsinger@mail.cho.org

© Springer International Publishing Switzerland 2017   209
T.K. Woodruff, Y.C. Gosiengfiao (eds.), *Pediatric and Adolescent Oncofertility*,
DOI 10.1007/978-3-319-32973-4_14

are infertile, or become so over time. Medical advances have improved life expectancy for TM patients over the past decades; consequently, there has been a shift to increased focus on decreasing morbidity and achieving a better QOL that inherently prioritizes attaining reproductive capacity.

Care for thalassemia has expanded aiming to allow patients to achieve social, vocational, and reproductive goals comparable to their healthy peers. Still, studies and programs addressing the pathogenesis and progression of their subfertility, education and early counseling, and implementation of means for fertility preservation are scarce. Women and men with TDT have a wide array of complications beyond the reproductive axis that can affect infertility treatment outcomes. These need to be addressed by a multidisciplinary approach when patients are consulted for family planning.

This chapter will review the pathogenesis and assessment of infertility, approach for fertility preservation, and pregnancy planning and management issues. The chapter will focus on TDT and will not discuss non-transfusion-dependent thalassemia (NTDT), as fertility problems are rare in this less iron-loaded thalassemia phenotype.

Pathophysiology and Evaluation of Fertility in TDT

Iron Overload, Hypogonadism, and Infertility

Iron-induced tissue damage in patients receiving chronic transfusions is a primary cause of endocrine disorders which can pose serious debilitating complications such as diabetes mellitus, short statue, delayed puberty, and disturbances of the reproductive system commonly noted in adolescent and adult TDT patients. Generally, the scope of complications is directly related to the extent of iron load. Regular transfusion therapy requires side-by-side iron chelation therapy to remove the excess iron: Deferoxamine (desferal) was the only agent available for many years. Though an effective chelator, it requires parenteral administration, resulting in poor compliance in over half of the patients. Subsequent introduction of oral chelation formulation, deferasirox and deferiprone, has increased treatment adherence, and a reduction in end-organ complications and endocrinopathies was reported [1, 2]. Oral chelation treatment has also allowed for treatment programs aimed to prevent iron burden and normalize iron stores via combination treatments and more aggressive chelation regimens. Such regiments were able to prevent some morbidities including hypogonadism, but are still not widely applied, partially since the chelation agents themselves carry unwarranted side effects [3, 4].

The major mechanism causing decline in fertility in TDT is often thought to be central hypogonadism due to the effect of iron deposition on the pituitary gonadotrope cells, which leads to disruption of gonadotropin production. Hypogonadotropic hypogonadism (HH) may present with slowly progressive puberty or arrested puberty and primary or secondary amenorrhea in females.

These are not uncommon complications in moderately or grossly iron-overloaded patients [5, 6]. In older patients, concerns of sexual dysfunction or reproductive issues will arise. A late-onset hypogonadism presenting in second or third decade of life, with low testosterone and oligospermia in males and a decline in ovarian reserve in females, was recently described [7, 8]. A large number of studies reported a high frequency of these problems [9–12], while later studies have shown that adequate iron chelation initiated at a young age allows for better sexual maturation [13]. However, more recent studies claimed that even in patients with regular iron chelation, the prevalence of hypogonadism is still high, reported at 27–55 % [7, 14–17]. The relationship of HH with reproductive status is not clear as gonadotropin levels are not always informative concerning ovarian or testicular function. An additional iron effect on the gonads may also exist, but the pathophysiology and association with the extent of iron overload have only been partially studied. Such a direct gonadal effect appears to occur more in men, disrupting spermatogenesis, while in women ovarian function is generally better preserved.

Mechanism of Iron Toxicity in Thalassemia

Transfusions invariably cause iron accumulation in the body. When iron exceeds the iron-carrying capacity of transferrin, it accumulates as nontransferrin-bound iron (NTBI) and its free form, labile pool iron (LPI). NTBI and LPI are capable of penetrating cells, primarily in the liver, heart, and endocrine organs. They catalyze the formation of free radicals, thereby disrupting the redox balance of the cells causing oxidative stress. Oxidative stress can cause progressive tissue damage through deleterious effects to mitochondria, lysosomes, lipid membranes, proteins, and DNA [18, 19]. Iron-mediated damage to various tissues probably depends on the length of exposure to iron, iron concentration, and tissue-specific sensitivity to damage [20]. A significant prooxidant/antioxidant imbalance exists in TDT patients, due to overproduction of free radicals secondary to the iron overload and reduced antioxidant defense mechanisms caused by alteration in serum trace elements and antioxidant enzyme levels [21, 22]. A decrease in the levels of antioxidants such as vitamins E and A, ascorbate, and beta-carotene and low zinc and selenium were well documented in several thalassemia studies, a result of a higher consumption rate as well as inadequate dietary intake [21, 23–25]. Several studies revealed an association of iron overload state and low antioxidant defense mechanism: Serum levels of vitamin E were inversely correlated with ferritin levels, suggesting major consumption of this antioxidant [20]. In addition, plasma malondialdehyde (MDA), a biomarker of oxidant stress, has been shown to correlate with iron toxicity in thalassemia [26], and a direct association of NTBI with measures of oxidative state and thalassemia heart disease was indicated [27].

Iron, Oxidative Stress, and the Reproductive System

In the reproductive literature, oxidative stress was shown to have a major role in male and female infertility [28–30]. The natural decline in female fertility and follicle aging are thought to result from oxidative stress. Mechanisms include an increase in reactive oxygen species (ROS) production, mitochondrial flaws, a compromised microenvironment, reduced enzymatic antioxidant defense mechanisms, and a decline in granulose cell production of steroid hormones, in particular estradiol [31–34].

In males, increase in ROS is considered a major contributory factor to infertility. ROS impose deleterious effects on the sperm membrane, nucleus, and proteins, thus impairing sperm quality, function, and overall fertilizing capacity [35, 36]. In seminal plasma, endogenous antioxidants such as glutathione (GSH); vitamins E, C, and A; folate; and carnitine were shown to have protective and repairing properties and a substantial effect on reproduction [37, 38]. However, when ROS are produced beyond the antioxidant capacity of seminal plasma, the pathogenic result is often cellular and sperm DNA damage [39]. Consequently, the assessment of total and seminal plasma oxidative profiles has been suggested as a tool to improve the evaluation of sperm reproductive capacity in infertile men [40]. Additionally, the use of antioxidant supplementation was studied and improved sperm qualities were demonstrated, though the overall effectiveness on fertility remains controversial [30, 35, 41, 42]. The effects of these approaches in thalassemia men have not been studied. Micronutrients, in particular zinc, are also known to impact male fertility; zinc takes part in generating sperm motility and has a positive effect on spermatogenesis [43].

Taken together, it is reasonable to assume that iron-induced disruption of the reproductive axis in TDT occurs through such mechanisms. This notion was investigated in a handful of studies described here:

Thalassemia Women

Increased levels of redox activity in the follicular fluid from a TM patient were demonstrated, suggesting that redox-active iron ions mediate free radical production, induce tissue injury, and possibly contribute to impairment of female reproduction [44]. Another study obtained histopathological evidence that deposition of hemosiderin occurs in the endometrial glandular epithelium of iron overload TM women, thus preventing blastocyst implantation. Notably, effective iron-chelating treatment with deferoxamine resulted in reduction or disappearance of the hemosiderin [45]. The iron overload effects on the reproductive system of TM women were recently reviewed [46].

Thalassemia Men

An increase in ROS in seminal plasma of TDT men and the presence of a compensatory mechanism for scavenging free radicals were suggested [47]. In addition, studies have shown sperm DNA damage, presumably a result from iron-induced oxidative injury [48–50]. In a recent study, the presence of both increased iron concentration and reduced GSH in the seminal plasma of TM patients compared to levels in normal controls was shown. Though a small sample size, a correlating effect of reduced sperm motility, an important measure of fertilization potential, was demonstrated [51]. In men, high seminal iron can reduce sperm motility to 10 % of normal levels, thereby significantly affecting reproductive potential [52]. In the same study, seminal zinc was low in patients with azoospermia. Plasma zinc levels are often low in TM patients adding to a compromised fertility [23, 40]. Though not well studied, it raises the need to monitor levels of plasma zinc and increase its intake in TDT males of reproductive age. The effects of administering selective antioxidants and replenishing low trace elements and vitamins on infertility in TM patients need further evaluation.

Pituitary Siderosis and Fertility in Thalassemia

The anterior pituitary may be very susceptible to iron-induced damage that results in defective gonadotropin secretion, a condition also known to occur in iron-loaded patients with the genetic disorder hemochromatosis [53]. In advanced cases the iron damage appears to be irreversible. Standard iron burden measures such as ferritin, liver iron concentration, and intensity of chelation have been used to measure total body iron and its association with gonadal dysfunction [9, 54, 55]. However, it cannot reliably assess pituitary hormone secretion capacity and reproductive potential [17, 56]. The development of MRI technology for pituitary iron quantitation brought about significant progress in determining pituitary siderosis, the relation to total body iron and detection of early stage endocrinopathies [57–60]. The association between gland siderosis and function was investigated in 50 TM patients using a T2-weighted signal intensity, and a significant correlation with hypogonadism was demonstrated [60]. The signal intensity was also shown to significantly correlate with pituitary height, indicating a decrease in the gland's size with an increase in siderosis [59]. It was shown that patients with transfusional iron overload begin to develop pituitary siderosis as early as the first decade of life; however, clinically significant pituitary volume loss was not observed until the second decade of life. Both pituitary iron overload and gland shrinkage were independently predictive of hypogonadism. Still, many patients with moderate to severe pituitary iron overload retained normal gland volume and function. This represents a potential therapeutic window to intensify iron chelation and other treatment modalities before irreversible gland shrinkage occurs [61].

Several studies have assessed the function of the hypothalamic-pituitary-ovarian axis utilizing a gonadotropin releasing hormone (GnRH) test and have demonstrated significantly lower baseline and peak luteinizing hormone (LH) and follicular-stimulating hormone (FSH) levels compared to those in the control group. The studies demonstrated an association of low LH and FSH levels with the severity of iron overload. Patients with severe iron overload had no response to GnRH bolus (apulsatile), suggesting irreversible hypothalamic-pituitary axis damage, while some response was observed in patients with less severe iron burden [12, 62, 63]. In another study, anterior pituitary function (GnRH stimulation test) correlated well with MRI results, but not with the pubertal status of patients [64]. Pituitary MRI for assessment of iron concentration and gland size in conjunction with standard hormone levels and fertility studies may be an important component of the evaluation of reproductive potential in TDT patients. Furthermore, more studies are needed to assess the effect of iron chelation therapy (various chelation agents and combination therapy) and its ability to reverse anterior pituitary malfunction.

Fertility Issues in Thalassemia Women

Conception and Obstacles for Attaining Pregnancy

Despite advances in the management of iron overload in TDT, abnormalities of ovulation are common and are estimated to occur in 30–80 % of adult women [56, 65, 66]. Nevertheless, over the past decades, an increasing number of pregnancies have been reported. In adequately transfused and well-chelated women, spontaneous pregnancies occurred, while others responded to hormone stimulation. The large variability in fertility potential and ability to induce pregnancies likely represents the wide range of iron overload states compounded by the chronological ages of TM women attempting to become pregnant. A summary of reported pregnancies in thalassemia women since the first report in 1969 to the year 2000 identified 335 pregnancies in 290 TM women and 22 TI women; the majority happened after 1990 [67].

More pregnancies in TDT women were reported in the subsequent 15 years, as summarized in Table 14.1. Of note, the average women age was higher than that in the earlier studies, and approximately 50–60 % of pregnancies required ovulation induction [68–71]. Based on these successful cases, ovarian function has been proposed to be preserved in women suffering from primary or secondary amenorrhea as they become able to conceive following stimulation therapy. However, not all will respond to such stimulation treatment. There is limited data on the frequency of failure of ovulation induction and on the length of time and number of attempts of hormonal stimulation required to achieve successful pregnancies.

Table 14.1 Successful pregnancies ($n=291$) reported in transfusion-dependent thalassemia women (2000–2015)

Number of pregnancies	Age (years)	Number (%) received ovulation induction	Ferritin (mean or range) µg/L		Delivery by CS (%)	Complications during pregnancy	Ref	Year
			Prepregnancy	Post-pregnancy				
3	23.6	0	735–1412	708–1160[b]	1 (33)	1 cardiac	89	2000
86	25.5–28.5	23 (27)	2000	2750	28 (32)	4 miscarriages 2 stillbirths	67	2004
24	19–38	12 (50)	1000–11,000	N/A	18 (75)	2 maternal deaths after delivery (cardiac failure) 7 cardiac 2 miscarriages	68	2005
1	28	0	3800	5800	1 (100)	None	90	2005
62[a]	N/A	0	N/A		12/45 (26)	5 cardiac 12 miscarriages	83	2006
1	38	0	67	1583	N/A	None	85	2008
5	31 ± 3.5	3 (60)	770–2100	N/A	4 (80)	1 GD, 1 cardiac arrhythmia 1 renal colic, 1 stillbirth	71	2008

(continued)

Table 14.1 (continued)

Number of pregnancies	Age (years)	Number (%) received ovulation induction	Ferritin (mean or range) µg/L		Delivery by CS (%)	Complications during pregnancy	Ref	Year
			Prepregnancy	Post-pregnancy				
11	N/A	11 (100)	2000	5000	7 (63)	1 thromboembolic episode / Premature labor	73	2009
58	29.5±4.5	33 (57)	1463±1,306	2692±1,629	52 (89)	4 miscarriages	84	2010
5	23–29	1 (20)	500–1000		5 (100)	None	97	2011
1	35	0	2430	2260	1 (100)	GD	93	2011
28	27	22[b](78)	N/A	N/A	N/A	4 GD / 4 cardiac	88	2013
4	27.9±3.7	1 (25)	236±1258	336±3054	3 (75)	1 miscarriage	96	2014
2	27	0	417	1196	0	None	94	2015

Two hundred ninety pregnancies were reported in prior ~15 years, 1985–2000 [14]

Cardiac complications: (1) cardiac death in patients who became pregnant despite preexisting cardiac dysfunction [68], (2) early congestive heart failure [89], (3) worsening measures of increase in LVEDD and LVESD, (4) decrease in SF and EF on echocardiogram

N/A not available, *GD* gestational diabetes

[a]NTDT patients possibly included

[b]In two of the three pregnancies, the patient continued iron chelation with deferoxamine throughout the pregnancy and maintained stable low ferritin levels [89]

Earlier studies, presumably conducted in heavily iron-overloaded patients, suggest impaired oocyte function contributing to infertility. Extensive iron deposition in the ovary has been implicated as a cause of ovarian failure [12, 44]. In two successful pregnancies, inability to fertilize the thalassemia woman's oocyte in vitro was alleviated by using donor oocytes and the husband's sperm [72]. In a more recent study, ovarian volume was significantly reduced to the range of that of postmenopausal women. This reduction was probably due to the lack of gonadotropin stimulation, but could also have been a direct result of iron on the ovarian tissue, particularly in thalassemia women with long-standing iron overload [8]. Another study demonstrated hemosiderin in the endometrial epithelium of three TM women [45].

Ovarian Reserve and Fertility Preservation

An important part of care for TM women is providing them with information about their reproductive state and initiating an overall plan for a prepregnancy care (see below). FSH and estradiol levels in the follicular phase in TDT women are not reliable markers for gonadal function evaluation, and hormone stimulation tests to assess gonadal function did not yield consistent results [62, 73, 74]. More advanced methods such as hormonal profile along with ovarian reserve testing (ORT) in TM women of reproductive age are scarce. A more recent study utilized antral follicle count (AFC), a strong predictor of ovarian reserve, and found it to be lower in TM compared to normal controls, in particular in TDT women 30 years and older [8].

Anti-Mullerian hormone (AMH), another sensitive marker of ovarian reserve, is applied often in fertility clinics. It represents the early primordial follicle pool in the ovary, and is therefore independent of gonadotropin effect [75–77]. It may therefore emerge as a more reliable marker for reproductive potential and predictor of success of assisted reproductive technology in thalassemia women. Two studies assessed AMH levels in TDT women, both describe low to a low-normal range compare to normal controls. However, a clear downward trend of AMH levels in older women, in the mid-30s and older, was noted [8, 77]. The two studies showed a reverse correlation between AMH and iron overload measures, NTBI or ferritin, that was independent of the patients' age. It appears that fertility declines in older TDT women who may have a faster drop in their ovarian reserve pool than age-matched normal women (Figs. 14.1 and 14.2). This suggests that duration of exposure to iron may increase the deleterious effects and exhaust the ovarian reserve, possibly through direct ovarian tissue effect (as discussed in earlier sections of this chapter). Therefore, it is important to initiate assessment, discussion, and consultation regarding patients' wishes and efforts to preserve fertility at a young age. Attempts to reduce iron overload through intensified chelation therapy may be helpful to restore some reproductive function in some cases. Notably, improvement in gonadal function was observed in one female who gave birth to two healthy children without hormonal stimulation after intense iron chelation treatment [3]. In addition, elective

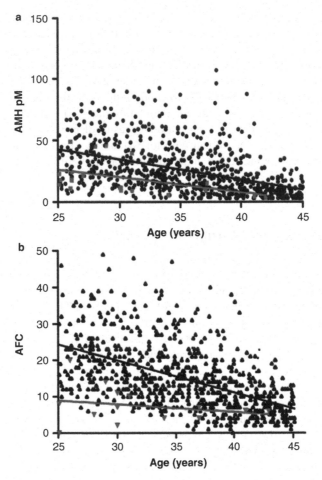

Fig. 14.1 AMH levels and AFC in TM women and normo-ovulatory controls. (**a**) AMH levels in the thalassemia women, 25 years and older (*n*=23, *red circles*), were compared with normal controls (●; *n*=759), showing that the slopes of the regression lines against age were not statistically different (*P*=0.56). The slope was significant for the normal controls (*P*<0.0001; 95 % CI, −1.867 to −1.406) and for the thalassemia patients (*P*<0.03; 95 % CI, −2.323 to −0.1142), implying an association with age. There was a 5.0pM (95 % CI, 13.4–26.8) difference between the group means. The levels in the thalassemia women were in the low-normal range of normal and dropped to lower levels in women older than 30 years. (**b**) Age-dependent AFC in thalassemia women and normal controls. AFC number includes all counted follicles 2–10 mm in size, in thalassemia women, and in the cohort of normal controls (*n*=769) (With permission from Singer, et al. *Blood*, 8 September 2011;118(10):2878–81)

cryopreservation of oocytes or ovarian tissue should be considered, while the oocytes and tissue are still attainable.

Over the past decade, there has been increasing interest in methods to expand the reproductive options of patients facing gonadotoxic therapies for various types of malignancies [78, 79]. There is, however, very limited such information for

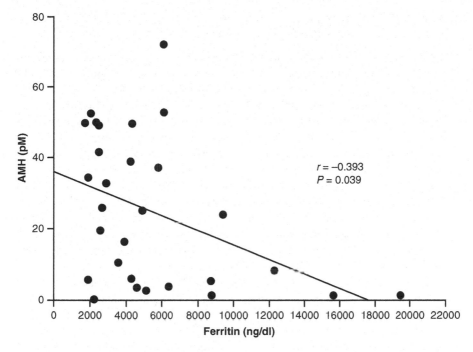

Fig. 14.2 Iron overload is associated with low AMH in women with TDT. Scatter plot with *fit line* of the untransformed serum ferritin and AMH levels in 29 women with transfusion-dependent beta-thalassemia. Age-adjusted Spearman correlation coefficient is shown (With permission from Chang H, et al. *BJOG.* 2011;118:825–83)

thalassemia patients. A recent successful ovarian tissue cryopreservation was demonstrated both in an adolescent thalassemia patient [80] and in a TDT woman prior to receiving gonadotoxic preconditioning treatment for hematopoietic stem cell transplantation (HSCT). Reimplantation of ovarian tissue resulted in IVF pregnancy and delivery of a healthy baby [81].

Prepregnancy Planning in Transfusion-Dependent Thalassemia Women

Prepregnancy counseling and planning are essential in order to minimize risk to the pregnant thalassemia woman and to the fetus. Apart from subfertility, other systemic and endocrine disorders, primarily cardiac disease, liver dysfunction, diabetes mellitus, and chronic viral infections, hamper fertility ability and pregnancy. Ideally, a multidisciplinary team comprised of a hematologist, reproductive medicine specialist, obstetrician, and cardiologist should be involved. In many cases, a psychologist is helpful also. Partner screening for carrier status of a thalassemia syndrome is essential and genetic counseling may be needed. The safety of pregnancy for mothers with TDT has been discussed in several reports [68, 73, 82–84]. A number of systems require prepregnancy evaluation and consideration during pregnancy:

Cardiac function. The cardiac load during pregnancy increases physiologically by about 25 %. In addition, most TM women require an increase in red blood cell transfusion to maintain high enough pre-transfusion hemoglobin levels. The increase in transfusion, coupled with discontinuing iron chelation throughout most of the gestational time due to concerns of teratogenicity can result in a significant increase in systemic and myocardial iron load (Table 14.1) [85]. In women with borderline cardiac function, these two factors can result in left ventricular dysfunction, serious cardiac complications, and even death. An evaluation of cardiac function by echocardiogram or by MRI and cardiac iron level by T2* MRI technology, if available, should be performed. The 2014 Thalassemia International Federation (TIF) guidelines for the management of TDT recommend having an ejection fraction >65 %, shortening fraction >30 % by echocardiogram, and T2* no less than 20 ms [86]. If cardiac function is low or cardiac iron load is high (T2* <20 ms), it is advised to intensify chelation to improve cardiac function before trying for a pregnancy. Occasionally, the use of iron chelation when faced with an increase in cardiac iron burden and cardiac failure during pregnancy is indicated.

Endocrinopathies. Patients need to be screened for early glucose intolerance or assure a well-balanced glucose range if diabetes mellitus has already developed. Screening for hypothyroidism and monitoring to assure a euthyroid state are important. Additionally, bone health and extent of osteopenia, osteoporosis, or chronic bone and joint pain need to be evaluated.

Viral infections. Screening for hepatitis B and C and HIV are important, and treatment for hepatitis C or HIV should be offered prior to pregnancy.

Psychological support. Thalassemia women face lifelong complications related to their disease that influence their self-esteem, sense of identity, social life, and family planning. TM women attempting to get pregnant have shown increased rates of anxiety and depression as compared to healthy pregnant controls [87]. Integrating psychological support in the multidisciplinary team that develops a program for a TM woman to become pregnant and follows her through her pregnancy is recommended.

Pregnancies: Management, Outcomes, and Complications

Cardiac Function Monitoring Cardiac hemosiderosis reduces myocardial contractility, causing compensatory hypertrophy that can compromise cardiac performance during pregnancy as the cardiac output rises significantly. Though minimal transient cardiac function changes have been shown in a large report [84], other smaller case studies have shown a more pronounced increase in left ventricular end-diastolic diameter (LVEDD) and left ventricular end-systolic diameter (LVESD) in TDT women compared to the expected normal physiological changes in pregnancy. Some were accompanied by a fall in ejection fraction and shortening fraction, likely due to diminished contractility [83, 88, 89] or overt heart failure and subsequent death [68]. As an increased number of pregnancies may now be expected, careful monitoring of cardiac function is important, even with normal prepregnancy echocardiograms, as iron overload can develop rapidly with discontinuation of chelation [85, 90]. Regular cardiac monitoring every 3 months has been suggested [67].

Transfusion and Iron Chelation Maintaining pre-transfusion hemoglobin of 10–11 g/dL through more frequent low volume blood transfusions is recommended. Data on the safety of iron chelation treatment during induction of ovulation treatment and during pregnancy is scarce. However, due to the concern of teratogenicity, a common practice is to discontinue chelation therapy during the ovulation induction days until the outcome is known, as well as during the first two trimesters of pregnancy (some patients chose to avoid chelation through the whole gestation period). In case reports, no teratogenicity with the use of deferoxamine was reported, and consideration should be given to offer it in second trimester or when a concern of change in cardiac function occurs [85, 89, 91, 92]. Withholding chelation with deferoxamine in such situations may result in further decline in cardiac function and possible heart failure during pregnancy or after delivery. There is limited data on newer oral chelators that are smaller molecules and may have a higher likelihood to cross the placenta. However, a case report of incidental use of deferasirox up to 22 weeks of gestation still resulted in the birth of a healthy baby [93].

Anticoagulation Due to an increased risk of thromboembolism in TDT women who underwent splenectomy, it is advised to use low-dose aspirin during pregnancy and postpartum [71, 89]. In a larger study, low molecular heparin was administered peripartum subsequent to aspirin during gestation without any increased bleeding tendency [84]. More detailed recommendation can be found in the 2014 TIF guidelines for the management of TDT [86].

Based on the above, it seems that, irrespective of spontaneous or induced ovulation, the current outcome of attempted pregnancies in TDT women, with proper multidisciplinary guidance and care, is optimistic. More than 500 pregnancies in TDT women have been reported; the majority delivered healthy term babies, while preterm babies were reported in 13–35 %, some related to multiple pregnancies [94]. Complications included a higher frequency of miscarriage, intrauterine growth retardation (IUGR), and low birth weight. Cesarean section is most often the chosen delivery method due to concerns of cephalopelvic disproportion resulting from maternal short stature and skeletal deformities and normal fetal growth [68, 70, 84, 88, 95–97]. Reports show a variable increase in iron load, which ranged from 10 to 100 % greater ferritin levels than preconception, likely related to the differences in the increase in blood transfusion during pregnancy. Some have noted a higher incidence of complications during pregnancy; these include: cardiac issues (compromised LV function, arrhythmias, and hypertension), gestational diabetes, impaired glucose tolerance, and renal colic (Table 14.1). There were no reports of increase in incidence of thrombosis or preeclampsia.

Fertility Issues in Thalassemia Men

While ovulation induction in TM women can result in successful pregnancies and births, successful paternity seems to occur less often in TM men, a discrepancy that is not well understood. It is estimated that more than one half of men with TM are affected by oligospermia, asthenospermia, and possibly compromised sperm quality [7, 17, 48, 62, 67]. However, great variability in TDT phenotypes in these studies likely affects these estimates. Additionally, emerging iron chelation treatments may positively impact this high prevalence. Infertility in TM men appears to have multiple causes, including HH, late-onset hypogonadism, abnormal spermatogenesis, and possibly nutrient deficiencies combined with an increase in oxidative stress that affects sperm qualities, as discussed above.

Assessment of Reproductive Potential

Hormonal Assessment

Several advances in diagnosis and treatment of male infertility have been made in recent years [98, 99]. In most sterile males in the general population, primary gonadal dysfunction will result in elevated LH and FSH levels; however, these are not useful predictors for fertility potential in thalassemia men, as their LH and FSH secretion will be compromised due to iron overload effects on the pituitary. Variable gonadotropin levels and age of onset of HH have been reported making the use of these hormone levels difficult for assessment of fertility potential [7, 17, 61]. Gonadal and fertility status is also difficult to predict by means of transfusion or chelation parameters, as no clear correlation was shown with HH [17, 100]. Levels of inhibin B, a hormone produced in sertoli cells in the testes that inhibits pituitary FSH secretion, seem to better reflect testicular function and spermatogenesis and show a more accurate predictive ability of male fertilization potential than FSH levels [101, 102]. Obtaining levels of inhibin B may have a better extrapolative value in TDT men, currently being studied.

Sperm Analysis

It has been suggested that sperm DNA integrity may be an important method to determine male fertility adding to the routine semen analysis of volume, sperm count, motility and morphology. There is evidence that sperm of infertile men contain more DNA damage than those of fertile men and that the DNA damage may have a negative effect on fertilization ability of these patients [39, 103, 104]. There are several methods to assess DNA loss of integrity and increased breakage. Among them, sperm chromatin structure assay (SCSA), terminal deoxynucleotidyl transferase-mediated assay (TUNEL), and single-cell gel electrophoresis assay (COMET) are commonly used [98, 103, 105]. High levels of sperm DNA fragmentation often correlate with poor seminal parameters such as reduced count and motility or abnormal morphology, but sperm DNA damage is also found in a small percentage of men with normal seminal parameters. Several investigators have applied this method for TDT men.

Paternity and Fertility Evaluation

A scarce study assessed fertility parameters or reported fatherhood in TDT men. Sperm abnormalities were frequent consisting of low sperm count, poor motility, and increased abnormal morphology, described in the majority of TM men (mostly in their mid twenties), more so in TM men with HH [50, 62, 67, 106]. In a study where oligospermia and asthenospermia were described in 50 % of TM men, lack of correlation with LH and FSH levels was noted, and the authors suggested that intense chelation with deferoxamine may have contributed to the sperm abnormalities [49]. In two studies that measured sperm DNA integrity, spermatozoa of TM men had a higher degree of DNA damage compared to controls. This increase in sperm DNA breakage was also shown to negatively correlate with sperm motility, an important measure of fertility potential [48, 49]. It should be noted that some of these men had significant iron overload, as measured by a median ferritin [48]. A more recent study demonstrated a normal DNA fragmentation in a small group of TDT men who had low iron overload and lacked findings of increased oxidative stress in their seminal plasma, suggesting a positive effect of consistent iron chelation [51]. There have been concerns about potential consequences of the use of DNA-damaged sperm with intracytoplasmic injections (ICSI) and IVF, as this technique overrides the process of natural selection during fertilization. However, the impact of sperm DNA damage on reproductive outcomes remains controversial and is unknown in thalassemia [39]. Similarly, the effect of different iron chelation agents on sperm quality parameters was not evaluated in thalassemia men. More prospective studies are needed to determine the clinical importance of abnormal sperm analysis on fertility in TDT men.

Induction of Spermatogenesis and Fertility Preservation

Induction of spermatogenesis in thalassemia males is more difficult and yields less success than the induction of ovulation in thalassemia females. In a study of both genders, 14 TM males with HH and infertility received gonadotropins for

6–24 months with variable outcomes. Although successful paternity did not occur, successful spermatogenesis with oligoasthenospermia occurred in six men and two men had successful paternity after in vitro fertilization (IVF) and ICSI. Male response to hormone stimulation was less favorable than that of the females [106]. Another study has also described a low response rate (10–15 %) to stimulation of spermatogenesis and noted the failure of several TM men who had previously fathered a child to respond later to stimulation treatment [67]. These small studies have a lower success rate of spermatogenesis subsequent to hormone stimulation than the success rate reported in men with hypogonadotropic hypogonadism due to other causes, estimated at ~80 % [107]. Though small-scale studies, it indirectly implies an important role of direct iron-induced impediment to spermatogenesis in thalassemia men, as discussed above.

For thalassemia men with a low testosterone level, the regular use of hCG instead of testosterone replacement is occasionally considered in order to avoid gonadotropin suppression and therefore possibly preserve spermatogenesis. However, this approach has not yet been studied in thalassemia. A common practice is to discontinue testosterone treatment and start biweekly hCG intramuscular injections approximately 6–12 months prior to planned pregnancy while monitoring semen analysis and testosterone levels.

Until further study on thalassemia male fertility preservation is conducted, patients can benefit from knowledge of their expected reproductive potential based on the above analysis. Additionally, early education and referral to a reproductive endocrinologist for discussion of sperm cryopreservation procedures should be considered. Advances in micromanipulation techniques such as ICSI and more recently physiological intracytoplasmic sperm injection (PICSI) can improve conception even in patients with poor sperm count and motility findings. Cryopreservation of testicular tissue is still experimental but may become an option in prepubertal boys [80].

References

1. Casale M, et al. Endocrine function and bone disease during long-term chelation therapy with deferasirox in patients with beta-thalassemia major. Am J Hematol. 2014;89(12):1102–6.
2. Pennell DJ, et al. Continued improvement in myocardial T2* over two years of deferasirox therapy in beta-thalassemia major patients with cardiac iron overload. Haematologica. 2011;96(1):48–54.
3. Farmaki K, Tzoumari I, Pappa C. Oral chelators in transfusion-dependent thalassemia major patients may prevent or reverse iron overload complications. Blood Cells Mol Dis. 2011;47(1):33–40.
4. Berdoukas V, et al. Iron chelation in thalassemia: time to reconsider our comfort zones. Expert Rev Hematol. 2011;4(1):17–26.
5. De Sanctis V. Growth and puberty and its management in thalassaemia. Horm Res. 2002;58 Suppl 1:72–9.
6. De Sanctis V, et al. Growth and endocrine disorders in thalassemia: the international network on endocrine complications in thalassemia (I-CET) position statement and guidelines. Indian J Endocrinol Metab. 2013;17(1):8–18.

7. De Sanctis V, et al. Late-onset male hypogonadism and fertility potential in thalassemia major patients: two emerging issues. Mediterr J Hematol Infect Dis. 2015;7(1):e2015047.
8. Singer ST, et al. Reproductive capacity in iron overloaded women with thalassemia major. Blood. 2011;118(10):2878–81.
9. Gabutti V, Piga A. Results of long-term iron-chelating therapy. Acta Haematol. 1996;95(1):26–36.
10. Borgna-Pignatti C, et al. Survival and disease complications in thalassemia major. Ann N Y Acad Sci. 1998;850:227–31.
11. Chatterjee R, et al. Prospective study of the hypothalamic-pituitary axis in thalassaemic patients who developed secondary amenorrhoea. Clin Endocrinol (Oxf). 1993;39(3):287–96.
12. Allegra A, et al. Hypogonadism in beta-thalassemic adolescents: a characteristic pituitary-gonadal impairment. The ineffectiveness of long-term iron chelation therapy. Gynecol Endocrinol. 1990;4(3):181–91.
13. Bronspiegel-Weintrob N, et al. Effect of age at the start of iron chelation therapy on gonadal function in beta-thalassemia major. N Engl J Med. 1990;323(11):713–9.
14. Skordis N, et al. The impact of iron overload and genotype on gonadal function in women with thalassaemia major. Pediatr Endocrinol Rev. 2004;2 Suppl 2:292–5.
15. Borgna-Pignatti C, et al. Survival and complications in patients with thalassemia major treated with transfusion and deferoxamine. Haematologica. 2004;89(10):1187–93.
16. Al-Rimawi HS, et al. Hypothalamic-pituitary-gonadal function in adolescent females with beta-thalassemia major. Int J Gynaecol Obstet. 2005;90(1):44–7.
17. Papadimas J, et al. beta-thalassemia and gonadal axis: a cross-sectional, clinical study in a Greek population. Hormones (Athens). 2002;1(3):179–87.
18. Esposito BP, et al. Labile plasma iron in iron overload: redox activity and susceptibility to chelation. Blood. 2003;102(7):2670–7.
19. Hershko C, Link G, Cabantchik I. Pathophysiology of iron overload. Ann N Y Acad Sci. 1998;850:191–201.
20. Livrea MA, et al. Oxidative stress and antioxidant status in beta-thalassemia major: iron overload and depletion of lipid-soluble antioxidants. Blood. 1996;88(9):3608–14.
21. Shazia Q, et al. Correlation of oxidative stress with serum trace element levels and antioxidant enzyme status in Beta thalassemia major patients: a review of the literature. Anemia. 2012;2012:270923.
22. Waseem F, Khemomal KA, Sajid R. Antioxidant status in beta thalassemia major: a single center study. Indian J Pathol Microbiol. 2011;54(4):761–3.
23. Claster S, et al. Nutritional deficiencies in iron overloaded patients with hemoglobinopathies. Am J Hematol. 2009;84(6):344–8.
24. Vogiatzi MG, et al. Bone disease in thalassemia: a frequent and still unresolved problem. J Bone Miner Res. 2009;24(3):543–57.
25. Chapman RW, et al. Effect of ascorbic acid deficiency on serum ferritin concentration in patients with beta-thalassaemia major and iron overload. J Clin Pathol. 1982;35(5):487–91.
26. Walter PB, et al. Oxidative stress and inflammation in iron-overloaded patients with beta-thalassaemia or sickle cell disease. Br J Haematol. 2006;135(2):254–63.
27. Piga A, et al. High nontransferrin bound iron levels and heart disease in thalassemia major. Am J Hematol. 2009;84(1):29–33.
28. Desai N, et al. Physiologic and pathologic levels of reactive oxygen species in neat semen of infertile men. Fertil Steril. 2009;92(5):1626–31.
29. Agarwal A, Said TM. Oxidative stress, DNA damage and apoptosis in male infertility: a clinical approach. BJU Int. 2005;95(4):503–7.
30. Makker K, Agarwal A, Sharma R. Oxidative stress & male infertility. Indian J Med Res. 2009;129(4):357–67.
31. Appasamy M, et al. Evaluation of the relationship between follicular fluid oxidative stress, ovarian hormones, and response to gonadotropin stimulation. Fertil Steril. 2008;89(4):912–21.

32. Tarin JJ. Potential effects of age-associated oxidative stress on mammalian oocytes/embryos. Mol Hum Reprod. 1996;2(10):717–24.

33. Tatone C, et al. Cellular and molecular aspects of ovarian follicle ageing. Hum Reprod Update. 2008;14(2):131–42.

34. Agarwal A, Gupta S, Sharma RK. Role of oxidative stress in female reproduction. Reprod Biol Endocrinol. 2005;3:28.

35. Agarwal A, et al. Effect of oxidative stress on male reproduction. World J Mens Health. 2014;32(1):1–17.

36. Zini A, San Gabriel M, Baazeem A. Antioxidants and sperm DNA damage: a clinical perspective. J Assist Reprod Genet. 2009;26(8):427–32.

37. Raijmakers MT, et al. Glutathione and glutathione S-transferases A1-1 and P1-1 in seminal plasma may play a role in protecting against oxidative damage to spermatozoa. Fertil Steril. 2003;79(1):169–72.

38. Atig F, et al. Impact of seminal trace element and glutathione levels on semen quality of Tunisian infertile men. BMC Urol. 2012;12:6.

39. Schulte RT, et al. Sperm DNA damage in male infertility: etiologies, assays, and outcomes. J Assist Reprod Genet. 2010;27(1):3–12.

40. Ebisch IM, et al. The importance of folate, zinc and antioxidants in the pathogenesis and prevention of subfertility. Hum Reprod Update. 2007;13(2):163–74.

41. Kobori Y, et al. Antioxidant cosupplementation therapy with vitamin C, vitamin E, and coenzyme Q10 in patients with oligoasthenozoospermia. Arch Ital Urol Androl. 2014;86(1):1–4.

42. Agarwal A, Prabakaran SA. Mechanism, measurement, and prevention of oxidative stress in male reproductive physiology. Indian J Exp Biol. 2005;43(11):963–74.

43. Marzec-Wroblewska U, et al. Zinc and iron concentration and SOD activity in human semen and seminal plasma. Biol Trace Elem Res. 2011;143(1):167–77.

44. Reubinoff BE, et al. Increased levels of redox-active iron in follicular fluid: a possible cause of free radical-mediated infertility in beta-thalassemia major. Am J Obstet Gynecol. 1996;174(3):914–8.

45. Birkenfeld A, et al. Endometrial glandular haemosiderosis in homozygous beta-thalassaemia. Eur J Obstet Gynecol Reprod Biol. 1989;31(2):173–8.

46. Roussou P, et al. Beta-thalassemia major and female fertility: the role of iron and iron-induced oxidative stress. Anemia. 2013;2013:617204.

47. Carpino A, et al. Antioxidant capacity in seminal plasma of transfusion-dependent beta-thalassemic patients. Exp Clin Endocrinol Diabetes. 2004;112(3):131–4.

48. Perera D, et al. Sperm DNA damage in potentially fertile homozygous beta-thalassaemia patients with iron overload. Hum Reprod. 2002;17(7):1820–5.

49. De Sanctis V, et al. Spermatozoal DNA damage in patients with B thalassaemia syndromes. Pediatr Endocrinol Rev. 2008;6 Suppl 1:185–9.

50. De Sanctis V, et al. Spermatogenesis in young adult patients with beta-thalassaemia major long-term treated with desferrioxamine. Georgian Med News. 2008;156:74–7.

51. Singer ST, et al. Fertility in transfusion-dependent thalassemia men: effects of iron burden on the reproductive axis. Am J Hematol. 2015;90(9):E190–2.

52. Skandhan KP, Mazumdar BN, Sumangala B. Study into the iron content of seminal plasma in normal and infertile subjects. Urologia. 2012;79(1):54–7.

53. Meyer WR, et al. Secondary hypogonadism in hemochromatosis. Fertil Steril. 1990;54(4):740–2.

54. Olivieri NF, Brittenham GM. Management of the thalassemias. Cold Spring Harb Perspect Med. 2013;3(6):1–14.

55. Telfer PT, et al. Hepatic iron concentration combined with long-term monitoring of serum ferritin to predict complications of iron overload in thalassaemia major. Br J Haematol. 2000;110(4):971–7.

56. Farmaki K, et al. Normalisation of total body iron load with very intensive combined chelation reverses cardiac and endocrine complications of thalassaemia major. Br J Haematol. 2010;148(3):466–75.
57. Christoforidis A, et al. MRI for the determination of pituitary iron overload in children and young adults with beta-thalassaemia major. Eur J Radiol. 2006;62(1):138–42.
58. Christoforidis A, et al. Correlative study of iron accumulation in liver, myocardium, and pituitary assessed with MRI in young thalassemic patients. J Pediatr Hematol Oncol. 2006;28(5):311–5.
59. Argyropoulou MI, Kiortsis DN, Efremidis SC. MRI of the liver and the pituitary gland in patients with beta-thalassemia major: does hepatic siderosis predict pituitary iron deposition? Eur Radiol. 2003;13(1):12–6.
60. Lam WW, et al. One-stop measurement of iron deposition in the anterior pituitary, liver, and heart in thalassemia patients. J Magn Reson Imaging. 2008;28(1):29–33.
61. Noetzli LJ, et al. Pituitary iron and volume predict hypogonadism in transfusional iron overload. Am J Hematol. 2012;87(2):167–71.
62. Safarinejad MR. Evaluation of semen quality, endocrine profile and hypothalamus-pituitary-testis axis in male patients with homozygous beta-thalassemia major. J Urol. 2008;179(6):2327–32.
63. Chatterjee R, Katz M. Reversible hypogonadotropic hypogonadism in sexually infantile male thalassaemic patients with transfusional iron overload. Clin Endocrinol (Oxf) 2000;53(1):33–42.
64. Berkovitch M, et al. Iron deposition in the anterior pituitary in homozygous beta-thalassemia: MRI evaluation and correlation with gonadal function. J Pediatr Endocrinol Metab. 2000;13(2):179–84.
65. Borgna-Pignatti C, et al. Growth and sexual maturation in thalassemia major. J Pediatr. 1985;106(1):150–5.
66. De Sanctis V, et al. Hypothalamic-pituitary-gonadal axis in thalassemic patients with secondary amenorrhea. Obstet Gynecol. 1988;72(4):643–7.
67. Skordis N, et al. Update on fertility in thalassaemia major. Pediatr Endocrinol Rev. 2004;2 Suppl 2:296–302.
68. Tuck SM. Fertility and pregnancy in thalassemia major. Ann N Y Acad Sci. 2005;1054:300–7.
69. Skordis N, et al. Fertility in female patients with thalassemia. J Pediatr Endocrinol Metab. 1998;11 Suppl 3:935–43.
70. Cohen AR et al. Thalassemia. Am Soc Hematol Educ Book. 2004;2004:14–34.
71. Mancuso A, et al. Pregnancy in patients with beta-thalassaemia major: maternal and foetal outcome. Acta Haematol. 2008;119(1):15–7.
72. Reubinoff BE, et al. Defective oocytes as a possible cause of infertility in a beta-thalassaemia major patient. Hum Reprod. 1994;9(6):1143–5.
73. Bajoria R, Chatterjee R. Current perspectives of fertility and pregnancy in thalassemia. Hemoglobin. 2009;33 Suppl 1:S131–5.
74. De Sanctis V, et al. Gonadal function in patients with beta thalassaemia major. J Clin Pathol. 1988;41(2):133–7.
75. Scheffer GJ, et al. Antral follicle counts by transvaginal ultrasonography are related to age in women with proven natural fertility. Fertil Steril. 1999;72(5):845–51.
76. Kwee J, et al. Evaluation of anti-Mullerian hormone as a test for the prediction of ovarian reserve. Fertil Steril. 2008;90(3):737–43.
77. Knauff EA, et al. Anti-Mullerian hormone, inhibin B, and antral follicle count in young women with ovarian failure. J Clin Endocrinol Metab. 2009;94(3):786–92.
78. Gracia CR, et al. Ovarian tissue cryopreservation for fertility preservation in cancer patients: successful establishment and feasibility of a multidisciplinary collaboration. J Assist Reprod Genet. 2012;29(6):495–502.

79. Senapati S, et al. Fertility preservation in patients with haematological disorders: a retrospective cohort study. Reprod Biomed Online. 2014;28(1):92–8.
80. Babayev SN, et al. Evaluation of ovarian and testicular tissue cryopreservation in children undergoing gonadotoxic therapies. J Assist Reprod Genet. 2013;30(1):3–9.
81. Revel A, et al. Micro-organ ovarian transplantation enables pregnancy: a case report. Hum Reprod. 2011;26(5):1097–103.
82. Karagiorga-Lagana M. Fertility in thalassemia: the Greek experience. J Pediatr Endocrinol Metab. 1998;11 Suppl 3:945–51.
83. Ansari S, Azarkeivan A, Tabaroki A. Pregnancy in patients treated for beta thalassemia major in two centers (Ali Asghar Children's Hospital and Thalassemia Clinic): outcome for mothers and newborn infants. Pediatr Hematol Oncol. 2006;23(1):33–7.
84. Origa R, et al. Pregnancy and {beta}-thalassemia: an Italian multicenter experience. Haematologica. 2009;94:1777–8.
85. Farmaki K, et al. Rapid iron loading in a pregnant woman with transfusion-dependent thalassemia after brief cessation of iron chelation therapy. Eur J Haematol. 2008;81(2):157–9.
86. Skordis N, Porter J, Kalakoutis G. Fertility and pregnancy in Guidelines for the management of Transfusion Dependent Thalassaemia (TDT). TIF, 3rd edition. 2014;9:158–69.
87. Messina G, et al. Pregnant women affected by thalassemia major: a controlled study of traits and personality. J Res Med Sci. 2010;15(2):100–6.
88. Thompson AA, et al. Pregnancy outcomes in women with thalassemia in North America and the United Kingdom. Am J Hematol. 2013;88(9):771–3.
89. Perniola R, et al. High-risk pregnancy in beta-thalassemia major women. Report of three cases. Gynecol Obstet Invest. 2000;49(2):137–9.
90. Butwick A, Findley I, Wonke B. Management of pregnancy in a patient with beta thalassaemia major. Int J Obstet Anesth. 2005;14(4):351–4.
91. Singer ST, Vichinsky EP. Deferoxamine treatment during pregnancy: is it harmful? Am J Hematol. 1999;60(1):24–6.
92. Vaskaridou E, et al. Deferoxamine treatment during early pregnancy: absence of teratogenicity in two cases. Haematologica. 1993;78(3):183–4.
93. Vini D, Servos P, Drosou M. Normal pregnancy in a patient with beta-thalassaemia major receiving iron chelation therapy with deferasirox (Exjade(R)). Eur J Haematol. 2011;86(3):274–5.
94. Merchant R, et al. A successful twin pregnancy in a patient with HbE-β-thalassemia in western India. J Postgrad Med. 2015;61(3):203.
95. Aessopos A, et al. Pregnancy in patients with well-treated beta-thalassemia: outcome for mothers and newborn infants. Am J Obstet Gynecol. 1999;180(2 Pt 1):360–5.
96. Al-Riyami N, Al-Khaduri M, Daar S. Pregnancy outcomes in women with homozygous beta thalassaemia: a single-centre experience from Oman. Sultan Qaboos Univ Med J. 2014;14(3):e337–41.
97. Pafumi C, et al. The reproduction in women affected by cooley disease. Hematol Rep. 2011;3(1):e4.
98. Natali A, Turek PJ. An assessment of new sperm tests for male infertility. Urology. 2011;77(5):1027–34.
99. Bann CM, et al. Cancer survivors' use of fertility preservation. J Womens Health (Larchmt). 2015;24:777–83.
100. Jensen CE, et al. Incidence of endocrine complications and clinical disease severity related to genotype analysis and iron overload in patients with beta-thalassaemia. Eur J Haematol. 1997;59(2):76–81.
101. Grunewald S, et al. Age-dependent inhibin B concentration in relation to FSH and semen sample qualities: a study in 2448 men. Reproduction. 2013;145(3):237–44.
102. Kumanov P, et al. Inhibin B is a better marker of spermatogenesis than other hormones in the evaluation of male factor infertility. Fertil Steril. 2006;86(2):332–8.

103. Bungum M, et al. Sperm DNA integrity assessment in prediction of assisted reproduction technology outcome. Hum Reprod. 2007;22(1):174–9.
104. Micinski P, et al. Total reactive antioxidant potential and DNA fragmentation index as fertility sperm parameters. Reprod Biol. 2011;11(2):135–44.
105. Erenpreiss J, et al. Sperm chromatin structure and male fertility: biological and clinical aspects. Asian J Androl. 2006;8(1):11–29.
106. Bajoria R, Chatterjee R. Hypogonadotropic hypogonadism and diminished gonadal reserve accounts for dysfunctional gametogenesis in thalassaemia patients with iron overload presenting with infertility. Hemoglobin. 2011;35(5–6):636–42.
107. Warne DW, et al. A combined analysis of data to identify predictive factors for spermatogenesis in men with hypogonadotropic hypogonadism treated with recombinant human follicle-stimulating hormone and human chorionic gonadotropin. Fertil Steril. 2009;92(2):594–604.

Chapter 15
Setting Up a Pediatric Oncofertility Practice

Karen Burns and Lesley Breech

Abbreviations

AMH	Anti-Mullerian hormone
BMT	Bone marrow transplant
CBDI	Cancer and Blood Diseases Institute
CCHMC	Cincinnati Children's Hospital Medical Center
CED	Cyclophosphamide equivalent dosing
EMT	Electronic medical record
FDA	Federal Drug Administration
FSH	Follicle-stimulating hormone
HIV	Human immunodeficiency virus
LH	Luteinizing hormone
NPC	National Physician Consortium
REI	Reproductive endocrinology
SDM	Shared decision making

K. Burns, MD, MS (✉)
Cancer and Blood Diseases Institute, Cincinnati Children's Hospital Medical Center,
3333 Burnet Ave., MLC 7015, Cincinnati, OH 45229, USA
e-mail: Karen.burns@cchmc.org

L. Breech, MD
Pediatric and Adolescent Gynecology, Cincinnati Children's Hospital Medical Center,
3333 Burnet Ave., MLC 2026, Cincinnati, OH 45229, USA

© Springer International Publishing Switzerland 2017
T.K. Woodruff, Y.C. Gosiengfiao (eds.), *Pediatric and Adolescent Oncofertility*,
DOI 10.1007/978-3-319-32973-4_15

Introduction

The rate of cure for childhood cancer is now over 80 % due to tremendous therapeutic advances over the past 50 years. Survivors now comprise approximately 1 of every 640 young adults aged 18–45 living in the United States (www.childrensoncologygroup.org). The number of childhood cancer survivors continues to grow. Today childhood cancer survivors are living well into adulthood. The goals of pediatric oncology treatment include achieving cure but also doing so in a way that minimizes a lifetime of late effects. One such late effect of therapy is the impact on fertility.

While the field of adult oncofertility is growing rapidly, pediatric oncofertility is relatively new. Pediatric patients present unique challenges not often encountered in the adult cancer arena. Patients under the age of 18 are not able to consent to treatment. Parents must consent with their child's best interest in mind. Many parents and patients have not yet considered future childbearing at the time of diagnosis. They may be prematurely forced to discuss the topic for the first time and under stressful conditions. Pediatric malignancies grow very rapidly, leaving a very short window between diagnosis and the initiation of possible gonadotoxic therapy. This results in a narrow time frame for a discussion of potential fertility preservation options. Finally, many pediatric malignancies occur prior to puberty. This limits the number of established fertility preservation options available to this population.

This chapter represents the experience of Cincinnati Children's Hospital Medical Center (CCHMC) in building an oncofertility program for pediatric, adolescent, and young adult patients. Our team comprises physicians and medical staff from the Cancer and Blood Diseases Institute (CBDI), Pediatric and Adolescent Gynecology, Pediatric Urology, and the University of Cincinnati Reproductive Endocrinology. CCHMC is a tertiary care center with >350 new patients in oncology and >100 bone marrow transplant patients per year. We are able to offer ovarian tissue cryopreservation for females as young as 1 month of age under an open IRB-approved study protocol. In collaboration with our REI team members, we also offer hormone therapy for postpubertal females, as well as oocyte/embryo cryopreservation for older adolescent and young adult females (over the age of 15). For males, testicular cryopreservation is available for patients at all ages under an open IRB-approved study protocol (at limited institutions), and sperm cryopreservation is available for postpubertal patients.

The Oncofertility Team

A successful pediatric oncofertility program involves a collaborative effort that crosses several disciplines. Our process flow is defined in a later section of this chapter. For now, we will begin by defining the key individuals on our team. Successful program development and implementation requires recognition of the valuable input of all stakeholders. Team members work closely together with the assistance and coordination of the fertility navigator throughout.

Primary Team Members

At our institution the fertility navigator role is performed by a registered nurse with experience in both pediatric oncology and pediatric and adolescent gynecology. She receives the initial consult and orchestrates communication between the multiple specialties, keeping timeliness and patient/family experience as the highest priorities. She is the core team member. She facilitates the actual consultation, ensures appropriate laboratory testing is performed, assists in the consultation, and arranges the indicated follow-up dependent upon the patient/family decision for intervention. At our institution, she also helps to navigate the research process and financial considerations. She is critical in assisting the patient/family through the oncofertility process as seamlessly as possible.

The pediatric oncologist on the oncofertility team is responsible for assessing the risk of infertility from the proposed treatment plan. He or she discusses the patient's treatment plan and timeline with their primary oncology/bone marrow transplant team. The pediatric oncologist will have knowledge of the cancer diagnosis as well as access to detailed treatment protocols. This allows an accurate and individualized risk assessment of the effect of treatment on future fertility for the patient.

Our pediatric and adolescent gynecologist plays a critical role in the consultation for female patients. He or she is able to meet with the patient and family to discuss the risk assessment and appropriate fertility preservation options. They are then able to perform select procedures at our freestanding pediatric hospital (in the case of ovarian tissue cryopreservation) or refer to the reproductive endocrinologist for rapid consultation (embryo and oocyte cryopreservation). The gynecology team also manages medical management, including hormone therapy for menstrual suppression during treatment.

Our pediatric urologist is likewise essential in the consultation process for male patients. He or she is able to meet with the patient and family to discuss the risk assessment and appropriate fertility preservation options. They are then able to refer the patient for testicular tissue cryopreservation in appropriate candidates or initiate a rapid sperm banking referral.

Many pediatric centers do not perform oocyte harvesting or oocyte/embryo cryopreservation, thus it is necessary to have a relationship with a reproductive endocrinologist familiar with oncofertility. They should be equipped to schedule urgent office visits to discuss the process of hormonal stimulation and oocyte harvest. Good communication is critical to maintaining the timeline agreed upon with the primary oncology team.

A research coordinator is also a valuable member of the team. Ovarian and testicular tissue cryopreservation are the only fertility preservation options available to prepubertal patients. Both methods of preservation are only performed under IRB-approved research protocols. The research coordinator ensures all proper research protocols are followed and informed consent has been obtained. He or she ensures appropriate documentation, record keeping, and follow-up are performed.

The team is not limited to the members detailed above. Other potential members might include a social worker to help identify community resources for financial aid, a member of the hospital ethics team to aid in complicated decisions, global health to ease cultural differences, and pastoral care to help patients and families work through religious concerns. A team psychologist can help families work through their thoughts about fertility preservation and the available options. Programs that plan to process their own specimens (testicular and ovarian tissue, oocyte, and embryo preservation) will also need to include team members from the laboratory who specialize in processing this tissue (Table 15.1).

Oncofertility Consultation Process

The oncofertility process begins when a patient initially presents to the oncology or bone marrow transplant (BMT) program for diagnosis and treatment of their underlying disease. The primary oncology/BMT team contacts the fertility navigator to initiate the fertility consult and risk assessment. Initial consultation can occur by

Table 15.1 Medical care team

Primary medical team	Address diagnosis and treatment plan with patient and family
	Introduce the concept of impaired fertility from necessary treatment
Pediatric oncology	Specific oncologist(s) with interest in oncofertility. Works with oncofertility team and primary medical team to determine risk of impaired fertility with proposed treatment plan. Works with primary medical team to form timeline
Pediatric and adolescent gynecology	Addresses risk of impaired fertility with patient and family. Discusses available fertility preservation options
	Performs surgery for ovarian tissue cryopreservation
Pediatric urology	Addresses risk of impaired fertility with patient and family. Discusses available fertility preservation options
	Performs surgery for testicular tissue cryopreservation
Oncofertility navigator	Orchestrates communication between multiple disciplines involved in consultation process
	Maintains timeline for fertility preservation procedures/treatment start date
	Participates in consultations with patient/family
	Helps navigate research process when applicable
Research coordinator	Ensures proper research protocols are followed and informed consent obtained for all research based fertility preservation options
Reproductive endocrinology	Provides services for oocyte harvesting and oocyte/embryo cryopreservation. Provides laboratory for semen collection/storage for sperm cryopreservation

phone and communication via the electronic medical record or by e-mail. By creating a separate specific e-mail address, the consulting team has an additional streamlined way to reach our team.

The goal of our oncofertility program is to see all patients new to the oncology and BMT division. However, we recognize that not every patient will be an appropriate candidate for a discussion on fertility preservation. A patient may be deemed ineligible for the following reasons:

- Diagnosed with malignancy but planned therapy consists of surgery/observation only
- Presents for phase I therapy or palliative therapy only
- Presented to CCHMC for second opinion/consult only (Table 15.2)

If a new patient meets one or more of these criteria, we will meet with the primary medical team to discuss whether or not it is appropriate to approach the family about fertility preservation options. Certainly some families who seem ineligible by criteria alone have many questions regarding future fertility. Patients who are acutely ill at the time of presentation and require immediate oncologic treatment will have the fertility consult delayed until the patient's medical condition is stable and timing is appropriate. This decision is always made in conjunction with the treating medical team. Patients who have previously had a fertility consult (relapse, transfer of care) may have an abbreviated consult to ensure all fertility preservation needs have been met.

Once a patient is classified as eligible, the fertility navigator contacts the oncofertility pediatric oncologist to perform the risk assessment. This physician will discuss the proposed treatment plan (surgery, radiation, chemotherapy) and timeline with the primary medical team. He or she calculates a patient-specific infertility risk assessment (low, intermediate, high). This is done using a cyclophosphamide equivalent dosing (CED) calculation and radiation/surgical risk assessment with published dose guidelines [1].

The risk assessment is then communicated back to the fertility navigator and documented in the electronic medical record. She advises the gynecology/urology team of the consultation. The fertility navigator facilitates timing of evaluation and testing for the patient to ensure all parameters are met in accordance with the fertility preservation and cancer treatment plan. In addition to the consultation with the

Table 15.2 Exclusion criteria

Exclusion criteria at time of presentation
Presented for second opinion/consult only
Presented for phase I/palliative therapy only
Diagnosed with malignancy however:
Surgery only
Observation only
Consult deferred at time of presentation
Acutely ill/urgent need to start cancer-directed therapy

provider and fertility navigator, the patient and family receive written information on the fertility preservation options available to them. Many families would like time to think about their decision prior to making a final choice. Thus, the fertility navigator reconnects with the family after 24–48 h and then begins to coordinate any necessary procedures or referrals. The consult is completed and documented in the electronic medical record using a standardized format. The primary medical team is updated regularly throughout the process to maintain good communication and best care for the patient (Fig. 15.1).

Laboratory Management

Assessment of fertility at the time of evaluation informs patients/parents and the team about current fertility potential and allows informed decision making regarding possible next steps. Our oncofertility team requests baseline laboratory studies on all patients who receive a consult. We request that these be drawn prior to starting chemotherapy. It allows a frame of reference for post-therapy values, as there can be some interpersonal variability in normal levels. For females, this includes baseline AMH, FSH, and LH. For males, we request baseline testosterone. Anyone who elects to have a cryopreservation technique is required to have infectious disease testing for HIV, hepatitis B, and hepatitis C drawn before the sample is frozen. It is important to use an FDA-approved lab (Table 15.3).

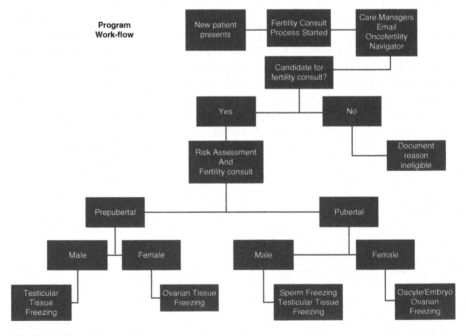

Fig. 15.1 Flow diagram of process

We do not have a laboratory for long-term storage of cryopreserved specimens at our institution. At this time, cryopreserved ovarian tissue at CCHMC is placed in shipping media and shipped offsite for storage. Patients who opt for oocyte and/or embryo cryopreservation receive those services (evaluation, hormonal management, and tissue processing) through an adult-based reproductive endocrinology (REI) facility. We maintain a strong collaborative relationship with the adult team to allow timely referrals as well as research and quality improvement work. Transportation for sperm banking services is sometimes difficult for patients due to timing and/or medical conditions prohibiting travel. A private, onsite room for semen collection (not the patient's hospital room) will help decrease anxiety and increase success rates.

With our current relationship with the Oncofertility Consortium/NPC, the ovarian tissue for cryopreservation is sent to Northwestern for research purposes. Through the cooperation we were able to create an account to obtain tissue media for immediate storage and processing. We initially sent the tissue to the REI lab with which we partner for oocyte/embryo management. However, this process proved challenging with OR timing changes, lab availability, and timely transport of tissue.

We have since moved the tissue processing and short-term storage in-house. We partnered with our pathology laboratory colleagues to identify appropriately trained staff, space, equipment, and surveillance of the transiently stored tissue and storage tanks. Our entire team was trained in good tissue practices to ensure proper management and handling of human ovarian tissue.

Minimizing transfer costs for cryopreserved tissue can be helpful. There is a transfer fee associated with shipping specimens to the long-term cryopreservation facility. It is a flat fee independent of the number of specimens that is passed along to the patient. Batching specimens helps to defray the cost to the patient by dividing it among multiple samples.

Financial Concerns

Unfortunately, since many insurance providers do not provide full coverage for fertility preservation services, it is important to include financial counseling as part of the initial consultation. Fees may vary by institution. In some cases, discounts may

Table 15.3 Laboratory testing

Female
AMH
LH
FSH
Estradiol
Male
Testosterone

be available for some or all of the services. It may be advantageous to attempt to process claims through the insurance carrier, before collecting any potential payment on the part of the patient. However, in order to store cryopreserved tissue for future use, payment is often due at the time of service. It is important to know the facilities and policies in your community to properly counsel families as they make their decision regarding fertility preservation.

Financial assistance is available through programs such as Sharing Hope (www.livestrong.org), Fertility Within Reach (www.fertilitywithinreach.org), and Verna's Purse (www.reprotech.com). Many assisted reproduction facilities offer discounted services for oncofertility patients as well. We have also found that combining fertility preservation procedure with other OR-related events (central line placement, etc.) when medically appropriate can help to bundle expenses and help to defray cost (Table 15.4).

Shared Decision-Making Tool

Most patients with a pediatric malignancy begin therapy very soon after diagnosis. The families receive a great deal of information in a very short and stressful time period. In addition to information about the diagnosis and therapy plan, they must

Table 15.4 Potential cost to patient

Consultation
Initial fertility consult at CCHMC
REI consultation for referred patients
Fertility preservation intervention
Sperm cryopreservation
Collection fee
Testicular tissue preservation
Transportation fee if not performed at local institution
OR/surgery/anesthesia cost if not covered under another procedure
Oocyte/embryo cryopreservation
Medication cost
Procedural costs in retrieving oocytes
Ovarian tissue cryopreservation
Transportation fee if not performed at local institution
OR/surgery/anesthesia cost if not covered under another procedure
Storage fees
Transportation to storage facility
Yearly storage fee
Future cost
Tissue reimplantation
In vitro fertilization

also process the information related to fertility risk and preservation. Employing written materials with the consultation may allow patients and families a resource for reviewing information in their decision making process. With the support of the Anderson Center for Health Systems Excellence at CCHMC, we developed a shared decision-making (SDM) tool. This gives the patient and family written information on risk and options in an easy to read format. It is easily reproducible so each family can keep their copy for future reference. The SDM tool is used to walk the family through the process of understanding the individualized risk to their child as well as the options available specifically to them. The tool also allows stratification of factors that will be important for patients and families to consider in making their decision. For example, factors such as timing, additional surgical risk, cultural importance of fertility, religious considerations, and cost are outlined in the tool.

Documentation

Patients who receive a fertility consult have the encounter formally documented in our electronic medical record (EMR). It becomes part of their official medical chart. We have created a separate category specific to our team (labeled fertility consult) so that it is searchable in the EMR. It is important to document the diagnosis, date of diagnosis, treatment plan, and expected risk of infertility from therapy. The note should also capture the patient age and pubertal status as this will significantly impact potential therapeutic options. The note should detail the discussion with the patient and family: fertility preservation options available to the patient and risk/benefit of each. Finally, the note must communicate the next steps in the fertility preservation plan. If a family is uncertain as to how they would like to proceed, the note will state a timeline for follow-up. In this circumstance a follow-up note will be needed to document the decision and next steps in the oncofertility process. There are many steps to a complete fertility consult; thus it may be helpful to link the notes in the EMR, if possible. Our EMR allows grouping notes for ease in locating information. We are also able to categorize our notes under a specific group title as mentioned above.

Finally, a clinical database of consults is helpful. This can be maintained by the fertility navigator. This allows the team to track patients for follow-up during and after their cancer-directed therapy. Many times new questions arise and/or new options become available throughout the course of therapy. For example, a patient with acute lymphoblastic leukemia may be classified as low risk of infertility due to therapy at diagnosis but then experiences a relapse and requires a bone marrow transplant. He or she is now at high risk of infertility from the planned therapy and may opt to choose a fertility preservation method. In another example, females at risk of premature ovarian insufficiency who did not have time to undergo oocyte or embryo cryopreservation prior to beginning therapy may elect to do so after completing therapy.

Communication and Institutional Awareness

Pediatric oncofertility is becoming more common but is still relatively rare in practice. Two of the greatest barriers are (1) not requesting the consult at all and (2) not initiating the consult in a timely manner. There are several ways one might address this issue:

- Initiating the consultation. An individual on the oncology team is designated as the person to initiate the consult on new patients. We have chosen to use our patient care manager (oncology navigator) for this role and added it to the checklist of our new diagnosis order set. This aligns the consult with our other new diagnosis consults and disease evaluation protocols. By relieving the primary oncologist from this obligation, it allows them to focus on their area of expertise – developing the best treatment plan for the malignancy.
- Medical provider education. Health-care professional education is key. Frequent in-service meetings for staff and physicians will increase awareness and knowledge. This in turn increases the volume of consultations. Our institution also has disease-specific team meetings. Having a presence at these meetings has helped to increase education and awareness.
- Ease of access. We have a designated e-mail: fertilityconsult@cchmc.org. Our patient care managers send new consult requests to this e-mail. It is checked several times per day by members of the fertility consult team. We also have a member of the fertility consult team on call at all times. The call number is listed along with the hematology/oncology/BMT call schedule. Consults may also be requested through the EMR.
- Visibility. With the increasing use of technology among today's health-care consumers, online access is critical. We have a designated fertility preservation landing page within the hospital website (www.cincinnatichildrens.org). The page is also embedded within the oncology pages. It is easily accessible through the hospital search function as well as independent search functions under the title "Comprehensive Fertility Care and Preservation Program."
- Peer-to-peer information. Nothing emphasizes the credibility of information like someone who has already navigated the same stressful or overwhelming experience. Web-based video testimonials from current and former patients are available on our website for patients, families, and providers to review.

Cultural Considerations

Our hospital has become an international referral center for many conditions. It is important for team members to appreciate the beliefs of the different cultures and religions surrounding fertility, children, and afterlife. We work closely with our Global Health Division to understand regional customs prior to performing consultations. In addition, we make every attempt to provide written information in the family's native language and use an interpreter for all interactions. We have found that the importance of having one's own biological child varies greatly by culture. By addressing this issue, we are able to properly acknowledge the future fertility concerns of our international families. This in turns educates our team and we gain a better understanding of fertility in each culture we encounter.

Reference

1. Green DM, Nolan VG, Goodman PJ, Whitton JA, Srivastava DK, Leisenring WM, Neglia JP, Sklar CA, Kaste SC, Hudson MM, Diller LR, Stovall M, Donaldson SS, Robison LL. The cyclophosphamide equivalent dose as an approach for quantifying alkylating agent exposure. A report from the Childhood Cancer Survivor Study. Pediatr Blood Cancer. 2014;61(1):53–67.

Chapter 16
Optimal Technique for Laparoscopic Oophorectomy for Ovarian Tissue Cryopreservation in Pediatric Girls

Erin Rowell

For parents of a girl facing treatment that poses a threat to future fertility, the option of removal of one ovary now exists to cryopreserve the ovarian tissue prior to beginning the potentially sterilizing medical treatment. This option has an even more powerful impact, given the recent pregnancy achieved by a woman in Belgium after reimplantation of strips of ovarian tissue which had been cryopreserved when she was 14 years old [1]. The state of the science is such that for both premenarchal and post-menarchal girls, there is more hope than ever that these girls can have a biologically related child in the future and possibly achieve natural pregnancy.

Preoperative Considerations

For the pediatric surgeon who is asked to perform the oophorectomy, it is important to remember that treatment of the potentially life-threatening medical condition is the primary goal, both for parents and the medical team. Many children need to undergo routine procedures for insertion of central venous access, biopsies of tumors, lumbar puncture, and bone marrow biopsy, and the oophorectomy procedure is combined under the same anesthesia whenever possible. Our policy is to treat the oophorectomy as an urgent case, which is expedited as much as possible, so as not to delay medical therapy. The laparoscopic oophorectomy procedure is preferred whenever possible, although some patients with intra-abdominal or intra-pelvic tumors will require an open incision and perhaps oophorectomy during an initial tumor resection or debulking (Fig. 16.1). If the laparoscopic oophorectomy is

E. Rowell, MD
Department of Surgery, Ann & Robert H. Lurie Children's Hospital of Chicago,
Chicago, IL, USA
e-mail: ERowell@luriechildrens.org

© Springer International Publishing Switzerland 2017
T.K. Woodruff, Y.C. Gosiengfiao (eds.), *Pediatric and Adolescent Oncofertility*,
DOI 10.1007/978-3-319-32973-4_16

Fig. 16.1 Large rhabdomyosarcoma arising from the bladder in a 5-year-old girl who required open oophorectomy during tumor debulking procedure

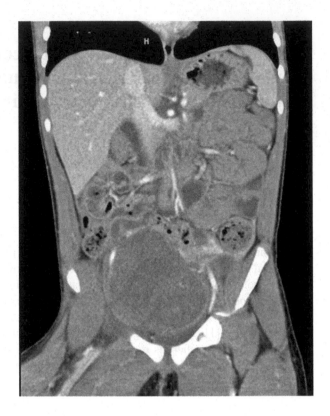

combined with another procedure, the medical procedure is typically conducted first, followed by the oophorectomy. The patient is asked to void just prior to entering the operating room, in order to avoid use of a Foley catheter.

Operative Technique

The details matter when removing an ovary for fertility preservation, even though the procedure itself is relatively straightforward. The laparoscopic approach typically involves a 10 mm umbilical port to accommodate the endoscopic retrieval bag, which facilitates quick removal of the ovary from the patient's body once the final ovarian arterial blood supply has been divided. Two additional 5 mm ports are needed for the dissection, which most often include left lower quadrant and suprapubic locations, for removal of the right ovary. This orientation is the same as that typically used for laparoscopic appendectomy, which is familiar to pediatric surgeons [2]. The procedure begins with clear visualization of the uterus and both ovaries. This requires careful lifting of the fallopian tubes to view the entire ovary for any cysts or masses (Fig. 16.2). If both ovaries are normal, then dissection of the right ovary typically ensues, due to the laparoscopic orientation as described. If the

Fig. 16.2 Laparoscopic view of both ovaries and uterus in a 7-year-old pediatric girl

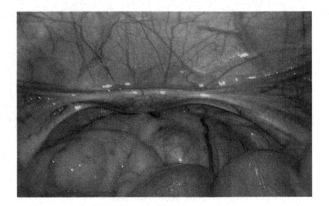

left ovary is appropriate for removal, then the suprapubic port is eliminated in favor of a right mid-abdominal 5 mm trocar. At times, both 5 mm ports are positioned in the left or right abdomen (opposite from the ovary), particularly in very young patients (Fig. 16.3).

In infants and pre-adolescent girls, the ligament of the ovary is long, the mesovarium is typically narrow, and the fallopian tube is located very close to the ovary, all of which increase the possibility of burn damage if the mesovarium is divided (Figs. 16.4 and 16.5). In these youngest girls, the mesovarium of the broad ligament between the ovary and the fallopian tube is grasped, and the fallopian tube is divided using the harmonic scalpel, at the isthmus, the location where it joins the uterus [4]. Our team prefers salpingo-oophorectomy in very young girls, since the excision of the ovary alone often requires handling the ovary or using the harmonic scalpel too close to the ovarian capsule, resulting in 2–3 mm of tissue burn damage that is visible microscopically. In peri-pubertal girls and in teenagers, the mesovarium may be wide enough to provide a safe plane of dissection between the ovary and fallopian tube, without need for concomitant salpingectomy (Fig. 16.6). The goal is complete dissection with no-touch technique of the ovarian capsule. Dividing the fallopian tube and working from a medial to lateral orientation, the broad ligament is divided (Fig. 16.7). The ovarian artery with the suspensory ligament of the ovary is divided last, which preserves the main arterial blood supply to the ovary during the entire dissection and until the last possible moment (Figs. 16.8 and 16.9). The ovary is then quickly placed in an endoscopic retrieval bag and removed through the umbilical incision. The operating room team is verbally coached that the blood supply will be divided so that the team is ready. A 5 mm piece of the ovary is sharply removed and then submitted to the anatomic pathology lab as a routine specimen. The ovary is then placed into the cryopreservation media as quickly as possible after division of the ovarian artery. Our goal is for the ovary to be placed in the cryopreservation media in less than 2 min after the severing of the ovarian arterial supply, which guarantees the healthiest follicles possible.

Placement of Laparoscopic Ports

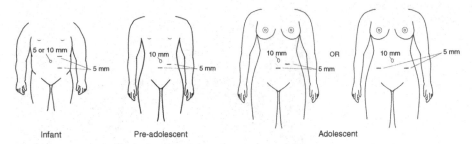

Infant   Pre-adolescent   Adolescent

Fig. 16.3 Laparoscopic trocars for oophorectomy, in infant, pre-adolescent and adolescent girls. The monitor is located at the foot of the bed

Fig. 16.4 Long ovarian ligament and narrow mesovarium in pediatric girl

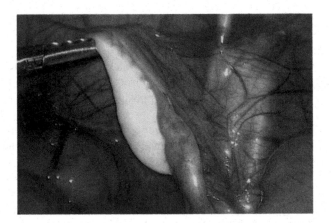

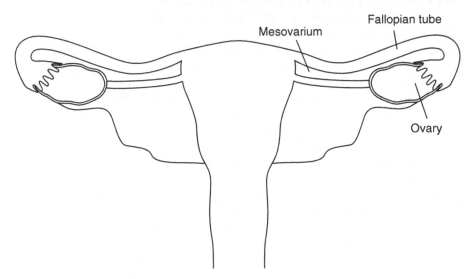

Fig. 16.5 Anatomic image of narrow mesovarium in a pediatric girl

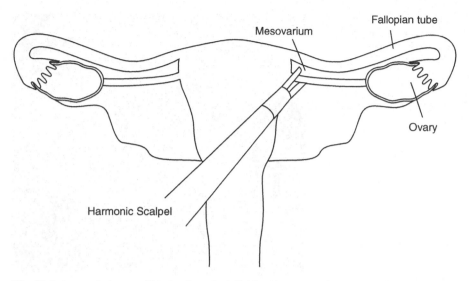

Fig. 16.6 Anatomic image of harmonic scalpel dividing the mesovarium at the isthmus, working from medial to lateral

Fig. 16.7 Intra-operative photo of mesovarium and small ovary in a 2 yo girl. The red arrow indicates the plane of incision for the mesovarium. This ovary measured 2 cm in size

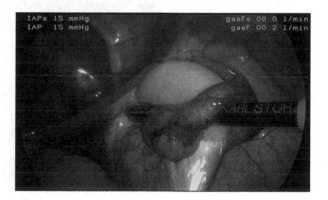

Particularly for the youngest pediatric patients with very small ovary size, the attention to detail during the oophorectomy ensures that the maximum amount of ovarian tissue is available for preservation. Even small areas where the heat source is too close to the ovarian capsule can have catastrophic burn effects on the tissue, damaging many follicles in the process. The maintaining of the ovarian arterial blood supply until the very end of the dissection is crucial in all patients but particularly in younger patients with smaller vessels. In the adult literature, the endo-GIA stapler has been used to divide the ovarian blood supply and surrounding tissue, thus eliminating the need for any heat source during the dissection [5]. However, in pediatric patients this can be problematic for several reasons: (1) need for a 12 mm trocar to accommodate the stapler and (2) small size of the pelvis in young girls which makes manipulation of the stapler difficult. Another report of

Fig. 16.8 The ovarian artery is the last structure to be divided. (marked with asterisk)

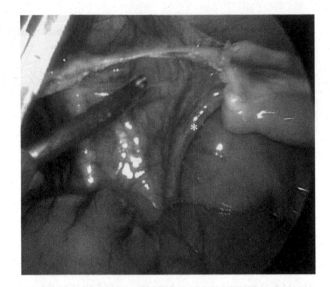

Fig. 16.9 Laparoscopic intra-operative photo of a small ovary in a 2 yo girl. The ovarian artery is the last structure to be divided

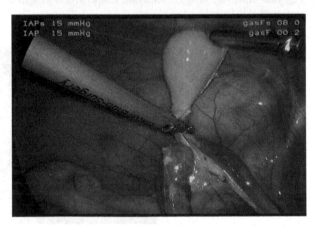

laparoscopic ovarian tissue collection in the pediatric age group describes partial oophorectomy of both ovaries, using a heat source to coagulate the cut surface of the ovary [3]. We do not recommend this approach because of simultaneous damage to both ovaries and to risk of hemorrhage from the bilateral raw surfaces of the ovary. Particularly in very young preadolescent patients, the ovaries are small and partial oophorectomy would risk damaging both the excised ovarian tissue and the remaining ovary left in situ.

Summary

The laparoscopic oophorectomy procedure is a safe, proactive option for pediatric girls facing medical treatment with a high risk of fertility loss. The recommended approach is mono-lateral oophorectomy or salpingo-oophorectomy, maintaining the major salpingo-oophorectomy, maintaining the major ovarian blood supply until the end of the dissection, and rapid placement of the tissue into the cryopreservation media.

References

1. Demeestere I, Simon P, Dedeken L, Moffa F, Tsepelidis S, Brachet C, et al. Live birth after autograft of ovarian tissue cryopreserved during childhood. Hum Reprod. 2015;30(9):2107–9.
2. Holcomb III G, Georgeson K, Rothenberg S, editors. Atlas of pediatric laparoscopy and thoracoscopy. Philadelphia: Saunders Elsevier; 2008.
3. Lima M, Gargano T, Fabbri R, Maffi M, Destro F. Ovarian tissue collection for cryopreservation in pediatric age: laparoscopic technical tips. J Pediatr Adolesc Gynecol. 2014;2:95–7.
4. Netter FH. Atlas of human anatomy. Summit: Novartis; 1989.
5. Roux I, Grynberg M, Linehan J, Messner A, Deffieux X. Ovarian cryopreservation after laparoscopic ovariectomy using the Endo-GIA stapling device and LAPRO-clip absorbable ligating clip in a woman: a case report. J Med Case Rep. 2011;5:48.

Chapter 17
The Fertility Preservation (FP) Consult

Barbara Lockart

The pace of pediatric oncology moves quickly, especially at the time of a cancer diagnosis. Families are overwhelmed by the diagnosis of a life-threatening illness in a previously healthy child and they are inundated with information. Counseling a family on FP may not be an initial priority at the time of diagnosis, and, fortunately, the majority of childhood cancer survivors are not at risk for infertility [4, 21]. For those patients receiving treatment which may harm future fertility, counseling regarding the impact of treatment on fertility and preservation options prior to initiation of cancer therapy is important. For patients at risk for compromised fertility, the evidence supports a discussion regarding the risk of infertility and FP options prior to treatment initiation is extremely important [17, 20].

Educating families regarding side effects of treatment is a responsibility of both nurses and physicians. Fertility preservation as a patient right is supported by the American Society of Clinical Oncologists (ASCO), the American Society for Reproductive Medicine (ASRM), the American Academy of Pediatrics (AAP), and the Association of Pediatric Hematology and Oncology Nurses (APHON). These professional organizations support patient access to FP prior to treatment, as well as the need for ongoing emotional and physical support once treatment is completed [1, 5, 9, 14]. Current recommendations from ASCO, ASRM, AAP, and the nursing committee of the Children's Oncology Group (COG) endorse offering sperm banking to all adolescent and young adult males receiving cancer treatment. Oocyte harvesting is no longer considered to be experimental and should be discussed prior to treatment initiation with adolescent and young adult female patients at high risk for infertility [1, 9, 10, 14]. Nonexperimental methods of FP may not be available to a patient because of age, urgency to start treatment, or disease process. In such cases, the healthcare team is obligated to explain to families that experimental methods

B. Lockart, DNP, APN/AC-PC, CPON
Solid Tumors & Fertility Preservation, Ann & Robert H. Lurie Childrens Hospital
of Chicago, Chicago, IL, USA
e-mail: BLockart@luriechildrens.org

© Springer International Publishing Switzerland 2017   251
T.K. Woodruff, Y.C. Gosiengfiao (eds.), *Pediatric and Adolescent Oncofertility*,
DOI 10.1007/978-3-319-32973-4_17

such as ovarian or testicular tissue cryopreservation may be an option for their child. Referral to an institution offering FP should be made as the family wishes.

The FP consult not only includes counseling with the patient and family but also with the oncology team, who are often unfamiliar with reproductive medicine technology. Conversely, reproductive medicine teams do not routinely encounter a critically ill pediatric or adolescent patient. The reproductive medicine team may require assistance in providing developmentally appropriate care to patient, as well as caring for the entire family at a time of great stress. Utilization of a nurse or patient navigator to facilitate the coordination of patient care between the primary oncology team and reproductive medicine specialists is key to successfully caring for patients and families throughout treatment and into survivorship.

The Primary Treatment Team

The FP referral is often initiated by the patient's primary oncology team, either as a standard component of the new diagnosis workup or at the request of the family. Despite professional guidelines from ASCO and the AAP, research shows that many patients, especially female patients, are not satisfied with FP discussions prior to treatment [6, 8, 22]. Barriers to FP include healthcare provider discomfort with patient sexuality, cultural and religious influences, lack of knowledge regarding FP options, and concerns regarding the cost of FP [18]. A fertility preservation consultant is able to provide the family with FP information and allows the oncology team to focus on supporting the family through the new diagnosis discussion.

The fertility preservation consultant must meet with the primary team prior to counseling the patient and family. Information regarding diagnosis, medical and surgical history, Tanner stage, relapse information, planned cancer treatment, as well as previous cancer treatment is vital to assess the patient's risk of infertility. Another key component to counseling families is information regarding religious or cultural influences, family literacy level, preferred language, and any discussions the treatment team had with families regarding FP. A consult order in the electronic medical record formalizes the referral process and allows the FP team to track the number of patients referred to the service.

Assessing Risk of Infertility

A comprehensive medical history and physical exam, including Tanner staging, should be performed. Review of the treatment plan to assess risk of infertility is vital. If the patient is eligible to enroll in a research study, determination of patient eligibility to participate based upon planned treatment is required and should be verified prior to discussing FP options with families. The risk of infertility must be weighed with the cost, potential delay in treatment, cultural and ethical concerns regarding assisted reproduction, and the health of the patient. The cyclophosphamide equivalent dose [13] has increasingly been used to estimate the potential risk of infertility due to alkylating agent exposure. When estimating the likelihood of infertility, previous chemotherapy, radiation, and surgeries must be included in the risk assessment.

Fertility preservation medical history
Family medical history
Genetic disorders
Cancer syndromes
Reproductive/sexual health
Biological children
Sexual transmitted infections
Sexual activity
Partners – male, female, both
Age at intercourse
Number of partners
Type of sex – oral, vaginal, anal
Puberty history – females
Tanner stage
Libido
Menstrual history
Age menstruating began
LMP
Frequency and duration of cycles
Pregnancies
Number
Terminations
Puberty history – males
Tanner stage
Nocturnal emissions – age
Erectile dysfunction
Libido

Counseling Children and Adolescents

Information families provide their children on the topics of sexuality and reproductive biology varies widely [15]. Healthcare providers counseling families on the topic of fertility preservation cannot assume either the parents or the patient possess an understanding of basic reproductive biology. Therefore, any discussion on fertility preservation must include an explanation of puberty, reproductive health, pregnancy, menopause, and hormone regulation. Information provided to the patient should be developmentally appropriate and determined by the patient's age, cognitive ability to grasp the topic, and maturity level. Initiation of fertility preservation or reproductive health following cancer treatment is more successful if a healthcare provider begins the discussion [22]. Open-ended questions such as "have you thought about being a mom or dad in the future" provide the patient the opportunity to express a vision of their future in a developmentally appropriate manner. Many pediatric hospitals employ child life therapists who are able to assist both the parents and the healthcare team to use developmentally appropriate language to explain reproduction and any FP procedures the patient might undergo.

There is never a "good time" to discuss the risk of infertility with a cancer patient, but waiting until after the initiation of treatment is not optimal and may mean FP is no longer feasible. The concepts of patient autonomy and informed decision making require the patient and family to be provided with the information needed to determine if fertility preservation is a viable option as early as possible. Armuand et al. [3] report adult female cancer patients not provided information on FP options described a loss of control and report a greater sense of loss than male cancer patients. The researchers also state healthcare providers' assumptions about a patient's desire for FP rob the patient of autonomy.

During the course of the diagnosis and treatment discussions, the healthcare team reviews all potential side effects of treatment. A fertility preservation counselor or patient navigator is often the best professional to provide the patient and family information on FP options as well as reproductive health during and following treatment. The impact of treatment on reproductive health and sexuality should also be included in the discussion. For example, a male patient at risk for retrograde ejaculation due to a reproperitoneal lymph node dissection should be informed of these side effects prior to surgery. Even patients whose treatment plan confers a low risk of infertility should be informed that treatment is unlikely to impact future reproductive health.

Parents of young child may prefer to discuss FP without their young child present and may seek guidance from the healthcare team on how and when to begin the discussion with their child. Ask the parents if they wish to discuss FP with their child or if a discussion led by the healthcare team is desired. Children can feel untethered if the adults around them are not providing information in an attempt to protect the child; therefore, it is important for the adults to structure the discussion, allow the patient to express concerns and fears, and have the parents and healthcare team respond to those concerns and fears. How adults respond to the child is more important than what is said [2]. A pediatric social worker or child life specialist may be helpful in providing the patient developmentally appropriate information.

It is best to begin with a basic explanation of reproduction, given in the patient and family's native language. Reassuring the patient that puberty and reproduction are a normal part of the human experience is vital. Quizzing the child is counterproductive and may inhibit any discussion on FP. Allowing the patient and family to ask questions is important, as well as giving them time to process the information provided. Patients may not be familiar with medical terms such as masturbation, oocyte, or testicles, requiring the healthcare provider to use slang terms to provide context to the discussion. Medications, stress, cognitive delays, language, fatigue, and cultural barriers may impact comprehension of the topic. The complex nature of the

Table 17.1 Guidelines for counseling families

Guidelines for counseling families
1. Set the environment to allow for a private discussion
2. Lead the discussion
3. Do not assume the patient or family has knowledge of reproductive biology
4. Allow time to process information and formulate questions
5. Do not allow the parent to speak for the child
6. Do not assume a patient's silence means a lack of interest in the topic

topic, as well as the seriousness of the cancer diagnosis, may necessitate several meetings with the family to adequately cover the topic. Do not assume that a child who is silent during the discussion is not paying attention or is not curious about the topic – embarrassment, fear, or anxiety may prevent him or her from engaging in a dialogue. Conversely, do not allow a parent to dominate the conversation or speak for the child (Table 17.1).

Adolescence is often divided into three distinct phases of development. Therefore, counseling adolescents on reproductive health and FP is quite different than younger children. Early adolescence is from 11 to 13 years, middle adolescence is 14–16 years, and then late adolescence is 17–21 years of age [19]. Cognitive, emotional, and developmental needs of each stage of adolescent development influence how sensitive information such as FP is communicated with the patient.

Physical development does not correspond to the emotional and cognitive changes occurring during this time. A physically mature 14-year-old may be a concrete thinker, not quite able to grasp the significance of the decision to proceed with FP. If desired, the adolescent should be given the opportunity to discuss reproductive health and FP without parents present. To avoid any conflict between the adolescent and parents, the healthcare provider asks the adolescent if he or she wishes to have a parent or both parents present during the FP consult visit. This establishes that the adolescent is the patient and not the parent(s) (Table 17.2).

Discussing Cost, Consent, and Disposal of Tissue in Event of Death

In addition to counseling families on risk of infertility and FP options, families need to be informed of the cost of FP, the consent process, and tissue disposal. These topics may be even more sensitive for families than FP. Children may worry about the cost of FP and decline due to concerns of cost or financial burden to the family. The decision on what happens to tissue or sperm in the event of the patient's death may be influenced by religion or culture. These are sensitive topics and for most families should not be discussed in the presence of a minor child. The healthcare provider must not allow assumptions regarding a family's socioeconomic level, culture, or religion to influence what information a family is given. A 2014 study examining adult male survivors of childhood cancer and their parents identified

Table 17.2 Sexual and developmental milestones of adolescents[a]

Early adolescence 10–14	Middle adolescence 15–17	Late adolescence 18–21
Puberty initiated	Puberty completed or near completion	Puberty completed
Sexual identity emerging	Recognition of sexual identity and desires	Accepting of sexual identity
Concern about being normal	Physical appearance and sexuality important	Sense of self-development
Masturbating or sexual exploration is common	Sexuality can be seen as expression of romantic interest	Comfortable with arousal and sexuality, may have multiple partners by this time
Socializing with peers in groups – group dates	Peers important, dates may now be individual	Romantic partner(s)
Parents important, but other adults – coaches, teachers, etc., significant	Relationships outside of family becoming more important	Life experiences beyond family – work, college
Beginning to develop executive functioning skills	More abstract thinking – able to interpret information	Logical and abstract thinking – able to plan for future, set goals

[a]Adapted from NSVRC.org [16]

many themes regarding FP decisions at the time of diagnosis. Cost of FP was not identified by any parent as a factor influencing their decision making at the time of diagnosis [20].

Consent for medical procedures and research is guided by both legal and ethical principles. In the United States, the age of consent is typically 18 years of age. An adolescent may be asked to provide assent for medical procedures. Participation in experimental and standard of care fertility preservation requires both parental consent and adolescent assent. Maintaining the adolescent's "independence and enabling supportive collaboration with parents" is vital [12]. When enrollment in a research study is sought, the adolescent patient's refusal to assent to the study should supersede the parent's consent to study enrollment [11]. Consent and assent documents must include what will be done with the tissue or sperm in the event of death. When a minor child reaches the age of 18, the tissue or sperm bank must consent the patient.

Fertility Preservation and Sexual Health Counseling After Treatment Is Completed

Optimal care of childhood cancer patients includes educating and informing them of sexual and reproductive health issues throughout their developmental stages and lifespan. Patients treated for cancer prior to the start of puberty should be monitored for precocious or delayed puberty. Anticipatory guidance includes discussing how treatment may or may not impact sexual development and fertility throughout all phases of treatment, including survivorship. For example, parents of a child diagnosed with cancer at the age of 4 may not be concerned about pubertal development until their child is approaching puberty. As the patient matures, information is provided in a developmentally appropriate manner. Patients should be given the opportunity to discuss sexual health and reproductive issues, including contraception, without parents present, regardless of the patient's age.

Ongoing monitoring of hormone levels such as testosterone or estradiol may be indicated for patients who received gonadotoxic treatment. The Children's Oncology Group Survivorship Guidelines provide recommendations for monitoring reproductive health of childhood cancer survivors post treatment. These guidelines may be incorporated into counseling patients [7]. Fertility preservation following cancer treatment may be appropriate after completion of cancer treatment for females who are at risk for premature menopause. Healthcare providers should review FP options following treatment with patients. Additionally, examining options such adoption, use of donor oocytes or sperm, or gestational carrier should be discussed with adult survivors of childhood cancers who are infertility due to treatment.

Conclusion

Counseling patients and families on the topic of FP starts at the time of diagnosis and continues throughout the care trajectory. Discussions include not only FP options available but also reproductive health and parenting options. Healthcare providers should not wait for families to initiate a conversation on the topic of FP. Reassurance that this is a normal part of the human experience and important to the care of any cancer patient is vital. For families struggling emotionally with concerns about their child's future fertility, utilizing other services such as social work, chaplain services, or child life therapists will provide both information and emotional support to families during a very difficult time.

References

1. American Society for Reproductive Medicine and Society for Assisted Reproductive Technology: Ethics Committees. Fertility preservation and reproduction in cancer patients. Fertil Steril. 2005;86(6):1622–8.
2. Anderson S, Barton D, Bell B, Beniquez L, Bodiford C, Butler E, Thibodeau J (2009) Hey, what do I say? A parent to parent guide on how to talk to children about sexuality. Planned Parenthood of New York City www.ppnyc.org.

3. Armuand GM, Wettergren L, Rodriguez-Wallberg KA, Lampic C. Women more vulnerable than men when facing risk for treatment-induced infertility: a qualitative study of young adults newly diagnosed with cancer. Acta Oncol. 2015;54:243–52.
4. Barton SE, Najita JS, Ginsburg ES, Leisenring WM, Stovall M, Weathers RE, Sklar CA, Robison LL, Diller L. Infertility, infertility treatment, and achievement of pregnancy in female survivors of childhood cancer: a report from the Childhood Cancer Survivor Study cohort. Lancet Oncol. 2013;14(9):873–81.
5. Bashore L, Carr B, Lockart B, Schmidt D (2012) Fertility preservation for pediatric, adolescent and young adult patients. Retrieved from www.aphon.org/files/public/onco-fertilitypaper.
6. Burns KC, Boudreau C, Panepinto JA. Attitudes regarding fertility preservation in female adolescent cancer patients. J Pediatr Hematol Oncol. 2006;28(6):350–4.
7. Children's Oncology Group. Long-term follow-up guidelines for survivors of childhood, adolescent, and young adult cancers and related health links Version 4. 2013.
8. Edge B, Holmes D, Makin G. Sperm banking in adolescent cancer patients. Arch Dis Child. 2006;91:149–52.
9. Fallat ME, Hutter J. Preservation of fertility in pediatric and adolescent patients with cancer. Pediatrics. 2008;121(5):1461–9. doi:10.1542/peds.2008-0593.
10. Fernbach A, Lockart B, Armus CL, Bashore LM, Levine J, Kroon L, Sylvain G, Rodgers C (2014) Evidence-based recommendations for fertility preservation options for inclusion in treatment protocols for pediatric and adolescent patients diagnosed with cancer. J Pediatr Oncol Nurs. 31(4):211–22. doi:10.1177/1043454214532025.
11. Giesbertz NAA, Bredenoord AL, van Delden JJM. Consent procedures in pediatric biobank. Eur J Hum Genet. 2014;23:1–6.
12. Grady C, Wiener L, Abdoler E, Trauernicht E, Zadeh S, Diekema DS, Wilfond BS, Wendler D. Assent in research: the voices of the adolescents. J Adolesc Health. 2014;54(5):515–20.
13. Green DM, Nolan VG, Goodman PJ, Whitton JA, Srivastava D, Leisenring WM, Neglia JP, Sklar CA, Kaste SC, Hudson MM, Diller LR, Stovall M, Donaldson SS, Robison LL. The cyclophosphamide equivalent dose as an approach for quantifying alkylating agent exposure. A report from the Childhood Cancer Survivor Study. Pediatr Blood Cancer. 2014;61(1):53–67.
14. Loren AW, Mangu PB, Nohr Beck L, Brennan L, Magdalinski AJ, Partridge AH, Quinn G, Wallace WH, Oktay K (2013) Fertility preservation for patients with cancer: American Society of Clinical Oncology clinical Practice Guideline Update. J Clin Oncol. Advance online publication. Retrieved from http://jco.ascopubs.org/cgi/doi/10.1200/JCO.2013.49.2678.
15. Martino SC, Elliott MN, Corona R, Kanouse DE, and Schuster MA. Beyond the "Big Talk": The Roles of Breadth and Repetition in Parent-Adolescent Communication About Sexual Topics. Pediatrics 2008;121;e612.
16. National Sexual Violence Resource Center. An overview of adolescent sexual development. 2014. Retrieved from www.nsvrc.org/saam.
17. Nieman CL, Kinahan KE, Young SE, Rosenbloom SK, Yost KJ, Volpe T, Zoloth L, Woodruff TK. Fertility preservation and adolescent cancer patients: lessons from adult survivors of childhood cancer and their patients. Cancer Treat Res. 2007;138:201–17.
18. Quinn GP, Vadaparampil ST. Fertility preservation and adolescent young/adult cancer patients: physician communication challenges. J Adolesc Health. 2009;44:394–400.
19. Shafii T, Burstein GR. The adolescent sexual health visit. Obstet Gynecol Clin N Am. 2009;36:99–117.
20. Stein DM, Victorson DE, Choy JT, Waimey KE, Pearman TP, Smith K, Dreyfuss J, Kinahan KE, Sadhwani D, Woodruff TK, Brannigan RE. Fertility preservation preferences and perspectives among adult male survivors of pediatric cancer and their parents. J Adolesc Young Adult Oncol. 2014;3(2):75–85.
21. Wasilewski-Masker K, Seidel KD, Leisenring W, Mertens AC, Shnorhavorian M, Ritenour CW, Stovall M, Green DM, Sklar CA, Armstrong GT, Robison LL, Meacham LR. Male infertility in long-term survivors of pediatric cancer: a report from the Childhood Cancer Survivor Study. J Cancer Surviv. 2014;8(3):437–47.
22. Yeomanson DJ, Morgan S, Pacey AA. Discussing fertility preservation at the time of cancer diagnosis: dissatisfaction of young females. Pediatr Blood Cancer. 2013;60:1996–2000.

Chapter 18
Ethical Issues in Pediatric and Adolescent Fertility Preservation

Lisa Campo-Engelstein and Diane Chen

Introduction

According to recent estimates, there are more than 270,000 survivors of pediatric cancer and long-term survivorship for pediatric cancer is around 80% [28]. Given the large number of survivors as well as the high survivorship rate, coupled with the fact that pediatric cancer survivors typically have a full lifetime ahead of them, it is increasingly important to examine their quality of life issues. Our goal in this chapter is to highlight some of the ethical issues that arise in the context of fertility preservation for pediatric cancer patients and survivors. Specifically, we explore assent/consent, best interest standard, parental and provider pressure, cost and insurance coverage, and experimental treatment.

Assent/Consent

There is general consensus that patients have a right to know about their health status, the available diagnostic and treatment options, and their associated risks and probable benefits and to choose freely among the options, including declining treatment [1]. Informed consent is the interactive process by which physicians and

L. Campo-Engelstein, PhD (✉)
Alden March Bioethics Institute, Department of Obstetrics & Gynecology, Albany Medical College, 47 New Scotland Avenue, MC 153, Albany, NY 12208, USA
e-mail: CampoeL@mail.amc.edu

D. Chen, PhD
Division of Adolescent Medicine, Ann & Robert H. Lurie Children's Hospital of Chicago, Northwestern University Feinberg School of Medicine,
225 East Chicago Ave, Box 10B, Chicago, IL 60611-2605, USA
e-mail: DiChen@luriechildrens.org

© Springer International Publishing Switzerland 2017
T.K. Woodruff, Y.C. Gosiengfiao (eds.), *Pediatric and Adolescent Oncofertility*,
DOI 10.1007/978-3-319-32973-4_18

patients communicate about a given clinical situation and treatment options, concluding with the patient providing treatment authorization or declining treatment. When the patient in question is a child or adolescent, a complicating factor can be uncertainly about decisional capacity. The ability to consent to or refuse treatment is based on the presumption of capacity, which refers to the cognitive and developmental ability to (1) understand treatment information, (2) appreciate the situation and likely consequences, (3) weigh treatment options, and (4) reach a decision [2, 3]. Among adults, capacity is assumed, unless through disability or disease, their decision-making ability is compromised. Children and adolescents, on the other hand, are presumed to lack capacity. Moreover, young people under the age of 18 are not considered legally able to give valid consent to medical treatment in the United States, with the exception of categorical issues such as birth control, abortion, and drug treatment and only on a state-by-state basis. In cases involving minors, parents can give proxy consent to medical procedures which are considered to be "in the best interests" of their child.

Despite this legal standard, the American Academy of Pediatrics has long maintained that children and adolescents should be involved in a process of assent to treatment "to the extent of their capacity" [1]. In their seminal study, Weithorn and Campbell [4] compared decision-making capacity among four age groups (9, 14, 18, 21 years) on outcome measures specifically designed to reflect the four legal standards of competency. At age 9, youth were less competent than adults in terms of ability to reason about and understand treatment options. However, these youth did not differ from adults in expressing a reasonable preference regarding treatment. By age 14, youth demonstrated the same level of competency as the two adult groups across the four competencies. Authors concluded that children as young as 9 years old appear able to participate meaningfully in personal healthcare decision-making.

Assent is a means of involving minors in treatment decisions. Like informed consent, assent is an interactive process, occurring between a minor and a physician, and involves developmentally appropriate disclosure of the minor's clinical situation and an assessment of the minor's willingness and preferences regarding treatment [1]. The commonly accepted definition of assent is as a minor's agreement to participate in a given treatment. Assent sets a lower standard of capacity than informed consent in that it does not require the depth of understanding or reasoning required to meet the informed consent standard [5]. Within the medical decisional capacity literature, there is consensus that all children and adolescents should be involved in discussions and decisions regarding their healthcare, appropriate to their understanding and maturity [6], and that as treatment decisions become increasingly subjective, youth should be afforded the opportunity for greater involvement [7].

Navigating consent and assent procedures for fertility preservation treatments in pediatric populations is very complex and generally viewed as a multistep process. The first part of the consent/assent process involves introducing the possibility of fertility preservation through gonadal harvesting and storage, which would occur at the time of cancer diagnosis. At this stage, the focus is on whether the proposed procedures to preserve fertility in children and adolescents serves their best interests

[8]. The second part of the consent process focuses on the disposition of the stored tissue, which is reserved for youth once they reach the age of majority. The focus at this stage is the desires of the now-grown youth to make their own decisions regarding reproduction [8].

Ideally, the decision to pursue fertility-preserving treatments would involve joint decision-making between parents and age-appropriate youth. During the consent/assent process, the procedure for procuring gonadal tissue, experimental nature of procedures, and the relevant physical and psychological risks should be discussed. If both parents and youth capable of giving assent agree to pursue fertility-preserving treatments, then treatment can be provided. Where issues arise is when there is disagreement between parents and youth. Because ovarian and testicular tissue cryopreservation in children is considered experimental, it is subject to federal regulations requiring parental consent for minors. Without parental consent, participation is not possible, even when a minor has the capacity to understand consequences of participation. On the other hand, parents may desire fertility-preserving treatments for their child in the context of their child's dissent. In this case, according to medical guidelines, if a minor is judged to have capacity, she or he is entitled to the same degree of autonomy as an adult patient [1]. Thus, the competent minor's decision should be binding [1]. In the case of immature minors with developing capacity or capacity to provide assent, disagreements between parents and youth should be mediated through consultation [1].

Best Interest Standard

When adults with decision-making capacity temporarily or permanently lose capacity, the healthcare proxy is supposed to rely on the substituted judgment standard, which means using the values of patient to determine what she would want if she had the capacity to make her own decisions. Because children, especially young children, may not have developed a robust value system, it is difficult and sometimes not possible to use the substituted judgment standard for them. Instead, parents/guardians and healthcare providers should use the best interest standard, which requires acting in the best interest of the child rather than looking at the value system of the child or the child's parents/guardians. Is pursuing fertility preservation in the best interest of a child with pediatric cancer?

Some ethicists argue that since children are not able to make certain decisions for themselves now, their parents/guardians should have an ethical responsibility to ensure that certain rights are protected so they can autonomously make their own decisions when they reach adulthood. Joel Feinberg refers to these as "rights-in-trust" [13] that will protect the child's right to an open future. Some have claimed that fertility preservation is a right in trust that allows children an open future, one that includes the possible genetic reproduction [15, 25]. Fertility preservation enhances children's future (adult) autonomy by providing them with the option of genetic reproduction, which may have been otherwise eliminated due to cancer treatment. Genetic parenthood is an important goal for many young cancer survivors [29], which is why it is especially important to preserve it.

In addition to promoting autonomy, fertility preservation for pediatric cancer patients also can prevent harm (the ethical principle of nonmaleficence). Adolescent cancer patients have reported that their fertility is connected to their sense of identity and lack of control over it causes distress [11]. Indeed, infertility can significantly affect mental health and this is particularly the case for women. Women experiencing infertility are twice as likely to be depressed as fertile women, and many of them report levels of psychological distress comparable to women with life-threatening conditions [32]. Some adult cancer survivors view fertility preservation as a symbol of optimism and source of "frozen hope" that contributes to their wellness and survivorship [20, 26, 30]. Fertility preservation in the pediatric population may function similarly: providing hope, easing anxiety regarding fertility, and upholding reproductive autonomy [8].

Some who may think fertility preservation is in the best interests of pediatric cancer patients may believe that not choosing fertility preservation is therefore necessarily unethical. McDougall, for example, argues that we should shift our framework from offering fertility preservation to pediatric and adolescent patients to making fertility preservation a rebuttable presumption based on the aforementioned benefits of fertility preservation [23]. Given that fertility preservation can augment future reproductive autonomy, one could argue that not pursuing fertility preservation is not only unethical but also equivalent to sterilization. A response to this claim is that not choosing fertility preservation should not be conflated with sterilization since the intentions behind these two actions are different and the former is an act of commission and the latter an act of commission. Furthermore, it is important to incorporate the medical facts here: fertility preservation, especially for experimental procedures, is not a guarantee of future genetic reproduction, and some cancer survivors who do not undergo fertility preservation are still able to genetically reproduce. Since fertility preservation does not assure genetic reproduction and it can carry medical risks, it may not make sense for all pediatric patients, especially if the patient is already very ill and there is no time to delay cancer treatment or if the fertility preservation procedure increases the risk of cancer spreading or recurring. In short, parents/guardians may have good reasons for choosing not to pursue fertility preservation for their children, and these decisions can be based on the best interest standard. McDougall recognizes that in some cases the potential harms of fertility preservation outweigh its benefits, but asserts that it should be the default option for postpubertal pediatric cancer patients who can safely use established methods [23].

Parental and Provider Pressure

One of the ethical issues for pediatric and adolescent fertility preservation is whether pediatric cancer patients feel pressured by their parents/guardians to undergo fertility preservation treatment and to use their frozen materials later on. Even when parents/guardians are acting in their child's best interest, by choosing fertility preservation treatment, they may be sending the message that they have an expectation to be genetic grandparents. The efforts and expenses of fertility preservation may lead children to believe they have an obligation to use their frozen materials. The pressure and guilt they may feel could inhibit their autonomy. For instance, children may feel like they have to use their frozen materials otherwise they will betray their parent/ guardians and their decision to pursue fertility preservation for them.

In addition to experiencing parental pressure, children may also feel pressured by healthcare providers to undergo fertility preservation treatment. Children may interpret healthcare providers' discussions about fertility preservation not as an option but as a mandate [24]. It is important to the tailor fertility preservation conversations with pediatric and adolescent patients to them and the specific challenges and concerns they face [31]. For instance, age-appropriate information should be available that explains fertility preservation as a possible treatment method.

In the case of pediatric and adolescent cancer patients, perceived parental and provider pressure can especially worrisome given the dominant social norm that associates womanhood with motherhood [24]. There is a strong cultural belief that girls and women innately desire genetic children [33] and women who do not are considered "deviant" [19]. Parent/guardians and healthcare providers suggesting and pursuing fertility preservation may indicate to pediatric and adolescent cancer patients that genetic motherhood is expected of them.

While certain degrees or types of parental pressure may not be healthy, it is probably not possible (or desirable) to completely avoid any parental influence on children. Parents' values strongly shape their children's values and these values often stay with them in adulthood [22]. Teasing apart parents' values and children's values may be challenging—a common problem in proxy decision-making. It is also worth noting that parental pressure is not unique the fertility preservation context. Parents invest time and money to overtly and covertly influence their children's decisions in a particular direction. Quinn et al. [25] provide the example of how parents contribute pretax dollars to education funds that can only be used for their children's college education. Parents contribute to these funds with the expectation that their child will attend college. Children's knowledge of these funds may make them feel pressured to attend college even if they do not want to. The examples of college funds and fertility preservation show that parents allocate their resources in ways that they believe are in the best interests of their children with the hopes that their children will follow the paths they have laid out for them. Although knowledge of college funds and fertility preservation treatment may cause some children to feel pressure, ideally the goal of these actions was to enhance the child's future autonomy by creating opportunities that can ensure them an open future.

Cost and Insurance Coverage

As has been discussed in the adult fertility preservation context, fertility preservation can be quite expensive and insurance companies generally do not cover it [9, 10]. Annual storage fees for frozen gametes can hundreds of dollars a year [34] and can quickly add up in the case of children since they will typically store their gametes for much longer than adults. Some have argued that insurance companies should cover fertility preservation because it is not different from other treatments for iatrogenic conditions currently covered for cancer patients [10]. For example, insurance covers other quality of life treatments such as breast reconstructive surgery following mastectomy and wigs for alopecia. Like these treatments, fertility preservation is not lifesaving but can dramatically improve quality of life; as previously mentioned, infertility can lead to depression, anxiety, and distress. Since much of medicine today focuses on improving quality of life for those with a variety of non-life-threatening conditions (e.g., poor vision, back pain, seasonal allergies, sexual dysfunction, etc.), it does not make sense to exclude fertility preservation on the basis that it is not life saving.

However, the question of whether fertility preservation for pediatric cancer patients is a just use of finite healthcare resources can be raised for other reasons. Some are concerned about the high costs of assisted reproductive technologies (ART): one cycle of IVF is on average $12,400 (Resolve) and estimates for ovarian tissue cryopreservation range from $5,000 to $30,000 [25]. While ART are indeed expensive on the individual level, on the broader social level, they are not: they account for only 0.06 % of the total healthcare expenditure in the United States [35]. Excluding fertility preservation from insurance coverage leads to the justice concern that only certain individuals will be able to afford it, probably the same demographic as the primary users of ART: white, educated, and middle and upper class [16]. While 14 states have mandates requiring insurance companies to cover infertility treatments, there are no similar laws for fertility preservation [9].

There is some anecdotal evidence that insurance companies have covered fertility preservation, but in such cases the individuals were typically aided by a patient navigator and/or were extremely medically savvy, again, individuals probably belonging to the same demographic as those using ART [10]. This is a justice issue, as fertility preservation is likely to be limited only to those who can pay out of pocket for it. Given the high cost of fertility preservation procedures, some nonprofit organizations like the Oncofertility Consortium and LIVESTRONG Fertility Discount Program (http://www.livestrong.org/we-can-help/fertility-services/) offer grants and discounted rates for fertility preservation procedures for cancer patients. However, these grants and discounts are usually limited to the initial fertility preservation and sometimes the storage fees, but generally do not include the cost of thawing and implanting the frozen gametes.

Experimental Treatment

Adult and postpubertal cancer patients have two established fertility preservation methods to choose from, gamete cryopreservation and embryo cryopreservation. In contrast, there are no established fertility preservation methods for prepubertal children; rather, the available method for prepubertal children is gonadal tissue (ovarian or testicular) cryopreservation, which is considered experimental for both girls and boys [23]. While some experts recommend removing the experimental label for ovarian tissue cryopreservation, its success (i.e., the birth of over two dozen babies through this method) is limited to postpubertal females [12].

Experimental treatment in general, especially in vulnerable populations like children, raises ethical concerns. In the case of experimental fertility preservation for pediatric cancer patients, there is the concern that the procedure exposes more risk than the possibility of benefit. Gonadal tissue cryopreservation involves surgical risks, which are small but can be serious, and the possibility of spreading the cancer, depending upon the type of cancer the patient has. Some parents/guardians and pediatric patients may find these risks too great in light of the uncertainty of whether gonadal tissue cryopreservation will lead to genetic children in the future. Yet there have been tremendous advancements in this area, and some experts are optimistic that experimental treatments will work in the future [17, 18]. McDougall argues that there is a strong case for parental discretion for prepubertal fertility preservation since the benefits are speculative and there are physical risks [23].

Psychological risk can also be present in experimental treatments. False hope is a type of psychological risk that occurs when patients are misled about the possibility of success for a particular treatment. False hope can be exacerbated in the case of experimental treatment since the experts are less certain of the likelihood of success for that treatment and since there may be a conflict of interest in recruiting people to participate in an experimental procedure and providing full disclosure. However, false hope can occur in any area of medicine and can be mitigated by good informed consent. Moreover, not preserving one's child's fertility can also lead to psychological risk in that the child may think her parents/guardians are not looking out for her best interests and her future reproductive autonomy [23].

Conclusion

Fertility preservation is an important quality of life consideration for many cancer patients, including children and adolescents. However, it is important to recognize some of the unique ethical issues that arise when dealing with this population. We have discussed some of the key ethical issues involved in fertility preservation for pediatric and adolescent cancer patients in this chapter. As the fields of pediatric and adolescent oncology and of fertility preservation continue to develop, it will be necessary to continually to reassess the ethical issues we have raised.

References

1. Informed consent, parental permission, and assent in pediatric practice. Committee on Bioethics, American Academy of Pediatrics. Pediatrics. 1995;95(2):314–7.

2. Parekh SA. Child consent and the law: an insight and discussion into the law relating to consent and competence. Child Care Health Dev. 2007;33(1):78–82.
3. Ruhe KM, et al. Decision-making capacity of children and adolescents-suggestions for advancing the concept's implementation in pediatric healthcare. Eur J Pediatr. 2014; 174(6):775–82.
4. Weithorn LA, Campbell SB. The competency of children and adolescents to make informed treatment decisions. Child Dev. 1982;53(6):1589–98.
5. Weithorn LA. Children's capacities to decide about participation in research. IRB. 1983;5(2):1–5.
6. Palmer R, Gillespie G. Consent and capacity in children and young people. Arch Dis Child Educ Pract Ed. 2014;99(1):2–7.
7. McCabe MA. Involving children and adolescents in medical decision making: developmental and clinical considerations. J Pediatr Psychol. 1996;21(4):505–16.
8. Cohen CB. Ethical issues regarding fertility preservation in adolescents and children. Pediatr Blood Cancer. 2009;53(2):249–53.
9. Basco D, Campo-Engelstein L, Rodriguez S. Insuring against infertility: expanding state infertility mandates to include fertility preservation technology for cancer patients. J Law Med Ethics. 2010;38:832–9.
10. Campo-Engelstein L. Consistency in insurance coverage for iatrogenic conditions resulting from cancer treatment including fertility preservation. J Clin Oncol. 2010;28:2184–1286.
11. Crawshaw MA, Sloper P. 'Swimming against the tide' – the influence of fertility matters on the transition to adulthood or survivorship following adolescent cancer. Eur J Cancer Care. 2010;19(5):610–20.
12. Donnez J, Dolmans MM, Pellicer A, Diaz-Garcia C, Sanchez Serrano M, Schmidt KT, Ernst E, Luyckx V, Andersen CY. Restoration of ovarian activity and pregnancy after transplantation of cryopreserved ovarian tissue: a review of 60 cases of reimplantation. Fertil Steril. 2013;99(6):1503–13.
13. Feinberg J, et al. The child's right to an open future. In: Aiken W, LaFollette H, editors. Whose child? Totowa: Rowman & Littlefield; 1980. p. 124–53.
14. Gardino S, Russell AE, Woodruff TK. Adoption after cancer: adoption agency attitudes and perspectives on the potential to parent post-cancer. Cancer Treat Res. 2010;156:153–70.
15. Jadoul P, Dolmans MM, Donnez J. Fertility preservation in girls during childhood: it is feasible, efficient and safe and to whom should it be proposed. Hum Reprod Update. 2010;93:1–14.
16. Jain T. Socioeconomic and racial disparities among infertility patients seeking care. Fertil Steril. 2006;85:876–81.
17. Loren AW, Mangu PB, Beck LN, Brennan L, Magdalinski AJ, Partridge AH, Quinn G, Wallace WH, Oktay K, American Society of Clinical Oncology. Fertility preservation for patients with cancer: American Society of Clinical Oncology clinical practice guideline update. J Clin Oncol. 2013;31(19):2500–10.
18. Luyckx V, Scalercio S, Jadoul P, Amorim CA, Soares M, Donnez J, Dolmans MM. Evaluation of cryopreserved ovarian tissue from prepubertal patients after long-term xenografting and exogenous stimulation. Fertil Steril. 2013;100(5):1350–7.
19. Kelly M. Women's voluntary childlessness: a radical rejection of motherhood? Women Stud Q. 2009;37.3(4):157–72.
20. Lee MC, Gray J, Han SH, et al. Fertility and reproductive considerations in premenopausal patients with breast cancer. Cancer Control. 2010;17:162–72.
21. LiveStrong. Parenthood options for women. http://www.livestrong.org/we-can-help/fertility-services/parenthood-options-women/. Accessed 18 Oct 2015.
22. Luster T, Okagaki L. Multiple influences on parenting: ecological and life-course perspectives. In: Luster T, Okagaki L, editors. Parenting: an ecological perspective. Hillsdale: Lawrence Erlbaum Associates; 1993. p. 227–50.
23. McDougall R. The ethics of fertility preservation for paediatric cancer patients: from offer to rebuttable presumption. Bioethics. 2015;29:639–45.

24. Petropanagos A, Campo-Engelstein L. Tough talk: discussing fertility preservation with adolescents and young adults with cancer. J Adolesc Young Adult Oncol. 2015;4(3):96–9.
25. Quinn GP, Stearsman DN, Campo-Engelstein L, Murphy D. Preserving the right to future children: an ethical case analysis. Am J Bioeth. 2012;12(6):38–43.
26. Quinn GP, Vadaparampil ST, Jacobsen PB, et al. Frozen hope: fertility preservation for women with cancer. J Midwifery Women Health. 2010;55:175–80.
27. RESOLVE, T.N.I.A. The costs of infertility treatment. [Cited 2 Nov 2014]. Available from: http://www.resolve.org/family-building-options/making-treatment-affordable/the-costs-of-infertility-treatment.html.
28. Ries LA, Harkins D, Krapcho M, et al. SEER cancer statistics review, 1975–2008. Bethesda: National Cancer Institute; 2008.
29. Schover LR. Motivation for parenthood after cancer: a review. J Natl Cancer Inst Monogr. 2005;34:2–5.
30. Shin D, Lo KC, Lipshultz LI. Treatment options for the infertile male with cancer. J Natl Cancer Inst Monogr. 2005;34:48–50.
31. Shnorhavorian M, Johnson R, Shear SB, Wilfond BS. Responding to adolescents with cancer who refuse sperm banking: when "no" should not be the last word. J Adolesc Young Adult Oncol. 2011;1(3):114–7.
32. Gardino SS, Rodriguez, Campo-Engelstein L. "Infertility, cancer, and changing gender norms." Journal of Cancer Survivorship 5.1 (March 2011).
33. Upchurch D, Lillard L, Constantijn WA, Panis. Nonmarital childbearing: influences of education, marriage, and fertility. Demography. 2002;39(2):311–29.
34. Mesen TB et al. Optimal timing for elective egg freezing. Fertil Steril. 2015;103(6):p.1551–6. e1–4.
35. Georgina M, et al. The economic impact of assisted reproductive technology: a review of selected developed countries. Chambers, Fertility and Sterility. 2009;91(6):2281–94.

Chapter 19
Optimizing the Decision-Making Process About Fertility Preservation in Young Female Cancer Patients: The Experience of the Portuguese Centre for Fertility Preservation

Cláudia Melo, Maria Cristina Canavarro, and Teresa Almeida-Santos

Introduction

Currently, cancer is no longer synonymous with death. Despite the increasing number of new cases of cancer per year in the last decades, the survival rates have also been increasing steadily [46]. Specifically in Portugal, in 2009, the cancer incidence rate was 426.5 cases per 100,000 individuals, which was the highest value ever registered [16]. However, Portugal is reported to be one of the European countries with the highest 5-year survival rates for several types of cancer (e.g., melanoma and colon cancer; [14]). The intervention in oncology therefore needs to be focused not only on the life preservation of patients but also on the promotion of their quality of life after the completion of cancer treatment [30]. Specifically, the patients' reproductive future needs to be taken into account by health professionals during the process of cancer diagnosis, mainly due to the risk of infertility and the duration of cancer treatments as well as the current characteristics of cancer patients.

Over the past years, there have been major advances in cancer treatment protocols. Currently, there are more aggressive regimens that are more effective against malignancies. However, these regimens also have more side effects, including the risk of fertility impairment [38]. Specifically in female patients, the treatment of

C. Melo (✉) • M.C. Canavarro
Faculty of Psychology and Educational Sciences, University of Coimbra,
Rua do Colégio Novo, Apartado 6153, 3001-802 Coimbra, Portugal

Unit of Psychological Intervention, Maternity Dr. Daniel de Matos, Coimbra Hospital and University Centre, Coimbra, Portugal
e-mail: claudiasmelosilva@gmail.com

T. Almeida-Santos
Faculty of Medicine, University of Coimbra, Coimbra, Portugal

Portuguese Centre for Fertility Preservation, Reproductive Medicine Department, Coimbra Hospital and University Centre, Coimbra, Portugal

© Springer International Publishing Switzerland 2017   269
T.K. Woodruff, Y.C. Gosiengfiao (eds.), *Pediatric and Adolescent Oncofertility*,
DOI 10.1007/978-3-319-32973-4_19

some types of cancer comprises hormonal therapy that can last for at least 5 years [23]. Given the normal ovarian reserve decline that registers significantly after the age of 32 [1], the combination of the impact of gonadotoxic cancer treatments and the postponement to later ages of attempts to become pregnant due to hormonal treatments may have a serious negative impact on female cancer patients' reproductive future [23].

Another important aspect to bear in mind is the characteristics of cancer patients at the present time. It is increasingly common to find cancer patients of reproductive age whose parental projects are not fully completed, mainly due to the increasing incidence of some types of tumors at young ages [29] and the current social trend of delaying childbearing until older ages [39]. This means that the reproductive future of many newly diagnosed cancer patients who are young and childless is at risk. However, despite the gonadotoxicity of cancer treatments, the possibility for these patients to have a biological child after surviving cancer is now a reality, mainly due to advances in fertility preservation (FP) methods. The decision-making process about FP is particularly demanding for female cancer patients for several reasons that are presented below.

The main aim of the present article was to describe the experience of the Portuguese Centre for Fertility Preservation in terms of the provision of support for the reproductive choices of young female cancer patients. To our knowledge, this is the first proposal of a prospective intervention model to counsel and support these patients with regard to their reproductive future.

Brief Notes on Female Fertility Preservation Methods

Retrospective data indicate that pregnancy after cancer can be safe for survivors and their offspring [43]. Research indicates that there does not seem to be an additional risk of death in survivors during subsequent pregnancies. The literature also suggests that the infants of cancer survivors do not have an increased risk of low birth weight, malformations [32], or cancer (in the absence of a genetic cancer syndrome) [6] when compared to the general population. However, pregnancy monitoring by a "high-risk obstetric service" ([38], p. 32) is recommended to supervise potential cancer treatment-related risks that are specifically associated with hormone-dependent tumors.

Taking into account the risk of future cancer-related infertility, both female and male FP techniques have been developed to attempt to ensure the possibility of cancer patients having biological children in the future. These methods comprise the cryopreservation of gametes before possibly gonadotoxic cancer treatments (e.g., chemo- or radiotherapy, surgery) and their subsequent use, after the recovery of the patient from the oncological disease, in case of fertility impairment [25].

Female FP methods consist of the cryopreservation of embryos, oocytes, or ovarian tissue.

Embryo cryopreservation comprises, first, the collection of oocytes from the female cancer patient (after an ovarian stimulation that can last 2 weeks) and, second, the in vitro fertilization (IVF) of these oocytes with sperm from the patient's partner. The obtained embryos are then stored. After cancer treatments, if the female patient is not able to conceive naturally, the patient and her partner can use their embryos to try to have a child. The cryopreservation of embryos is a well-established technique [25], and data have shown good success rates (i.e., the clinical pregnancy rate per transfer of frozen embryos is 22.3 % on average; [19]). However, this method has drawbacks that should be considered. First, ovarian stimulation may imply the postponement of the beginning of cancer treatments and may have an impact on the growth of hormonal tumors, a risk that remains unclear in the research [25]. Second, this method does not maintain the reproductive autonomy of the female patient because it can only be performed in female patients who are married or in civil unions, and only the couple can use the previously cryopreserved embryos. It is important to note that in Portugal, since July 2015, embryo cryopreservation has been considered an unviable FP method given the related ethical, moral, and legal issues.

Cryopreservation of oocytes also involves ovarian stimulation and its disadvantages, as previously described. However, in this procedure, the collected oocytes are stored without being fertilized. After cancer treatments, if the female's reproductive function is affected, it is possible to collect sperm from her partner and perform an IVF with the previously cryopreserved oocytes [25]. Since 2013, this has been considered a well-established technique [2] due to the increasing number of live births resulting from oocyte cryopreservation (i.e., there have been more than 1000 children born through IVF with frozen oocytes; [13]).

Cryopreservation of ovarian tissue comprises the extraction of an ovary (partially or totally) through laparoscopy and the subsequent dissection and freezing of the ovarian cortex into small fragments. To reestablish the reproductive function of the female patient after the cancer treatments, the ovarian tissue slices are implanted, one by one, in the remaining ovary in the patient's uterus. It is hoped that this transplantation can restore the activity of the ovary that was subjected to the impact of the oncological treatment. This is a recent and still experimental technique [25], but clinical and research results have been improving in recent years (i.e., there are now more than 40 babies born through transplantation of frozen ovarian tissue; [17]). Despite its experimental label, this FP method has some cons that should be considered. This procedure does not require as much time as ovarian stimulation does, so it can be performed in patients who need to begin their cancer treatments as soon as possible. Moreover, in the case of a successful ovarian tissue transplant, there is no need to perform IVF and embryo transplant in the future to achieve pregnancy [25].

In conclusion, reproductive medicine now provides techniques that attempt to ensure the biological parenthood of cancer patients who plan to undergo treatments that may threaten their fertility. In this context, oncofertility is rising as an imperative research and clinical field that involves an "integrated network of clinical resources [to] focus on developing methods to spare or restore reproductive function in patients diagnosed with cancer" ([44], p. 2).

The Decision-Making Process About Female FP

The decision-making process about FP is complex in female cancer patients for two main reasons. First, and according to the description in the previous section, female FP techniques are invasive, and one of these techniques is still considered experimental. Second, in the decision-making process about female FP, it is necessary to consider several clinical (e.g., type of cancer, time until the beginning of cancer treatments, ovarian reserve), sociodemographic (e.g., age, marital status), and FP technique-related (e.g., success rates, medical procedures, risks, duration of the techniques, maintenance of the reproductive autonomy) variables. Often, there is little time to consider these variables [10, 25].

Although this may be a difficult and emotionally overwhelming process for recently diagnosed young adult female cancer patients [31], some data in the literature suggest the importance of this decision in these women's lives.

Research with Female Cancer Patients

Young female cancer patients seem to value the opportunity to make a decision about FP [33, 36]. These patients report the desire to receive as much information about fertility treatments and FP interventions as possible around the time of the diagnosis so they can play an active role regarding this decision [33]. This is particularly important because studies reveal that more informed patients who have the opportunity to make a decision about FP together with health professionals have lower decisional-conflict levels [24, 33], make higher-quality decisions [33], have greater satisfaction with their care after the decision [24], and have better psychological adjustment to the diagnosis [33] than patients who are less informed and do not have the opportunity to be part of this decision-making process. A study by Peate and colleagues [33] that evaluated women with breast cancer of reproductive age (21–40 years old) reported that a lack of information increases anxiety and negatively influences the quality of the decision-making experience. However, this study also revealed that the presence of anxiety levels in female breast cancer patients do not appear to be correlated with their fertility knowledge or with their desire for information, suggesting that fertility-related information should be provided to all women regardless of their emotional well-being.

Research with Female Cancer Survivors

Results on the motivations for parenthood among female cancer survivors and the impact of cancer-related infertility and of the FP decision in these women's psychological adaptation in survivorship suggest the key role of the FP decision before cancer treatment in these women's lives.

Research reveals that female cancer survivors have more positive motivations for childbirth than healthy women do (e.g., [48]). Despite the fear of a cancer recurrence after a pregnancy, these survivors associate having a child with happiness and a fulfilling life [18], value the family, and feel very competent to educate a child [41]. Through a systematic literature review, Gonçalves et al. [21] reported that childbearing seems to be an important issue for young female breast cancer survivors, even for those who are against having children after cancer due to the potential risks associated with some types of tumors.

The diagnosis of cancer-related infertility has been shown to have a negative impact on the individual adaptation of these survivors in terms of the experience of high levels of anxiety [28, 41], depression [8], sexual dysfunction [9, 37], disruptions to intimate relationships [37], and feelings of loss and anger [37, 40]. Moreover, infertile survivors also must address menopausal symptoms, such as vaginal dryness and hot flashes, which can have a negative impact on their quality of life [9]. Some female cancer survivors even describe the experience of being infertile as being as painful as the cancer diagnosis itself [18]. According to results reported by Canada and Schover [5], social parenting (i.e., adoption) does not completely resolve this distress.

Young adult female cancer survivors evaluate the opportunity to make a decision about FP before the cancer treatments as important because this experience can make them feel positive, peaceful, happy, and hopeful and can give them a reason to live [20, 47]. Many survivors report that one good thing about FP is that it is one of the few decisions that they can make themselves; it allows them to feel in control of an uncontrollable situation [20]. Furthermore, this decision-making process seems to have a positive impact on the adaptation of these female patients in survivorship. Letourneau and colleagues [26] preformed a retrospective study with 1041 female cancer survivors of reproductive age (18–40 years old) who had previously submitted to fertility-threatening treatments and found higher levels of life satisfaction and quality of life and lower levels of regret in relation to the FP decision in women who were counseled by a specialist in reproductive medicine about FP before cancer treatments than in women who did not receive this consultation. These results were found regardless of the decision of the female patients about FP.

Despite the importance that the decision-making process about FP seems to have for young female cancer patients, these women note significant gaps in the information provided by their oncologists about the risks of a pregnancy in survivorship, the infertility risk associated with cancer treatments and possibilities to spare their fertility [4]. Moreover, the literature reveals a lack of or delayed referral of these patients to a fertility specialist consultation to make a decision about the preservation of their fertility (e.g., [20]). These two factors can prevent these patients from having a choice in this matter [4] because these cancer patients cite their oncologists as a critical source of support and information in the cancer diagnosis and treatment process [36]. The literature has also reported the key role of written information and web-based tools in the improvement of FP decision-making outcomes [34, 42].

Taking this situation into account, the guidelines for intervention of several oncology societies around the world (e.g., the American Society of Clinical

Oncology, Clinical Oncology Society of Australia [COSA], European Society for Medical Oncology, the European Society of Breast Cancer Specialists) emphasize the responsibility of all health professionals in oncology to inform all cancer patients about the risk of cancer treatment-related fertility and to refer them in a timely manner to a specialist in reproductive medicine to make a decision about FP [7, 12, 27, 35]. Specifically in Portugal, updated and general guidelines for intervention in oncology, with recommendations for the discussion with young adult cancer patients about their reproductive future, are needed (i.e., the existing guidelines are from 2009 and are specific to breast cancer patients; [15]).

The Prospective Intervention Model of the Portuguese Centre for Fertility Preservation

The PCFP of the Reproductive Medicine Department of the Coimbra Hospital and University Centre is the sole public center in Portugal that provides all the available FP options (i.e., cryopreservation of sperm, embryos, oocytes, and ovarian tissue) to patients facing treatments that may threaten their reproductive function. It was officially created in 2010 to meet the reproductive needs of patients whose fertility is at risk. Despite the availability since the 1990s of male FP in several Portuguese public institutions, female FP techniques were not previously available in Portuguese public practice. Thus, it is clearly important to attempt to ensure the potential for biological parenthood among female patients.

In the present day, the PCFP team is constituted by seven doctors, two embryologists, a psychologist, and a pharmacist. Its main goal is to support informed reproductive decisions through the life course of female cancer patients who are risk of cancer treatment-related infertility. To achieve this aim, in the last 4 years, the team has worked through different but complementary pathways that are described below.

Clinical Practice

The PCFP provides reproductive monitoring and counseling to female cancer patients from all over the country who are planning to undergo treatments that may threaten their fertility.

These patients can be referred to the PCFP by their oncologists or can ask for a consultation. Regardless of the situation, the first appointment at the center is scheduled in the 24–48 h following the request.

In their first visit to the PCFP, female cancer patients are supported in making a decision about FP. They undergo (1) a medical appointment with a specialist in reproductive medicine, where they are informed about the available FP options in terms of medical procedures involved, costs, risks, and success rates, and the adequacy of each method to each situation is discussed, taking into account sociodemographic, clinical, and reproductive variables; (2) medical exams to assess their baseline reproductive function; and (3) an appointment with the psychologist. The psychologist plays an important role in this process because this health professional assesses the psychological adaptation of the patient to the recent cancer diagnosis, the patient's attitudes toward the risk of future infertility, and their understandings and expectations of FP and discusses the pros and cons of each FP option (this appointment is also important to identify information that needs to be better clarified by the oncologist or the specialist in reproductive medicine). This process is always performed in collaboration with the patient's oncologist, which is essential to ensure that the decision about FP does not interfere with the cancer treatments. In this first visit to the center, the amount of time the patient has to make the final decision is defined, taking into account several variables, such as the date provided by the oncologist for the beginning of the gonadotoxic cancer treatments.

If the patient, together with the health professionals involved, decides to preserve her fertility, the next step is to perform the chosen technique. It is important to note that throughout the medical procedures involved, medical and psychological support is provided to patients according to their needs.

After this process, all patients are followed up regardless of whether they preserve their fertility. First, during the cancer treatments, the patients' follow-up is performed by phone calls made by the psychologist of the team every 6 months. These are important opportunities for the PCFP team to stay updated about the clinical situation of the patients and for the patients to maintain contact with the team that is available to support their reproductive decisions in the future. These phone calls are also important to provide emotional support and to identify patients in need of regular appointments with a psycho-oncologist. Second, after the completion of the cancer treatments, the patients are followed through visits to the PCFP every 6 months. As in the first visit to the center, in these follow-up visits, the patients undergo (1) a medical appointment where they are counseled about their reproductive health and decisions (e.g., the possibility of becoming pregnant naturally, the use of cryopreserved material in case of previous FP, implementation of assisted reproduction techniques [ART]); (2) medical exams to monitor their reproductive function after the cancer treatments and to assess the impact of the cancer treatments in ovarian function, taking into account the baseline assessment of the first visit to the PCFP; and (3) an appointment with the psychologist. The psychologist plays an important role in this process because this health professional assesses the patients' psychological adaptation to survivorship, their understandings and attitudes toward survivorship, and their expectations and plans about their parental project, provides emotional support in case of an infertility diagnosis, and supports decisions regarding the use of the cryopreserved material to achieve pregnancy (in case of previous FP) and attitudes about ART and even third-party techniques and adoption. It is important to note that the goals of each medical and psychological appointment in the follow-up phase are variable according to each patient, taking into account the patient's sociodemographic, reproductive, and clinical variables.

As of October 2015, 149 female cancer patients of reproductive age ($M = 31.08$; $DP = 5.43$; 18–42 years old) were counseled in the PCFP to make decisions about FP. Most of them were single (52 %) but were involved in an intimate relationship (66 %) and did not have a child at the time of the FP decision (83 %). Breast cancer was the most prevalent diagnosis in these female patients (62 %). Although the majority of the patients had preserved their fertility (12 patients cryopreserved embryos or zygotes before July 2015, 67 cryopreserved oocytes, and 27 patients cryopreserved ovarian tissue; note that some women used more than one FP technique), 55 women decided to not use any FP method. However, it is important to highlight that whatever their final decision about FP was, these female cancer patients revealed high levels of satisfaction with their decision-making process about FP and the clinical monitoring provided by the PCFP (these results were obtained from an online anonymous questionnaire that all female patients were asked to complete; 83 % response rate). Specifically with regard to the psychological support provided, in the same questionnaire, patients revealed the importance of this appointment for their decision-making process: "the psychologist was truly important to help me and my husband to talk about my cancer and about our fears. Infertility is one of them. The psychologist helped us to think about our priorities and about what we were capable and up to do to preserve the fertility"; "important to help me anticipate me in the future and what I would think about my decision about FP"; "essential to translate the technical information provided by the doctor into simpler words… Really important for me to understand everything that every technique could involve in terms of physical procedures and emotional too"; "it was really important to express all the emotions that I was feeling through the last days of diagnosis and oncological appointments. It is overwhelming to make this important decisions so quickly and so vulnerable. The psychologist helped me to address my worries and to be capable to be rational to think about FP".

The number of female cancer patients counseled in the PCFP for FP has been increasing in the past few years. So far in 2015, 47 women have been counseled; this is the year with the highest number of requests for an appointment in this center (there were 43 patients in 2014, 26 patients in 2013, 19 patients in 2012, 8 patients in 2011, and 10 patients counseled in the PCFP for an FP decision in 2010).

It is important to note that this intervention model has also been applied in PCFP to pre- and postpubertal girls. In these cases, the decision-making process and the follow-up consultations are developed with the participation of the parents (or other legal representatives of the child/adolescent), taking into account that the patients are underaged. At the time of the decision-making about FP, the psychologist consults with the child/adolescent alone, the parents, and the family together to discuss the topics described for the counseling of female adult patients. Talking about these reproductive health issues with underage girls is a great challenge. It needs to be done through language adapted to their age, their level of comprehension, and their emotional maturity. The use of specific communication tools, such as figures, toys, and videos, is important to make these patients interested and motivated to make a decision about FP. Parents and underaged patients also revealed high levels of satisfaction with this intervention model through the online anonymous questionnaire.

Adaptation and Development of Information Resources for Shared Decision-Making About FP

Although most of the female cancer patients are referred to the PCFP by their oncologists (92 %), some of them ask for a consultation on their own. Thus, one aim of the PCFP team is to attempt to better inform patients, health professionals, and the general population about the impact of cancer in fertility and the techniques of FP.

To achieve this goal, the team has adapted and developed several decision-making tools regarding FP to these target populations. First, some materials of the Oncofertility Consortium®, including the iSaveFertility application, the Myoncofertility website, and Repropedia, have been translated and adapted into European Portuguese. These tools are very helpful because they provide high-quality and organized information to the general population and to health professionals, leading to easier decision-making processes. Moreover, it is important to highlight that all these materials, together with the fact sheets and brochures developed by the PCFP team for the female cancer patients who are counseled in the center, are very helpful in clinical practice. These resources are explored at the psychologists' appointments with the patients, and the patients are advised to consult these resources at home and ask the team any questions. Thus, in the decision-making process about FP, patients are guided to have access to important information through specific and recommended tools.

Second, the development of the PCFP website has already begun. This native language online resource will include information and tools developed specifically for the Portuguese general population, patients, and health professionals. Moreover, it will include a tool to easily and rapidly ask for an appointment in the PCFP.

Beyond the development and adaptation of these decision-making tools and in collaboration with the Portuguese Society for Reproductive Medicine, the PCFP team also organized the first course about FP for health professionals in October 2013 at the 5th Portuguese Congress of Reproductive Medicine. This course was evaluated by the participants as extremely important for their clinical practice. Other courses are being scheduled for 2015, not only for health professionals but also for the general population and cancer patients.

Research Projects

It is also important to highlight that research projects are being implemented by some members of the PCFP team, particularly with regard to the decision-making process about FP in female cancer patients, the impact of this decision for future individual adaptation, the impact of cancer treatments on patients' reproductive function, and the FP techniques themselves. These projects are being developed in collaboration with several departments of the University of Coimbra, and most of them are funded by Portuguese organizations such as the Portuguese Foundation for

Science and Technology and the Portuguese League Against Cancer. More recently, in 2015, a proposal for a major research project in the field of pediatric oncofertility was developed, and an application for funding was submitted (proposal under evaluation).

Oncofertility Consortium® Global Partner

In 2013, the PCFP became a partner of the Oncofertility Consortium®. This is an interdisciplinary consortium that was established in 2007 at the Northwestern University of Chicago "to expand research in fertility loss in cancer patients, accelerate clinical translation of fertility preservation techniques and address the complex health care and quality of life issues that concern young cancer patients whose fertility may be threatened by their disease or its treatment" ([3], p. 5).

Participation in this intercultural network with 17 global partners ([3], p. 5) allows the PCFP to collaborate with medical specialists and scientists from several countries who are working in the oncofertility field and to share methodologies, tools, and experiences of clinical research and practice. In this context, and as described, the PCFP has already translated and adapted some information and decision-making tools of the Oncofertility Consortium® to European Portuguese and has provided the community with tools that the PCFP team has developed that can be used and disseminated by the other global partners. This exchange of materials leads to a major dissemination across the globe of useful resources and information about the reproductive health of cancer patients.

Discussion

This article presents the experience of the CPFP throughout the last 5 years in supporting the reproductive decisions of Portuguese young female cancer patients. In particular, it describes the first proposal of a prospective model of intervention and support of these patients in terms of their reproductive future.

Decisions in clinical practice have changed in recent years. A shift has occurred from the paternalistic model of practice to a new paradigm of shared decision-making. Paternalistic physician practices, characterized by full authority to make medical decisions for their patients, have been replaced by shared decision-making with patients. In this new paradigm, patients are integrated into clinical decisions, and they should obtain the best medical information to make their decisions about their treatment. The shared decision-making model includes increased autonomy for the patient and respect for patients' beliefs, goals, and priorities [11, 45].

In terms of cancer patients and reproductive decisions such as FP, there are clinical international guidelines that highlight the need for the inclusion of patients in this decision and the need to provide them with information about their fertility risks and about FP options as early as possible to give them the opportunity to decide (e.g., [27]). This decision-making process is particularly demanding for female patients [10]. Nevertheless, the literature reveals that this is an important opportunity for these patients that improves their individual adaptation to the diagnosis and their well-being in survivorship (e.g., [26, 33]). Thus, not informing these patients and preventing them from making their own decision about FP can have a negative impact on their quality of life later in survivorship. However, female cancer patients often lack information about their reproductive future and about the opportunity for FP [4]. In this context, CPFP has worked for the last 5 years to promote the reproductive decisions of Portuguese female cancer patients, not only to support their FP decision-making process but also to provide these patients with reproductive follow-up and counseling throughout the course of the disease and in survivorship.

CPFP is the sole Portuguese center that offers all the female FP techniques and is the only one that has a prospective and multidisciplinary intervention model to support the reproductive decisions of female cancer patients. To our knowledge, there are no international guidelines about the intervention and support of reproductive decisions in female cancer patients and future survivors. Therefore, the CPFP has developed and implemented the first proposal of a prospective model for intervention and support for young female cancer patients in terms of their reproductive decisions.

This model has two main innovative characteristics: three phases of intervention and counseling of young female cancer patients and the integration of a multidisciplinary team, highlighting the role of the psychologist in supporting these patients' decisions. First, the intervention model that CPFP proposes is prospective, providing counseling and support to patients in three main phases: (1) before the beginning of cancer treatments, (2) during cancer treatments, and (3) after the completion of cancer treatments. Second, it emphasizes the importance of a multidisciplinary intervention, highlighting the role of psychologists in supporting these patients' decisions along with specialists in reproductive medicine, oncologists, and other health professionals. It is important to highlight that this model was developed and implemented in collaboration with the team of the unit of psychological intervention of a central Portuguese maternity ward, which is particularly experienced in providing psychological support to patients in the context of other reproductive decisions (e.g., infertility diagnosis, prenatal diagnosis, pregnancy in the context of a human immunodeficiency virus diagnosis, voluntary interruption of pregnancy). The psychologist seems to play an important role in the three phases of the intervention for the provision of emotional support and for counseling with regard to reproductive decisions. It is important to note that at the time of the FP decision, the presence of psychopathology symptoms is frequent (e.g., high levels of anxiety and depression) given the recent cancer diagnosis and the anticipation of the cancer treatments [22]. Anxiety and depressive symptoms can have a considerable impact on cognitive functioning and, subsequently, on the decision-making process. Thus, we must bear in mind that these symptoms may influence patients' FP decisions, possibly leading them to undervalue this decision at that time. Psychological support seems crucial at this phase to identify these particularly emotionally vulnerable patients and to try to help them decrease their anxiety levels and support them in making an informed and conscious decision while anticipating how they will live with it the future. The same process can occur in survivorship, where psychopathology symptoms are also frequent [22].

In addition to clinical activity, the CPFP team has also been working on the development and implementation of several types of information aids for the general population, patients, and physicians as well as scientific events to attempt to enhance knowledge about oncofertility in Portugal. Some members of the CPFP team are also working on research projects with funding from relevant Portuguese organizations to increase the quality of FP techniques and to better understand the importance of this decision to these patients. Becoming a Global Partner of the Oncofertility Consortium® network was also extremely important for the CPFP because it allows the CPFP team to be part of a community of researchers and clinicians from all over the world, to exchange knowledge, skills, and experience and to develop and implement the European Portuguese versions of some information aids that were previously developed and that are very useful for the Portuguese population.

Throughout its 5 years of existence and activity, the CPFP has contributed to informing and supporting female cancer patients about their reproductive decisions, namely, about FP. Patients from public institutions from all over the country are referred for consultations to this center to make decisions about FP, and the number of patients counseled has been increasing. This increase can be associated with oncofertility information dissemination and increasing awareness that CPFP has promoted through the development of the previously described resources.

There are some reproductive and clinical characteristics of the patients referred to the center that should be noted. First, although most of the patients referred to the center for FP decisions did not have children, 27 % were already mothers; nevertheless, they wanted to be referred to make their decision. Thus, this cannot be a criterion for oncologists to avoid discussing these options with patients. Second, it is important to highlight that the most prevalent diagnosis in the female cancer patients counseled in this center has been breast cancer. This may be because this is the most prevalent cancer diagnosis in young women, but it may also be that gynecologists may be more aware of fertility issues than other specialists who treat other types of cancer. Thus, this increased awareness should be generalized to all specialties. Lastly, it is important to note that despite the experimental label of the ovarian tissue cryopreservation method, this procedure has been performed on 27 patients, which can be explained by the fact that this technique does not require as much time as oocyte cryopreservation. This situation calls attention to the importance of the early referral of patients to make a decision about FP so they can have access to all the techniques and choose the one they prefer without time pressure and without the need to postpone the beginning of cancer treatments.

Implications for Research and Clinical Practice

Future research should be conducted to confirm the value of the proposed intervention model and its components and to help to create national and international guidelines for the support of high-quality reproductive decisions by young female cancer patients and survivors.

Furthermore, more studies are needed about the FP decision-making process of recently diagnosed female cancer patients. The few existing international studies (only three, to our knowledge) have some limitations that should be considered, such as the cross-sectional design, the sample size, the focus on women with breast cancer, and the small spectrum of variables assessed. Despite the existence of more research with survivors about their fertility concerns and decisions, these studies have some limitations, such as the heterogeneous samples in terms of time since diagnosis and the age of the patients at the time of diagnosis; furthermore, most of the research is qualitative. Moreover, the literature on survivors lacks information about the impact of the FP decision in individual adaptation in survivorship and the attitudes of cancer survivors about ART and third-party techniques.

Specifically in Portugal, to our knowledge, there are no studies about the FP decision-making process of female cancer patients and survivors. It would be important to develop research to understand the information needs of Portuguese patients about FP and their reproductive future and to study the profiles of patients who decide to preserve their fertility and those who decide not to preserve. This research would make it possible to understand the factors that influence the FP decision. Likewise, there is no research about the knowledge, practices, and attitudes of Portuguese oncologists about oncofertility. This research would be essential to help physicians to communicate fertility issues with their patients and to develop resources that are specifically developed to meet their patients' needs.

In terms of implications for clinical practice, this article highlights the importance of a prospective and multidisciplinary approach to support the reproductive decisions of young female cancer patients, who reveal high levels of satisfaction with it. In particular, the inclusion of psychologists in the teams and the communication between oncologists and specialists of reproductive medicine seem essential for this intervention. Moreover, doctors from all specialties should have knowledge and awareness of fertility issues to inform patients and to refer them to fertility centers in time to make a decision about FP before cancer treatments. Taking into account the international guidelines on oncofertility and the experience of the CPFP, all patients should be informed about the infertility risk of cancer treatments and FP options so they can have the opportunity to make a decision about their FP. Specifically in Portugal, clinical guidelines about the referral of patients to FP centers should be developed.

Acknowledgments This study is part of the *Fertility preservation in female cancer patients: Decision-making process of patients, individual adaptation after cancer treatments and practices of oncologists* research project, which is part of the Relationships, Development and Health Research Group of the R&D Cognitive and Behavioral Center for Research and Intervention of the

University of Coimbra (PEst-OE/PSI/UI0730/2014). Cláudia Melo is supported by a scholarship from the Portuguese Foundation for Science and Technology (SFRH/BD/84677/2012).

We would like to thank Teresa Woodruff, director of the Oncofertility Consortium®, for her generosity and for her vital assistance and input in discussions about several topics related to intervention with cancer patients regarding their reproductive future.

We are also grateful to all cancer patients who participated anonymously in the online survey about their level of satisfaction with their experience at the Portuguese Centre for Fertility Preservation. These opinions are very important to better understand patients' perceptions of their clinical experience and were fundamental in consolidating the model of intervention that we propose in the present publication.

Finally, we would like to thank the clinical staff of the Reproductive Medicine Department (all the doctors, the embryologists, the nurses, and the clinical secretaries) who collaborate to provide better support for these patients' needs.

References

1. American College of Obstetricians and Gynecologists Committee on Gynecologic Practice and Practice Committee. Female age-related fertility decline. Fertil Steril. 2014;101:633–4. doi:10.1016/j.fertnstert.2013.12.032.
2. American Society for Reproductive Medicine. Mature oocyte cryopreservation: a guideline. Fertil Steril. 2013;99(1):37–43. doi:10.1016/j.fertnstert.2012.09.028.
3. Ataman L, Rodrigues J, Marinho R, Caetano J, Chenin M, Alves da Motta E, Serafini P, Suzuki N, Furui T, Takae S, et al. Creating a global community of practice for oncofertility. J Glob Oncol. in press. 2015. doi:10.1200/JGO.2015.000307.
4. Balthazar U, Deal A, Fritz M, Kondapalli L, Kim J, Mersereau E. The current fertility preservation consultation model: are we adequately informing cancer patients of their options? Hum Reprod. 2012;27(8):2413–9. doi:10.1093/humrep/des188.
5. Canada A, Schover L. The psychosocial impact of interrupted childbearing in long-term female cancer survivors. Psycho-Oncology. 2012;21:134–43. doi:10.1002/pon.1875.
6. Cardonick E, Gilmandyar D, Somer R. Maternal and neonatal outcomes of dose-dense chemotherapy for breast cancer in pregnancy. Obstet Gynecol. 2012;120:1267–72. doi:10.1097/AOG.0b013e31826c32d9.
7. Cardoso F, Loibl S, Pagani O, Graziottin A, Panizza P, Martincich L, Gentilini O, Peccatori F, Fourquet A, Delaloge S, Marotti L, Penault-Llorca F, Kotti-Kitromilidou AM, Rodger A, Harbeck N. The European Society of Breast Cancer Specialists recommendations for the management of young women with breast cancer. Eur J Cancer. 2012;48:3355–77. doi:10.1016/j.ejca.2012.10.004.
8. Carter J, Rowland K, Chi D, Brown C, Abu-Rustum N, Castiel M, Barakat R. Gynecologic cancer treatment and the impact of cancer-related infertility. Gynecol Oncol. 2005;97:90–5. doi:10.1016/j.ygyno.2004.12.019.
9. Carter J, Chi D, Brown C, Abu-Rustum N, Sonoda Y, Aghajanian C, Levine DA, Baser RE, Raviv L, Barakat R. Cancer-related infertility in survivorship. Int J Gynecol Cancer. 2010;20:2–8. doi:10.1111/IGC.0b013e3181bf7d3f.
10. Chang H, Suh C. Fertility preservation for women with malignancies: current developments of cryopreservation. J Gynecol Oncol. 2008;19(2):99–107. doi:10.3802/jgo.2008.19.2.99.
11. Charles C, Gafni A, Whelan T. Decision-making in the physician-patient encounter: revisiting the shared treatment decision-making model. Soc Sci Med. 1999;49:651–61.
12. Clinical Oncological Society of Australia. Fertility preservation for AYAs diagnosed with cancer: guidance for health professionals. In: Cancer council Australia. 2012. Retrieved from http://wiki.cancer.org.au/.
13. Cobo A, Serra V, Garrido N, Olmo I, Pellicer A, Remohí J. Obstetric and perinatal outcome of babies born from vitrified oocytes. Fertil Steril. 2014;102:1006–15. doi:10.1016/j.fertnstert.2014.06.019.

14. De Angelis R, Sant M, Coleman M, Francisci S, Baili P, Pierannunzio D, Trama A, Visser O, Brenner H, Ardanaz E, Bielska-Lasota M, Engholm G, Nennecke A, Siesling S, Berrino F, Capocaccia R. Cancer survival in Europe 1999–2007 by country and age: results of EUROCARE-5 – a population-based study. Lancet Oncol. 2014;15:23–34. doi:10.1016/S1470-2045(13)70546-1.

15. Direção Geral de Saúde – Programa Nacional para as Doenças Oncológicas. Recomendações nacionais para diagnóstico e tratamento do cancro da mama. In: Direção Geral de Saúde. 2009. Retrieved from http://www.dgs.pt.

16. Direção Geral de Saúde – Programa Nacional para as Doenças Oncológicas. Doenças oncológicas em números 2014. In: Direção Geral de Saúde. 2014. Retrieved from http://www.dgs.pt.

17. Donnez J, Dolmans M. Transplantation of ovarian tissue. Best Pract Res Clin Obstet Gynaecol. 2014;28(8):1188–97. doi:10.1016/j.bpobgyn.2014.09.003.

18. Dow K. Having children after cancer. Cancer Pract. 1994;2(6):407–13.

19. Ferraretti A, Goossens V, Kupka M, Bhattacharya S, Mouzon J, Castilla J, Erb K, Korsak V, Andersen A. Assisted reproductive technology in Europe, 2009: results generated from European registers by ESHRE. Hum Reprod. 2013;28(9):2318–31. doi:10.1093/humrep/det278.

20. Garvelink M, Ter Kuile M, Bakker R, Geense W, Jenninga E, Louwé L, Hilders CG, Stiggelbout A. Women's experiences with information provision and deciding about fertility preservation in the Netherlands: 'Satisfaction in general, but unmet needs'. Health Expect. 2013. doi:10.1111/hex.12068.

21. Gonçalves V, Sehovic I, Quinn G. Childbearing attitudes and decisions of young breast cancer survivors: a systematic review. Hum Reprod Update. 2013;20(2):279–92. doi:10.1093/humupd/dmt039.

22. Hewitt M, Greenfield S, Stovall E. Committee on cancer survivorship: from cancer patient to cancer survivor. Washington, DC: The National Academies Press; 2006. URL: http://www.nap.edu/catalog/11468/from-cancer-patient-to-cancer-survivor-lost-in-transition.

23. Hickey M, Peate M, Saunders C, Friedlander M. Breast cancer in young women and its impact on reproductive function. Hum Reprod Update. 2009;15(3):323–39. doi:10.1093/humupd/dmn064.

24. Kim J, Deal A, Balthazar U, Kondapalli L, Gracia C, Mersereau J. Fertility preservation consultation for women with cancer: are we helping patients make high-quality decisions? Reprod Biomed Online. 2013;27(1):96–103. doi:10.1016/j.rbmo.2013.03.004.

25. Lee S, Schover L, Partridge A, Patrizio P, Wallace W, Hagerty K, Beck L, Brennan L, Oktay K. American Society of Clinical Oncology recommendations on fertility preservation in cancer patients. J Clin Oncol. 2006;24(18):2917–31. doi:10.1200/JCO.2006.06.5888.

26. Letourneau J, Ebbel E, Katz P, Katz A, Ai W, Chien A, Melisko ME, Cedars MI, Rosen M. Pretreatment fertility counseling and fertility preservation improve quality of life in reproductive age women with cancer. Cancer. 2012;118(6):1710–17. doi:10.1002/cncr.26459.

27. Loren A, Mangu P, Beck L, Brennan L, Magdalinski A, Partridge A, Quinn G, Wallace WH, Oktay K. Fertility preservation for patients with cancer: American Society of Clinical Oncology clinical practice guideline update. J Clin Oncol. 2013;31:1–12. doi:10.1200./jco.2013.49.2678.

28. Loscalzo M, Clark K. The psychosocial context of cancer-related infertility. In: Woodruff T, Snyder K, editors. Oncofertility: fertility preservation for cancer survivors. New York: Springer; 2007. p. 180–90.

29. Makin G, Meyer S. Oncology. In: McIntosh N, Helms P, Smyth R, Logan S, editors. Forfar and Arneil's textbook of pediatrics. New York: Churchill Livingstone; 2008. p. 991–1038.

30. McCabe M, Bhatia S, Orffinger K, Reamn G, Tyne C, Woolins D, Hudson M. American Society of Clinical Oncology Statement: achieving high-quality cancer survivorship care. J Clin Oncol. 2013;31(5):631–40. doi:10.1200/JCO.2012.46.6854.

31. Mersereau J, Goodman L, Deal A, Gorman J, Whitcomb B, Su H. To preserve or not to preserve: how difficult is the decision about fertility preservation? Cancer. 2013;119:4044–50. doi:10.1002/cncr.28317.

32. Pagani O, Partridge A, Korde L, Badve S, Bartlett J, Albain K, Gelber R, Goldhirsch A. Pregnancy after breast cancer: if you wish, ma'am. Breast Cancer Res Treat. 2011;129:309–17. doi:10.1007/s10549-011-1643-7.

33. Peate M, Meiser B, Friedlander M, Zorbas H, Rovelli S, Sansom-Daly U, Sangster J, Hadzi-Pavlovic D, Hickey M. Decision-making preferences, and treatment intentions in young women with breast cancer: an Australian fertility decision aid collaborative group study. J Clin Oncol. 2011;29(13):1670–77. doi:10.1200/JCO.2010.31.2462.

34. Peate M, Meiser B, Cheah B, Saunders C, Butow P, Thewes B, Hart R, Phillips KA, Hickey M, Friedlander M. Making hard choices easier: a prospective, multicentre study to assess the efficacy of a fertility-related decision aid in young women with early-stage breast cancer. Brit J Cancer. 2012;106:1053–61. doi:10.1038/bjc.2012.61.

35. Peccatori F, Azim H, Orecchia R, Hoekstra H, Pavlidis N, Kesic V, Pentheroudakis G. Cancer, pregnancy and fertility: ESMO clinical practice guidelines for diagnosis, treatment and follow-up. Ann Oncol. 2013;24(Suppl 6):vi160–70. doi:10.1093/annonc/mdt199.

36. Peddie V, Porter M, Barbour R, Culligan D, MacDonald G, King D, Horn J, Bhattacharya S. Factors affecting decision making about fertility preservation after cancer diagnosis: a qualitative study. BJOG. 2012;119:1049–57. doi:10.1111/j.1471-0528.2012.03368.x.

37. Perz J, Ussher J, Gilbert E. Loss, uncertainty, or acceptance: subjective experience of changes to fertility after breast cancer. Eur J Cancer Care. 2014;23(4):514–22. doi:10.1111/ecc.12165.

38. Royal College of Physicians, The Royal College of Radiologists, Royal College of Obstetricians and Gyneacologists. The effects of cancer treatment on reproductive functions: guidance on management. Report of a Working Party. London: RCP; 2007.

39. Schmidt L, Sobotka T, Benzten J, Andersen A. Demographic and medical consequences of the postponement of parenthood. Hum Reprod Update. 2012;18(1):28–43. doi:10.1093/humupd/dmr040.

40. Schover L. Psychological aspects of infertility and decisions about reproduction in young cancer survivors: a review. Med Pediatr Oncol. 1999;33:53–9.

41. Schover L, Rybicki L, Martin B, Bringelsen K. Having children after cancer: a pilot survey of survivors' attitudes and experiences. Cancer. 1999;86:697–709.

42. Stacey D, Légaré F, Col N, Bennett C, Barry M, Eden K, Holmes-Rovner M, Llewellyn-Thomas H, Lyddiatt A, Thomson R, Trevena L, Wu J. Decision aids for people facing health treatment or screening decisions. Cochrane Database Syst Rev. 2014;1. doi:10.1002/14651858. CD001431.pub4.

43. Surbone A. Counseling young cancer patients about reproductive issues. In: Surbone A, Peccatori F, Pavlidis N, editors. Cancer and pregnancy. New York: Springer; 2008. p. 237–45.

44. Woodruff T. The Oncofertility Consortium: addressing fertility in young people with cancer. Nat Rev Clin Oncol. 2010;7(8):466–75. doi:10.1038/nrclinonc.2010.81.

45. World Health Organization. Where are the patients in decision-making about their own care? WHO Press; 2008. Available from: http://www.who.int/management/general/decisionmaking/WhereArePatientsinDecisionMaking.pdf

46. World Health Organization. World cancer report 2014. Lyon: WHO Press; 2014.

47. Yee S, Abrol K, McDonald M, Tonelli M, Liu K. Addressing oncofertility needs: views of female cancer patients in fertility preservation. J Psychosoc Oncol. 2012;30(3):331–46. doi:10.1080/07347332.2012.664257.

48. Zanagnolo V, Sartori E, Trussardi E, Pasinetti B, Maggino T. Preservation of ovarian function, reproductive ability and emotional attitudes in patients with malignant ovarian tumors. Eur J Obstet Gynaecol Reprod Biol. 2005;123(2):235–43.

Chapter 20
Fertility Preservation in Japanese Children and Adolescents with Cancer

Yoko Miyoshi and Nao Suzuki

As the survival rate of pediatric and adolescent patients with cancer has shown marked improvement, the late effects of anticancer therapy on survivors of childhood/adolescent cancer have also been recognized as a critical issue in Japan. The Long-Term Follow-Up Guidelines for Survivors of Childhood and Adolescent Cancers were prepared by pediatric oncologists and endocrinologists with the aim of improving the management of various issues. Nevertheless, avoiding subfertility after anticancer therapy is still the responsibility of the individual treating pediatric oncologists who lack adequate coordination with reproductive medicine specialists. Thus, appropriate preventive measures for possible loss of fertility are often unavailable to young cancer survivors. Young patients with cancer may not receive any information about fertility after anticancer therapy. Also, follow-up for the primary disease is discontinued in quite a few patients, so that children and adolescents who survive cancer commonly face the crucial matter of infertility in adulthood without support.

In 2012, we established the Japan Society for Fertility Preservation (JSFP) (President: Nao Suzuki, MD, PhD) in order to promote measures for oncofertility in Japan. The JSFP holds a symposium every year, with the aim of promoting multidisciplinary coordination among medical and nonmedical professionals in the field of oncofertility. The JSFP has also established an Internet website to distribute the latest information concerning oncofertility. The JSFP initially developed a network based at Gifu University for oncofertility-related medical coordination that also involved the Gifu Prefectural Government (Gifu-Patients and Fertility Specialists established by Professor Kenichiro Morishige and

Y. Miyoshi, MD
Department of Pediatrics, Osaka University Graduate School of Medicine, Osaka, Japan

N. Suzuki, MD, PhD (✉)
Department of Obstetrics and Gynecology, St. Marianna University School of Medicine, Kawasaki, Japan
e-mail: nao@marianna-u.ac.jp

© Springer International Publishing Switzerland 2017
T.K. Woodruff, Y.C. Gosiengfiao (eds.), *Pediatric and Adolescent Oncofertility*,
DOI 10.1007/978-3-319-32973-4_20

Associate Professor Tatsuro Furui: GPOFs). Subsequently, regional oncofertility medical service coordination networks are being developed in many regions around Japan based on GPOFs, in order to provide coordinated and integrated medical care for oncofertility within a particular region. At a December 2014 meeting of the Cancer Control Promotion Council, which is the top Japanese organization for cancer control policies and programs, Dr. Suzuki provided a Statement of Opinion seeking national programs for fertility preservation in pediatric and adolescent patients with cancer. In May 2015, Dr. Suzuki and colleagues submitted a Letter of Request to Minister Shiozaki (the Minister of Health, Labour and Welfare) seeking the establishment of a clinical practice coordination system that will allow pediatric and adolescent patients with cancer to preserve the potential for future pregnancy and childbirth. Specifically, we made the following two suggestions: (1) the government should urgently launch projects for preservation of the reproductive function of young cancer patients and for the alleviation of physical and psychological distress due to loss of fertility, and (2) the government should take measures to establish a regional medical collaboration system among local governments, key hospitals, and community clinics that provides sustainable oncofertility services within each region.

In collaboration with Dr. Suzuki and utilizing a 2014 Scientific Research Grant from the Ministry of Health, Labour and Welfare, Dr. Miyoshi (a pediatric endocrinologist and a member of JSFP) organized a working panel to compile evidence about the fertility of long-term survivors who developed cancer during childhood or adolescence and to develop a reproductive medicine network. This project has attracted the attention of the central government and has received a research grant from the Ministry of Health, Labour and Welfare as a cancer control promotion project. The activities of this project gained considerable appreciation in the first year. Key hospitals involved in the fields of pediatric oncology, pediatric endocrinology, child health and development, and reproductive medicine are participating in this project, and a medical practice team has been set up that consists of pediatric oncologists, pediatric endocrinologists, gynecologists, obstetricians, urologists, reproductive medicine specialists, medical oncologists, and psychologists. We have conducted a questionnaire survey targeting doctors who were involved in the care of pediatric/young adult patients with cancer and survivors of cancer during childhood or adolescence so that current issues could be determined. The working panel has also been involved in other activities, including a field survey of pregnancy and childbirth and a cohort study on gonadal function and fertility in female survivors of pediatric gynecologic cancer, as well as providing a consulting desk for patients and other clinical improvements and performing a basic study to establish a method for cryopreservation of immature testicular tissue. Furthermore, the working panel collaborated with the JSFP to host the "2015 Symposium on Cancer and Reproduction: Discussion of Childhood Cancer and Fertility" in February 2015 in Osaka. This symposium provided the first opportunity for information exchange among Japanese doctors, nurses, psychotherapists, counselors, and patients. During the symposium, discussion focused on the latest topics, such as ovarian tissue cryopreservation, uterus transplantation, and oocyte donation.

The JSFP has prepared a booklet for young breast cancer patients that explains fertility preservation and provides guidance about medical care and reproductive medicine for patients with this cancer who want to become pregnant and give birth. We have also posted a list of medical institutions providing reproductive medicine and a list of children's hospitals where consultation about fertility preservation is possible on our website. Nevertheless, not enough has been done to support fertility preservation in pediatric cancer patients. Our questionnaire for pediatric endocrinologists revealed that fertility preservation procedures were only implemented at a very few institutions, although every institution is concerned about techniques for fertility preservation. Cryopreservation of sperm has come to be implemented for male patients at some institutions, while cryopreservation of immature testicular tissue is still experimental. Thus, it is expected that the above basic research will provide useful findings. Doctors frequently refrain from retrieving oocytes in girls with cancer, taking into the consideration physical and mental burden of the oocyte retrieval procedure on the patient. As of May 2015, ovarian tissue cryopreservation for pediatric/young adult female patients has been implemented after receiving ethics committee approval at only 1 institution. In order to implement oocyte cryopreservation for pediatric/young adult cancer patients, the following issues need to be solved: (1) the method of providing an explanation and obtaining consent from girls, (2) validation of the safety of long-term cryopreservation, (3) establishment of a system for long-term storage, (4) providing psychological support for pediatric patients as they grow, and (5) coordinating oncofertility procedures with anticancer therapy.

To achieve further progress in oncofertility in Japan, it is necessary to establish medical practice coordination systems among healthcare departments and specialists in various fields and to energetically implement educational activities. At present, the commitment to preserving the fertility of pediatric/young adult cancer patients is just beginning in Japan.

Chapter 21
Managing Fertility Preservation in Childhood Cancer Patients in Brazilian Scenario

Jhenifer Kliemchen Rodrigues, Bruno Ramalho de Carvalho, Ana Carolina Japur de Sá Rosa e Silva, Simone França Nery, Jacira Ribeiro Campos, Ricardo Mello Marinho, João Pedro Junqueira Caetano, Ricardo Marques de Azambuja, Mariângela Badalotti, Álvaro Petracco, Maurício Barbour Chehin, Joaquim Lopes, and Fernando Marcos dos Reis

---

J.K. Rodrigues (✉)
In Vitro Consultoria, Belo Horizonte, MG, Brazil

Latin America Oncofertility Network – Oncofertility Consortium, Belo Horizonte, MG, Brazil
e-mail: jhenifer.kr@invitroconsultoria.com.br

B.R. de Carvalho
Latin America Oncofertility Network – Oncofertility Consortium, Belo Horizonte, MG, Brazil

A.C.J. de Sá Rosa e Silva • J.R. Campos
Medical School of Ribeirão Preto, University of São Paulo, Ribeirao Preto, SP, Brazil

Latin America Oncofertility Network – Oncofertility Consortium, Belo Horizonte, MG, Brazil

S.F. Nery
Federal University of Minas Gerais, Belo Horizonte, MG, Brazil

R.M. Marinho • J.P.J. Caetano
Pró-Criar Medicina Reprodutiva, Belo Horizonte, MG, Brazil

Medical Sciences Faculty, Belo Horizonte, MG, Brazil

Latin America Oncofertility Network – Oncofertility Consortium, Belo Horizonte, MG, Brazil

R.M. de Azambuja • M. Badalotti • Á. Petracco
Fertilitat Centro de Medicina Reprodutiva, Porto Alegre, RS, Brazil

Latin America Oncofertility Network – Oncofertility Consortium,
Belo Horizonte, MG, Brazil

M.B. Chehin
Huntington Medicina Reprodutiva, Sao Paulo, SP, Brazil

Latin America Oncofertility Network – Oncofertility Consortium, Belo Horizonte, MG, Brazil

J. Lopes
Cenafert, Salvador, BA, Brazil

Latin America Oncofertility Network – Oncofertility Consortium, Belo Horizonte, MG, Brazil

F.M. dos Reis
Federal University of Minas Gerais, Belo Horizonte, MG, Brazil

Latin America Oncofertility Network – Oncofertility Consortium, Belo Horizonte, MG, Brazil

© Springer International Publishing Switzerland 2017
T.K. Woodruff, Y.C. Gosiengfiao (eds.), *Pediatric and Adolescent Oncofertility*,
DOI 10.1007/978-3-319-32973-4_21

Introduction

The preservation of fertility in young and adolescent population is a matter of great relevance at the present time. For many young children, there are many psychological stress factors that affect them in the context of their lives at the time of illness, and the risk of losing their fertility is a major concern. The ability to preserve fertility can contribute positively to the emotional aspects of the disease and its treatment. In adulthood, reproductive capacity is for most individuals, one of the main determinants of their quality of life [5, 15].

In United States of America, the incidence of cancer up to 14 years of age is estimated at about 17 cases per 100,000 boys and 15 cases per 100,000 girls every year [21]. According to Brazilian National Cancer Institute data, between 1983 and 2005, 54.5 % of childhood cancers occurred in males and 45.5 % in females in Brazil [3].

Despite this increase in childhood cancer diagnosis, there has been a significant increase in posttreatment survival. However, while childhood and adolescent cancer therapies improve long-term survival, such treatments may lead to abnormal pubertal development infertility and gonadal failure. It is essential that clinicians are aware of the available options for gamete cryopreservation whether they are well established or experimental.

Dealing with fertility preservation upon diagnosis of cancer is challenging for a young adult patient. This issue is even more complex for pediatric patients where decision-making generally falls to the parents, but high cancer survival rates increase the possibility of survivors needing to confront infertility later in life.

The scope of potential fertility issues for pediatric cancer patients is difficult to predict. Both genders are susceptible to negative impact on the hormone production and gonads. These effects can be reversible or permanent. Many pediatric clinicians are aware that radiation and chemotherapy can affect fertility, but few of them are aware of gender differences in toxicity, and few consult with specialists regarding fertility preservation [17].

The present chapter summarizes the Brazilian scenario of cancer childhood oncofertility.

Fertility Preservation for Cancer Patients

In a scenario where cancer mortality falls more dramatically than its incidence, another picture is built up where women at the height of their careers, or without a stable relationship, increasingly choose to postpone motherhood. In the United States of America, statistics on births point to the downward trend of 1–2 % per year among women aged 20–29 and an upward trend to 3 % in their 30s, with births among women aged 35–39 reaching nearly 50 births/1,000 individuals in 2013 (the highest rate in the country since 1963) [19]. Similarly, in Brazil, higher live births rates are observed among women aged 30–39 years, and there is a clear fall of the numbers among younger women [24].

Looking at the two situations and understanding that the incidence of many cancers increases with increasing age, it is assumed that there will be more cancer diagnoses in women who did not have children or finished their offsprings, and consequently there will be more cancer survivors interested in future procreation.

Although still few cases, there is an observed increase in cases over time. The number of referrals has increased, already very close number of referrals to the sum of all referrals made in previous years in some of the big centers of Reproductive Medicine in Brazil. This is likely due to women's increased access to information on the possibility of preserving their gametes before the antineoplastic treatment, as well as repeat diffusion actions of oncofertility among clinical oncologists, oncology surgeons, gynecologists, urologists, mastologists, and other health professionals.

The best way to raise oncologist's awareness about the importance of discussing oncofertility should begin with the identification of those patients who would potentially benefit fertility preservation strategies before chemotherapy or radiation therapy. Considering an estimated 10% of female cancer cases occur before the age of 45, with a survival rate of about 85% [21], and passing the yearly statistics of cancer around the world [4, 12, 13, 21], we could share with the oncologists the deduction that oncofertility strategies could benefit more than 15,000 women in Brazil, 66,000 women in the United States of America, 160,000 women in Europe, and 830,000 women worldwide every year.

As recently suggested by the founder of the Global Oncofertility Consortium, Teresa Woodruff [37], there is a great expectation that, in a near future, oncofertility assumes the role of modifying culture on cancer treatment, bringing innovation while opening the world's eyes to procreation perspective as a quality of life factor for cancer survivors.

Childhood Cancer and Fertility Preservation

In Brazil, cancer is already the leading cause of death (7% of total) due to illness among children and adolescents from 1 to 19 years old, for all regions. It is estimated that approximately 12,600 new cases of cancer occur in children and adolescents in Brazil each year in 2016 and 2017. The Southeast and Northeast regions will present the highest number of new cases, 6,050 and 2,750, respectively, followed by the South 1,320), Midwest (1,270) and North (1,210) [4].

In Brazil, the most common types of cancer in children are carcinomas and other epithelial malignancies (28%), leukemia (15%), bone tumors (14%), lymphoma and other reticuloendothelial tumors (10%), soft tissue sarcomas (7%), renal tumors (6%), central nervous system and miscellaneous intracranial tumors, and intraspinal neoplasms (6%) [3].

Between 2005 and 2009, the overall incidence of cancer in children aged under 14 increased about 0.5% per year, a consistent trend in the country since mid 1970s. However, the mortality rate for childhood cancer has decreased by more than a half over the past three decades, from 4.9 per 100,000 in 1975 to 2.1 per 100,000 individuals in 2009 [35]. The good results of anticancer treatments in children can also be translated by mean cumulative survival rate in 5 years, which now exceeds 80 % [3, 21]. Thousands of girls and adolescents with cancer receive successful anticancer treatments annually, and then we may already have at least one childhood or adolescence cancer survivor in each group of 570 adults in reproductive age [20].

Ovarian cortex cryopreservation is the fertility preservation strategy of greater relevance in oncological patients in childhood. Sixty births have already been well documented in literature [11], at orthotopic or heterotopic sites, reinforcing the near inclusion of this strategy in the routine of specialized services in reproductive medicine around the world. Although it is still considered experimental [23], the advantage of allowing the preservation of thousands of viable primordial follicles could be held in the absence of the hypothalamic-pituitary-ovarian axis activation [6, 27], and it should be applied to specific groups of patients, such as prepubertal girls [7, 28].

The major restriction to the use of ovarian cryopreservation is the presumed risk of recurrence of cancer, originated from metastasis in ovarian tissue reused. Although there are no reports in humans, this hypothesis should be highlighted for the patient and their caregivers and is fundamental to clarify that the risks may vary according to the type of tumor, as not all tumors are likely to develop metastatic foci in the ovaries [29, 36]. The literature reports efforts to develop efficient techniques for isolation of primordial, primary and secondary follicles, and their maturation in vitro. There are only reports of births after cultivation of secondary follicles in mice [40], but studies with primate and human follicles have shown promising results [2, 30, 38, 39, 41].

Depending on the age and on the stage of pubertal development, different fertility preservation options can be offered; ovarian tissue cryopreservation is always an option, especially if ovarian failure is highly probable. For those patients in a postpubertal stage oocyte cryopreservation, applying a random start ovulation induction can also be offered. In general, postpubertal girls and their parents are more likely to agree with fertility preservation procedures; younger kids and their parents are not usually receptive to fertility matters and frequently refuse to accept, especially when laparoscopy is indicated for ovarian biopsy.

The precocity of referral also influences the procedures that are offered. For ovulation induction, the patients need nearly 9–12 days until retrieval of mature oocytes, and sometimes, depending on ovarian response, more than one retrieval is necessary. In case ovarian tissue cryopreservation is indicated in combination with oocyte cryopreservation, the ideal is to proceed ovarian biopsy and then ovulation induction and oocyte pick up, because the punctures and the hematomas make the tissue unfeasible for storage. In cases of precondition chemotherapy before bone marrow transplantation (BMT) in none oncological patients, when we have 2 months or more available, oocyte pickup may be done before ovarian biopsy without prejudice of the tissue.

An important and delicate issue is the process of obtaining informed consent for fertility preservation in children and incapable. That is because the subject is a difficult context in the age group or the lack of awareness for such a decision. Still, because the techniques considered most appropriate for sexually immature individuals, they are considered experimental in younger populations [26], as discussed in the previous paragraphs.

In such cases, parents or legal guardians often make the decision on behalf of the patient, assisted by a multidisciplinary team. It is observed commonly the exclusion of patient of decisions to be made around the antineoplastic treatment. The reasons for that are exclusive focus on healing, without valuing the quality of life after survival; the discomfort of parents in dealing with issues related to sexual life of the child as an adult; and the desire to protect children and adolescents against anxiety generated by sensitive issues such as sexuality and procreation [18]. However, it should be noted that the American Academy of Pediatrics recommends assistants to give the child over the age of 7 the opportunity to discuss the issue and even refuse to preserve fertility, even if it is a desire of parents [1, 32].

Experience of Brazilian Oncofertility Consortium Centers Members

Brazil is a country of an emerging economy that has a Public Health System which, although still needs improvements in many ways, offers a comprehensive care to any patient with cancer. At the present, there are 276 hospitals enabled in cancer treatment. All states have at least one hospital enabled in oncology, where the cancer patient can find medical access to more complex surgeries and treatments.

However, in fertility preservation in Brazil, the procedure's cost is an important obstacle. In the Brazilian Public Health System, infertility, in general, is not considered as a disease; thus, the patient has to pay for the ovulation induction drugs and for the procedure itself. There are few centers that offer assisted reproduction techniques for free.

The practice of fertility preservation for cancer patients it is still being built even in the private clinics. Not many doctors are aware of the options for gametes preservation, and few know that the procedure should be done before the start of the treatment. Fertility preservation is generally more discussed in more developed regions where the hospitals and universities are aware of the concept of oncofertility.

Oncofertility has been increasingly discussed in Brazil through meeting events related to cancer and fertility, and information has been widespread also through the Internet. The eight current center members of the Brazilian Oncofertility Consortium have contributed to many discussions, participation, and promotion of events on the topic of oncofertility and fertility preservation.

At Pró-Criar Medicina Reprodutiva, located in Belo Horizonte, State of Minas Gerais, they have received an increasing number of young men and women with cancer diagnosis for discussion of fertility preservation. Most of them choose to cryopreserve oocytes and sperm, and a reduced number makes the choice to cryopreserve ovarian tissue. The clinic have provided this technique as an experimental treatment, including children and adolescents, with no cost, as a research project, in partnership with the Faculty of Medical Sciences of Minas Gerais, approved by a Research Ethics Committee. This increase in number of patients looking for gamete preservation has not happened with children or adolescents in pre- or peripubertal periods. The clinic has seen patients who have undergone treatment for cancer, chemo- and radiation therapy, and even marrow transplant, whose parents did not have the opportunity to discuss alternatives to preserve fertility before the start of treatment. Rare cases received information before the cancer treatment. In only one peripubertal case was held freezing of ovarian tissue samples. In a few other cases, the clinic was approached by oncologists, but the children had no medical condition for a laparoscopy. The clinic aims to assist the cancer patient in up to 24 h for a consultation and, in case of male, for also a sperm banking.

Genesis – Centro de Assistência em Reprodução Humana, located in Brasília, Federal District, had its first two ovarian stimulation cycles for cryopreservation of oocytes of oncologic patients in 2010. Since then, there were eight cases between 2012 and 2014 and seven cases until July 2015. Of the 17 performed cycles, one breast cancer patient developed the empty follicle syndrome and therefore did not cryopreserve oocytes. Considering the others, an average of 11.6 metaphase II oocytes has been cryopreserved for each women (nonpublished data).

Huntington Medicina Reprodutiva, located in São Paulo, State of São Paulo, has been conducting fertility preservation in cancer patients for over 10 years, initially with the freezing of embryos and sperm. The freezing of oocytes started 8 years ago, and they are currently introducing in the routine the freezing of ovarian tissue. They understand that preserving gametes for pre pubescent girls can be offered, respecting the ethical and medical dilemmas in question. It was tried in 2014 to cryopreserve ovarian tissue unsuccessfully in two girls aged 8 and 10 years with diagnostic of bilateral borderline ovarian tumor, but during surgery, there was full commitment of the ovaries, and it was not possible to preserve the tissue. The clinic created a fast and integrated system of care where any cancer patient can be attended to by a doctor within 48 h and can start any kind of procedure in this same time. Also, the entire team is trained to assist this type of patient. The nurses receive special training and do partly the role of patient navigator, facilitating multidisciplinary care, which contributes to more humane and comprehensive care to the patient.

Fertilitat Centro de Medicina Reprodutiva, located in Porto Alegre, State of Rio Grande do Sul, regularly freeze semen samples for male young patients who need go under radio- or chemotherapy, before the start of the treatment. For women, the clinic offers the cryopreservation of mature oocytes and ovarian tissue. So far, no male or female child has had gamete samples cryopreserved because the clinic was not sought for that yet. The clinic also has no experience with fertility preservation in children. The youngest patient that has frozen oocytes was 19 and did the procedure because she was a bearer of Turner syndrome. The youngest female cancer patient was 23 and had ovarian cancer, and the younger boy who has frozen semen sample was 14 and had testicular tumor.

Cenafert – Centro de Medicina Reprodutiva, located in Salvador, State of Bahia, also does not have experience in cryopreserving gametes for child cancer patients. They work exclusively with adults. A recent case was a patient with lymphoma who cryopreserved embryos despite the clinic's suggestion to the couple to cryopreserve oocytes. She also used the agonist of GnRH. After chemotherapy, she maintained a good ovarian reserve and got pregnant spontaneously.

Ribeirão Preto Medical School/University of São Paulo, located in Ribeirão Preto, State of São Paulo, work with the Public Health System. The Clinical Hospital of Ribeirão Preto Medical School is one of the centers where the patient does not need to pay for fertility treatment; however, the patient must cover the cost of medication. Although fertility preservation options are all available for the oncological patients, adults and children, not every patient can afford it.

At the beginning of this fertility preservation program, the oncopediatric doctors have more often referred the children for fertility preservation counseling. The Fertility Preservation Program at Ribeirão Preto Medical School for young children and adolescents is the same offered for adults. But, one of the more important factor associated to ovarian failure after oncologic treatment is age, in a protective manner; thus, these patients are more likely to maintain their natural fertility after chemotherapy. Also, ovarian biopsy for cryopreservation may have a negative impact in ovarian reserve, besides the experimental character of this technique. So it is very important to individually evaluate a child or an adolescent for fertility preservation; all these points should be put to stakeholders, in order to guide their decision.

The Assisted Reproduction Laboratory of the Federal University of Minas Gerais offers semen cryopreservation for both adult and young people who already ejaculate and can collect the material, regardless of age (with the informed consent of the person and when under 18, also of a legal guardian). If semen collection is not possible, sperm can be obtained from urine (in cases of retrograde ejaculation) or through the epididymis punching and/or testicular biopsy. The urology service inside the hospital is their partner in this mission, and they are working to extend this partnership to other oncology, hematology, and pediatrics departments. The service also offers embryo and mature oocyte cryopreservation for woman.

All the centers feel there is a lack of information for oncologists about available fertility preservation techniques, even those still considered experimental. Also it is difficult for these professionals to discuss this issue in a very difficult time for the family. The centers' members of the Brazilian Oncofertility Consortium have been working together to change this reality, through the dissemination of updated information to physicians of various specialties, other health professionals, and laypeople giving lectures at conferences and courses, radio interviews, newspaper, and television and most recently publishing the book in Portuguese *Fertility Preservation: a new frontier in Reproductive Medicine and Oncology* (Preservação da Fertilidade: Uma nova fronteira em Medicina Reprodutiva e Oncologia) with the support of Oncofertility Consortium.

Conclusion

Preservation of fertility in prepubertal children is not yet a reality of clinical practice in Brazil. The demand of the youth population is still very small in the whole country. Sometimes the service is searched directly by the family, without medical referral, for clarification on fertility preservation, which demonstrates an understanding and awareness of the patient/family. However, this knowledge is not universal and is usually vague and sometimes misleading and obtained through nonscientific media. Moreover, in many cases the maintenance of fertility is not even considered for the disease that often represents the risk of death. The family concern is generally the cure. It is a role of the physician to address this issue with the patient and his family at the right time, whenever possible, before the reproductive capacity commitment.

Not all doctors guide their patients to seek fertility preservation services despite the recommendations of the American Society of Clinical Oncology. What could be the explanations for this fact? Not being sufficiently sensitized to the issue of fertility preservation in this group of patients? Why not be part of their routine? Or simply by not remembering this possibility in due course? Perhaps the ethical issues related to the preservation of fertility in underage individuals by the greater complexity may present as a limiting factor for some professionals. The difficulties are not only ethical and social but also technical, especially the difficulty in indicating invasive and experimental procedure for a child.

Doctors should be encouraged to work in promoting quality of life issues with their patients throughout the diagnostic and therapeutic process. Among the numerous actions involving this purpose, one of them should be the approach to fertility preservation possibility with all patients at risk of their commitment, wherever this is possible and viable option [5, 14, 31].

The medical and scientific communities are aware and dedicated to the study of solutions to this problem. The literature up to the present time presents some results on non-gonadotoxic treatments (improvements in some protocols such as chemotherapy for acute lymphoblastic leukemia without cyclophosphamide and other alkylating agents), gonadal hormone protection (still experimental), germ cell transplantation (may be an option in the future), xenograft testicular tissue (various strategies unsuccessfully), autograft germ cell (successfully study in primates), autograft of testicular tissue (underdevelopment in humans, including cancer patients at high risk of infertility, but seems to be a promising option especially for noncancer patients), in vitro maturation of germ cells and follicles (possible option for the future showing already promising results), in vitro differentiation of embryonic stem cells (spermatogenesis in vitro has been demonstrated and can be an option for the future, especially for people with the syndrome of "Klinefelter" and "Sertoli cell only"), and immature testis culture in three-dimensional system (success differentiation to the spermatid stage in mice). In short, so far the most promising option for fertility preservation in prepubertal boys on stage seems to be the cryopreservation of testicular tissue obtained by testicular biopsy ("testicular tissue banking") and for girls the option of ovarian tissue cryopreservation. However, this is still an experimental method, since the cryopreserved testis tissue transplantation techniques have not been established in human and transplantation techniques of ovary still considered experimental. Both require more studies to be implemented in clinical routine. One of the ethical questions related to these cases would be: can an experimental technique that has potential benefits and possible risks be offered to minors? This and many other questions are yet to be answered. What are the clinical indications and the ideal time to perform testicular and ovary biopsies? What are the best strategies to monitor contamination by malignant cells? What are the best cryopreservation protocols for differentiation of male and female germ cells in vitro? What are the best strategies and culture conditions for human spermatogenesis and folliculogenesis in vitro [5, 8, 16, 22, 34]?

Fertility preservation options will only be offered to patients if the knowledge of oncology providers leads them to appropriately identify patients at risk and if they have appropriate resources to support their patients in fertility preservation decision-making.

Optimal care of pediatric cancer patients undergoing gonadotoxic therapy should include enrollment in available clinical trials that will continue to refine knowledge of the effects of therapy on fertility for both male and female patients. Patients and families need information at diagnosis regarding the potential impact of therapy on fertility as well as referral to appropriate specialists for fertility preservation when desired. Studies and resources that allow potentially fertility-sparing interventions such as ovarian cryopreservation will not only need to be expanded, but adequate education and support for oncology providers who screen for patients at risk will be key. For patients that did not undergo fertility-sparing procedures prior to treatment, careful monitoring of reproductive function is warranted, and current technologies will still allow many of those patients to parent their own biological children.

At this time, it seems there are more issues and questions than answers. But we believe that in the near future, effective and safe strategies to benefit children who are in fertility impairment risk will be implemented. And this must be one of the public health service targets in our country.

References

1. American Academy of Pediatrics, Committee on Bioethics. Informed consent, parental permission, and assent in pediatric practice. Pediatrics. 1995;95:314–17.
2. Amorim CA, Van Langendonckt A, David A, Dolmans MM, Donnez J. Survival of human preantral follicles after cryopreservation of ovarian tissue, follicular isolation and in vitro culture in a calcium alginate matrix. Hum Reprod. 2009;24:92–9.
3. Brasil. Instituto Nacional de Câncer. Coordenação de Prevenção e Vigilância de Câncer. Câncer da criança e adolescente no Brasil: dados dos registros de base populacional e de mortalidade. / Instituto Nacional de Câncer. Rio de Janeiro: INCA; 2008.
4. Brasil. Ministério da Saúde. Instituto Nacional de Câncer José de Alencar Gomes da Silva (INCA) [Internet]. Estimativa 2014: incidência de câncer no Brasil. Rio de Janeiro: INCA; 2014. http://www2.inca.gov.br/wps/wcm/connect/inca/portal/home. Acesso em 30 de abril de 2015.

5. Camargos AF, et al. Anticoncepção, endocrinologia e infertilidade: soluções para as questões da ciclicidade feminina. Belo Horizonte: Coopmed; 2011. p. 941–7.

6. Campos JR, Rosa-e-Silva JC, Carvalho BR, Vireque AA, Silva-de-Sá MF, Rosa-e-Silva AC. Cryopreservation time does not decrease follicular viability in ovarian tissue frozen for fertility preservation. Clinics (Sao Paulo). 2011;66:2093–7.

7. Carvalho BR, Rodrigues JK, Campos JR, Silva AA, Marinho RM, Rosa e Silva ACJS. Strategies to preserve the reproductive future of women after cancer. JBRA Assist Reprod. 2014;18(1):16–23.

8. Di Pietro ML, Teleman AA. Cryopreservation of testicular tissue in pediatrics: practical and ethical issues. J Matern Fetal Neonatal Med. 2013;26(15):1524–7.

9. Donnez J, Dalmans MM, Demylle D, Jadoul P, Pirard C, Squifflet J, Martinez-Madrid B, Van Langendonckt A. Livebirth after orthotopic transplantation of cryopreserved ovarian tissue. Lancet. 2004;364:1405–10.

10. Donnez J, Dolmans MM, Pellicer A, Diaz-Garcia C, Sanchez Serrano M, Schmidt KT, Ernst E, Luyckx V, Andersen CY. Restoration of ovarian activity and pregnancy after transplantation of cryopreserved ovarian tissue: a review of 60 cases of reimplantation. Fertil Steril. 2013;99(6):1503–13.

11. Donnez J, Dolmans MM. Ovarian cortex transplantation: 60 reported live births brings the success and worldwide expansion of the technique towards routine clinical practice. J Assist Reprod Genet. 2015;32(8):1167–70.

12. Ferlay J, Shin H, Bray F, Forman D, Mathers C, Parkin DM. Estimates of worldwide burden of cancer in 2008: GLOBOCAN 2008. Int J Cancer. 2010;127:2893–917.

13. Ferlay J, Steliarova-Foucher E, Lortet-Tieulent J, Rosso S, Coebergh JWW, Comber H, Forman D, Bray F. Cancer incidence and mortality patterns in Europe: estimates for 40 countries in 2012. Eur J Cancer. 2013;49:1374–403.

14. Fernbach A, Lockart B, Armus CL, Bashore LM, Levine J, Kroon L, Sylvain G, Rodgers C. Evidence-based recommendations for fertility preservation options for inclusion in treatment protocols for pediatric and adolescent patients diagnosed with cancer. J Pediatr Oncol Nurs. 2014;31(4):211–22.

15. García A, Herrero MB, Holzer H, Tulandi T, Chan P. Assisted reproductive outcomes of male cancer survivors. J Cancer Surviv. 2015;9:208–14.

16. Goossens E, Tournaye H. Male fertility preservation, where are we in 2014? Ann Endocrinol. 2014;75:115–7.

17. Goodwin T, Oosterhuis BE, Kiernan M, et al. Attitudes and practices of pediatric oncology providers regarding fertility issues. Pediatr Blood Cancer. 2007;48:80–5. In: Woodruff TK, Snyder KA. Oncofertility: fertility preservation for cancer survivors. Springer; 2007.

18. Gracia CR, Gracia JJE, Chen S. Ethical dilemmas in oncofertility: an exploration of three clinical scenarios. Cancer Treat Res. 2010;156:195–208.

19. Hamilton BE, Martin JA, Osterman MJK, Curtin SC. Births: preliminary data for 2013. Natl Vital Stat Rep. 2014;63(2). http://www.cdc.gov/nchs/data/nvsr/nvsr63/nvsr63_02.pdf.

20. Henderson TO, Friedman DL, Meadows AT. Childhood cancer survivors: transition to adult-focused risk-based care. Pediatrics. 2010;126:129–36.

21. Howlader N, Noone AM, Krapcho M, Garshell J, Miller D, Altekruse SF, Kosary CL, Yu M, Ruhl J, Tatalovich Z, Mariotto A, Lewis DR, Chen HS, Feuer EJ, Cronin KA, editors. SEER Cancer Statistics Review, 1975–2012, National Cancer Institute. Bethesda. http://seer.cancer.gov/csr/1975_2012/. Acesso em 15 de setembro de 2015.

22. Jahnukainen K, Stukenborg J-B. Present and future prospects of male fertility preservation for children and adolescents. J Clin Endocrinol Metab. 2012;97(12):4341–51.

23. Loren AW, Mangu PB, Beck LN, Brennan L, Magdalinski AJ, Partridge AH, et al. Fertility Preservation for Patients With Cancer: American Society of Clinical Oncology Clinical Practice Guideline Update. J Clin Oncol. 2013;31(19):2500–10.

24. MS/SVS/DASIS/SINASC – Sistema de Informações sobre Nascidos Vivos. Disponível em: http://tabnet.datasus.gov.br/cgi/deftohtm.exe?sinasc/cnv/nvuf.def. Acesso em 15 de setembro de 2015.

25. Oehninger S. Strategies for fertility preservation in female and male cancer survivors. J Soc Gynecol Investig. 2005;12:222–31.
26. Patrizio P, Caplan AL. Ethical issues surrounding fertility preservation in cancer patients. Clin Obstet Gynecol. 2010;53:717–26.
27. Poirot CJ, Vacher-Lavenu MC, Helardot P, Guibert J, Brugières L, Jouannet P. Human ovarian tissue cryopreservation: indications and feasibility. Hum Reprod. 2002;17:1447–52.
28. Rosa e Silva ACJS, Carvalho BR, Rosa e Silva JC, Sá MFS. Ovarian function preservation after cancer. In: Moorland MT, editor. Cancer in female adolescents. 1st ed. New York: Nova Science Publishers; 2008. p. 139–53.
29. Rosendahl M, Greve T, Andersen CY. The safety of transplanting cryopreserved ovarian tissue in cancer patients: a review of the literature. J Assist Reprod Genet. 2013 Jan;30(1):11–24.
30. Rodrigues JK, Navarro PA, Zelinski MB, Stouffer RL, Xu J. Direct actions of androgens on the survival, growth and secretion of steroids and anti-Müllerian hormone by individual macaque follicles during three-dimensional culture. Hum Reprod. 2015;30(3):664–74.
31. Saias-Magnan J, et al. Préservation de la fertilité masculine. Oncologie. 2013;15:225–30.
32. Shah DK, Goldman E, Fisseha S. Medical, ethical, and legal considerations in fertility preservation. Int J Gynecol Obstet. 2011;115:11–5.
33. Shaw JM, Bowles J, Koopman P, Wood EC, Trounson AO. Fresh and cryopreserved ovarian tissue samples from donors with lymphoma transmit the cancer to graft recipients. Hum Reprod. 1996;11:1668–73.
34. Shirazi MS, Heidari B, Shirazi A, Zarnani AH, Jeddi-Tehrani M, Rahmati-Ahmadabadi M, Naderi MM, Behzadi B, Farab M, Sarvari A, Borjian-Boroujeni S, Akhondi MM. Morphologic and proliferative characteristics of goat type a spermatogonia in the presence of different sets of growth factors. J Assist Reprod Genet. 2014;31:1519–31.
35. Siegel R, Naishadham D, Jemal A. Cancer statistics, 2013. CA Cancer J Clin. 2013;63(1):11–30.
36. Sonmezer M, Shamonki M, Oktay K. Ovarian tissue cryopreservation: benefits and risks. Cell Tissue Res. 2005;322:125–32.
37. Woodruff TK. Oncofertility: a grand collaboration between reproductive medicine and oncology. Reproduction. 2015;150(3):S1–10.
38. Xu J, Lawson MS, Yeoman RR, Pau KY, Barrett SL, Zelinski MB, Stouffer RL. Secondary follicle growth and oocyte maturation during encapsulated three-dimensional culture in rhesus monkeys: effects of gonadotrophins, oxygen and fetuin. Hum Reprod. 2011;26:1061–72.
39. Xu M, Barrett SL, West-Farrell E, Kondapalli LA, Kiesewetter SE, Shea LD, Woodruff TK. In vitro grown human ovarian follicles from cancer patients support oocyte growth. Hum Reprod. 2009;24:2531–40.
40. Xu M, Kreeger PK, Shea LD, Woodruff TK. Tissue-engineered follicles produce live, fertile offspring. Tissue Eng. 2006;12:2739–46.
41. Xu M, West-Farrell ER, Stouffer RL, Shea LD, Woodruff TK, Zelinski MB. Encapsulated three-dimensional culture supports development of nonhuman primate secondary follicles. Biol Reprod. 2009;81:587–94.

Index

© Springer International Publishing Switzerland 2017

T.K. Woodruff, Y.C. Gosiengfiao (eds.), *Pediatric and Adolescent Oncofertility*,
DOI 10.1007/978-3-319-32973-4

Lightning Source UK Ltd.
Milton Keynes UK
UKOW06n1434090717

304921UK00002B/6/P